HEALTHCARE PROFESSIONAL GUIDES

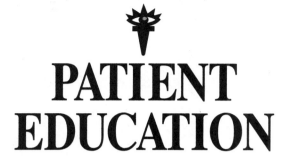

PATIENT EDUCATION

PATIENT EDUCATION

Springhouse Corporation
Springhouse, Pennsylvania

Staff

Senior Publisher
Matthew Cahill

Editorial Director
Patricia Dwyer Schull, RN, MSN

Clinical Manager
Judith A. McCann, RN, MSN

Art Director
John Hubbard

Senior Project Editor
Kathy E. Goldberg

Editor
Patricia A. Wittig

Clinical Project Manager
Helene K. Nawrocki, RN, MSN

Clinical Editors
Stanley W. Nawrocki, RN, CEN; Beverly Ann
Tscheschlog, RN; Marybeth Morrell, RN, CCRN,
Collette Bishop Hendler, RN, CCRN

Copy Editors
Cynthia C. Breuninger (manager), Karen C.
Comerford, Stacey A. Follin, Brenna H. Mayer,
Pamela Wingrod

Designers
Arlene Putterman (associate art director),
Elaine Ezrow, Joseph John Clark, Jacalyn
Facciolo, Susan Hopkins Rodzewich, Jeff
Sklarow, Mary Stangl

Illustrators
Julie Devito, John Gist, Bob Jackson, BJ Krim,
Bob Neumann, Judy Newhouse

Typography
Diane Paluba (manager), Joyce Rossi Biletz,
Phyllis Marron, Valerie Rosenberger

Manufacturing
Deborah Meiris (director), T.A. Landis, Otto
Mezei

Production Coordinator
Margaret A. Rastiello

Editorial Assistants
Beverly Lane, Mary Madden

Indexer
Barbara Hodgson

Contents

Advisory board

Foreword

The title of this book, *HealthCare Professional Guides: Patient Education,* refers to a major theme in health care today: patients' need to be informed about all aspects of their illness and treatment. This theme fits well with our society's emphasis on self-determination. More and more patients are asking for, if not demanding, a significant role in their own health care; they want to become partners in their care.

Another trend in health care is the increasing emphasis on preventive medicine. Studies have shown that many of our current medical problems could be diminished by behavioral changes and lifestyle modifications. In order to make such changes, patients need to understand the relationship between behavior and illness. And patients dealing with chronic diseases need to be aware of the symptoms they can expect and the measures they can take to relieve these symptoms and minimize exacerbations.

In addition, because many patients are being sent home earlier or are never admitted to a health care facility, they're responsible for more and more of their own care. They need to know about their disease process, the diagnostic tests involved, and the treatments they must undergo.

For all of these reasons, education is paramount and today's health care providers need to be consummate teachers. Whether you're a nurse, nurse practitioner, physician's assistant, physical therapist, or any other member of the health care team, *Patient Education* can help you accomplish that task confidently and effectively.

Organized by body system and enhanced by numerous illustrations and charts, this book explains not only *what* to teach but *how* to teach — even in problem situations, such as when faced with a combative patient. Chapter 1 explicates the relationship between effective teaching and learning, illuminating the concepts of cognitive and emotional development, learning styles, teaching methods, and outside factors that influence learning. And, because people do not act on knowledge alone, the chapter reminds you of the need to understand the value system in which your patient operates and to take care not to let your own values and beliefs intrude on the learning process. With this foundation, you'll be well positioned to develop your skills as a teacher and to present your medical knowledge within the patient's context.

In the subsequent chapters — each one devoted to a broad category of chronic conditions — information is presented in a clear and concise manner that's readily accessible. Each entry follows the same easy-to-use format: a brief introduction about the disorder, a bulleted list of teaching topics, and summaries of the diagnostic workup, treatments and, when appropriate, self-care and home care measures.

Throughout the book, you'll find graphic designs that call your attention to special pointers that you can teach a patient to improve his comfort and recovery and even save him money ("Tips and timesavers"), to alert him to dangers associated with certain diseases or procedures ("Warning"), and to inform him about the disorder itself ("Insight into illness"). In addition, a valuable appendix provides national sources of information and support for patients with various disorders or conditions.

HealthCare Professional Guides: Patient Education provides you with the relevant tools to carry out your role as a teacher. Adopting its teaching strategies will help you — and any health care professional — better serve patients and increase their participation in their own healing.

Willard P. Green, PhD
Dean, School of Health Professions
Allegheny University of the
    Health Sciences
Philadelphia

How to teach patients

Today, the need for patient teaching is greater than ever before because of the shrinking health care budget, shorter hospital stays, and growing consumer awareness of health care issues and services. Patients need to know about their illnesses, their diagnostic tests and treatments, and their home care regimens.

What is patient teaching?

Patient teaching is something the health care professional does formally, with planning and deliberation. But you also do it informally whenever you take time to answer a patient's question. You do it through a variety of methods, including explanation, demonstration, role playing, and teamwork.

THE PATIENT AS PARTICIPANT
In the past, the teaching efforts of health care professionals focused on gaining the patient's passive compliance with the prescribed regimen. Today, the thrust of teaching has shifted toward promoting the patient's active involvement in his care.

Patient teaching is an active process that aims to produce an observable change in the patient's behavior or attitude. The key words here are *active*, *process*, and *change*.
• *Active* reflects the need for the patient's involvement.
• *Process* signals an ongoing series of actions or events that aim to help the patient learn how to maintain or improve his current health status.

• *Change* refers to gaining new knowledge, skills, values, or beliefs.

WHO BENEFITS FROM PATIENT TEACHING?
Although the patient is the main beneficiary of effective teaching, he isn't the only one — the entire health care system gains.

With shorter hospital stays, patients have less time to learn about their health care. What's more, many are discharged from the hospital even though they require continued care at home — and must learn the skills they need to care for themselves safely and effectively after discharge. This, of course, increases the demand for teaching.

Also, patients may undergo batteries of diagnostic tests and procedures as outpatients, which often increases their teaching needs. And patients who undergo same-day surgery need to know about postoperative care measures crucial to their safety and comfort.

Moreover, as medical advances have helped to extend life expectancy, the number of chronically ill patients has increased. Because many of these patients live independently and assume responsibility for their own care, they need to become willing partners in planning it.

The patient who has been taught about his condition and treatment is better prepared to leave the hospital early. And the patient who's better able to understand and implement his home care plan has allowed more efficient use of personnel and equipment.

How to teach effectively

To be an effective teacher, you must control the learning environment, assess your patient's learning needs, create a teaching plan, supply instructional materials, and enlist the help of other health care team members. You must also use appropriate teaching techniques and evaluate their outcome.

You also need to look at your "classroom" to be an effective teacher. If you care for patients primarily in their homes, the "classroom" may well be an inviting and comfortable place for learning. This doesn't hold true if you work mainly in a hospital or clinic. Its staff, rules, and rituals may seem alien to the patient, making him feel especially vulnerable. This creates a barrier to learning that you must overcome to teach effectively.

Assessing learning needs

Much of the teaching process rests on accurately assessing the patient's readiness and ability to learn. Understanding the developmental stages of personality can aid your assessment. Of course, you'll also have to assess the patient's learning needs on an ongoing basis.

RELATING DEVELOPMENTAL STAGES TO TEACHING AND LEARNING

You can assess your patient's developmental stage using models of psychosocial and intellectual (cognitive) development. All aspects of development are continuous, concurrent, and interrelated. Just as a person follows a pattern of physical growth and development, he also follows patterns of emotional, psychological, and cognitive development. These patterns conform to stages.

The characteristics of growth, or developmental tasks, within the stages have been described by Erikson,

Piaget, and Knowles, among others. The patient's level of physical, emotional, and psychological development influences his readiness, willingness, and ability to learn.

Erikson's developmental stages

Psychoanalyst Erik Erikson describes the physical, emotional, and psychological stages of development and relates specific issues, or developmental work or *tasks,* to each stage. For example, if an infant's physical and emotional needs are met sufficiently, he completes his task — developing the ability to trust others.

A person who's stymied in an attempt at task mastery may proceed to the next stage but carries within him the remnants of the unfinished task. For instance, if a toddler isn't allowed to learn by doing, he develops a sense of doubt in his abilities, which may complicate later attempts at independence. (See *Erikson's stages of development.*)

Piaget's cognitive stages

Much of your teaching depends on cognitive abilities — sharing information with the patient and looking for signs that he understands it. As a result, you need to understand cognitive stages.

Child psychologist Jean Piaget describes the mechanism — cognition — by which the mind processes new information. Piaget proposes that a person assimilates, or understands, whatever information fits into his established view of the world. When information doesn't fit, the person must reexamine and adjust his thinking to accommodate the new information. Piaget describes four stages of cognitive development and relates them to a person's ability to accommodate and assimilate new information.

Sensorimotor stage

During the sensorimotor stage, which extends from birth to about age 2, the child learns about himself and his environment through motor and

Erikson's stages of development

Infant
Trust vs. mistrust
Needs maximum comfort with minimal uncertainty to trust himself, others, and environment

Toddler
Autonomy vs. shame and doubt
Works to master physical environment while maintaining self-esteem

Preschooler
Initiative vs. guilt
Begins to initiate, not imitate, activities; develops conscience and sexual identity

School-age child
Industry vs. inferiority
Tries to develop a sense of self-worth by refining skills

Adolescent
Identity vs. role confusion
Tries integrating many roles (child, sibling, student, athlete, worker) into a self-image under role model and peer pressure

Young adult
Intimacy vs. isolation
Learns to make personal commitment to another as spouse, parent, or partner

Middle-age adult
Generativity vs. stagnation
Seeks satisfaction through productivity in career, family, and civic interests

Older adult
Integrity vs. despair
Reviews life accomplishments, deals with loss and preparation for death

reflex actions. Thought derives from sensation and movement. The child learns that he's separate from his environment and that aspects of his environment — such as his parents or favorite toys — continue to exist even though they may be outside the reach of his senses.

Your teaching, then, for a child in this stage should be geared to the sensorimotor system. You can modify behavior by using the senses: a frown, a stern or soothing voice — these serve as appropriate techniques to elicit desired behavior.

Preoperational stage
This stage begins about the time the child starts to talk and continues to about age 7. Applying his new knowledge of language, the child begins to use symbols to represent objects. Early in this stage, he also personifies objects. He's now better able to think about things and events that aren't immediately present. But he's unable to think through a series of actions; he still must perform them. Oriented to the present, the child has difficulty conceptualizing time. His thinking is influenced by fantasy — the way he'd like things to be — and he assumes that others see situations from his viewpoint. He assimilates information and then changes it in his mind to fit his ideas.

Because of the child's vivid fantasies and undeveloped sense of time, you'll be challenged to present information in a time frame that allows for questions and learning without fostering rumination. Using neutral words, body outlines, and equipment that a child can touch will give him an active role in learning.

Concrete stage
During this stage, which appears around the time the child enters first grade and lasts into early adolescence, accommodation increases. The child develops an ability to think abstractly and to make rational judgments about concrete or observable phenomena, which in the past he could understand only through physical manipulation. However, for these thought processes to occur, concrete objects must be within his sight or grasp. Giving this child the opportunity to ask questions and to explain things back to you allows him to mentally manipulate information.

Formal operations stage
This stage brings cognition to its final form during adolescence. A person reaches this stage when he no longer requires concrete objects to make rational judgments. At this point, he's capable of hypothetical and deductive reasoning. Teaching for the adolescent may be wide-ranging because he is able to consider many possibilities from several perspectives.

Knowles and the adult learner
Educator Malcolm Knowles used Piaget's and Erikson's work to study the adult learner. Knowles proposed that the adult learner brings life experiences to learning, incorporating and complementing the cognitive abilities of Piaget's adolescent.

According to Knowles, the individual undergoes the following changes as he matures:
● His self-concept moves from dependency to self-direction.
● He accumulates a growing reservoir of experience that becomes a resource for learning.
● His learning readiness becomes increasingly oriented to the tasks of his various social roles.
● His time perspective changes from one of postponed knowledge application to immediate application.
● His orientation to learning shifts from subject-centered to problem-centered.

If you examine personal and cognitive development and compare teaching approaches, you can see that children tend to be dependent as learners, whereas adults need to be independent and exercise control. For example, you'll usually teach an adult patient with migraine headaches some method of relaxation. Because an adult has more control over his time than a child does, you can let him decide which method fits his lifestyle and self-image. Of the possible methods, progressive muscle relaxation, which usually requires 10 to 20 minutes to perform, may not appeal to a busy executive. A deep-breathing exercise may be more effective because it conforms to his time constraints.

Implications for teaching

Accurately assessing your patient's developmental stage can direct your planning and impel your teaching. For instance, recognizing a 16-year-old's concern about his appearance and standing among his peers may promote your rapport with him and eliminate some learning barriers.

Keep in mind that chronological age and developmental stage aren't always related. Throughout life, people move sequentially through developmental stages, but most people also fluctuate somewhat among stages, often in response to outside stressors. These stressors, which may include illness and hospitalization, can cause a person to regress temporarily to an earlier stage. Sometimes a person may not achieve the task expected of his chronological age. So you'll need to address your patient at his current developmental stage, not at the stage you'd expect him to be because of his chronological age.

ONGOING ASSESSMENT

Assessing a patient's learning needs doesn't stop with the preteaching assessment; it's an ongoing process. Each time you talk with a patient, check his chart, or attend a meeting with the health care team, you gather information that can help you assess the patient's learning needs and abilities.

To help determine your patient's learning needs, consider the following sources of information: patient interviews, family interviews, written records (such as the patient's chart), and meetings with other health care team members.

Be aware of your attitude

Your own attitude may affect not only the information you collect from a patient and his family but also your interpretation of the patient's learning needs. Your feelings and values, like everyone else's, are shaped by your experiences. But as a health care professional, you can't allow your feelings to interfere with the objective assessment each patient deserves.

Being aware of your feelings can help you recognize, anticipate, and avoid problems. As you obtain information, ask yourself whether your response to the patient seems to be affecting your assessment of his learning needs in a negative way. If so, check your assessment findings with other health care team members.

Meet with other health care providers

Formal and informal interviews with the patient's doctor, nurses, and other health care team members will expand and validate your preteaching assessment. Find out what your colleagues learned from their interviews with the patient and his family. Do their impressions support or contradict your findings?

Also find out what other health care team members have told the patient and his family about his condition and his treatment plan. By clarifying these facts, you can avoid dispensing conflicting information.

Assessing readiness to learn

Various factors affect a patient's readiness to learn: his emotional state, stage of adaptation to his illness, emotional maturity, life experiences, and the goals he and his family want to reach. Answer these questions to assess your patient's readiness to learn:
• What information, if any, is the patient emotionally ready to learn?
• How well is he adapting to his illness?

• Is he emotionally mature enough to take responsibility for learning?
• Have the patient's experiences prepared him to learn the concept or skill you're planning to teach?
• Do the patient and his family have realistic learning goals?

Most patients show that they're ready to learn by asking questions or participating in care. If possible, time your teaching to take advantage of your patient's readiness to learn. Not only will learning be more effective, but your teaching will proceed more easily.

Assessing willingness to learn

A patient becomes willing to learn when he recognizes a gap between what he knows and what he wants to know. Conversely, if a patient doesn't want to learn about and comply with a particular treatment regimen, he won't — especially if it means giving up long-held habits or beliefs without any evident reward. For example, an overweight diabetic patient who "feels fine" may be unwilling to learn and follow a modified diet to control his illness.

When assessing the patient's willingness to learn, try to determine his attitude about the subject you're planning to teach. Does he think this information will benefit him, or does he consider it a waste of time? Take into account his health beliefs, sociocultural background, and religious beliefs. These factors can affect his willingness to learn by influencing his attitude toward health and illness.

HEALTH BELIEFS
A patient's health beliefs determine his response to illness or the threat of illness. For example, a patient who says, "A yearly checkup is important to me" may believe his actions can help prevent certain health problems. His health beliefs tend to enhance his willingness to learn.

Another patient who says, "I'm afraid to see my doctor; he might find that something's wrong with me" may believe his actions can have a negative effect by forcing him to confront a condition that frightens or confuses him.

By assessing your patient's health beliefs, you can determine how he makes health care decisions and predict his compliance with the treatment plan — essential information for planning an effective teaching strategy. (See *How health beliefs affect willingness to learn.*)

Typically, a patient's willingness to learn increases if he believes he's susceptible to a specific illness or that the illness would have a serious effect on his lifestyle. Besides, if a patient believes his actions can prevent the illness or that taking action is less dangerous than incurring the illness, he'll be more willing to learn about and comply with treatment.

SOCIOCULTURAL BACKGROUND
From one generation to the next, families pass on values, beliefs, and customs that help determine how their members respond to various circumstances. In many cultures, for instance, emotional expression is more acceptable for women than for men.

Ask your patient about his sociocultural background. Where were his parents or ancestors born? How long has his family lived in this country? Does he speak a second language at home? Then, consider how his sociocultural background has shaped his response to illness. Imagine, for example, you're caring for a 51-year-old hypertensive patient whose parents immigrated to the United States from Ireland. In this patient's family, men may be expected to present a strong, rugged image — a factor that may influence his willingness to learn the relaxation techniques his doctor prescribes.

When you assess a patient's sociocultural background, try to determine its impact on his current lifestyle.

How health beliefs affect willingness to learn

Research demonstrates that a patient learns better when she wants to learn. That's why it's important to assess your patient's health beliefs — they usually reveal what she wants, or is willing, to learn. Knowing her health beliefs helps you to predict her response to illness or the threat of illness. This, in turn, will help you tailor your teaching plan to meet her needs. In the chart below, you'll read how an illness — in this case, breast cancer — helps clarify how health beliefs affect a patient's willingness to learn.

PATIENT'S STATEMENT	PATIENT'S HEALTH BELIEF	EDUCATOR'S ASSESSMENT
"I worry a lot about getting breast cancer. It runs in my family."	She has a greater-than-average chance of getting breast cancer.	Patient's perceived susceptibility to breast cancer promotes her willingness to learn.
"If I had breast cancer, my whole life would change."	Breast cancer would affect all aspects of her life.	Patient's perception of the seriousness of breast cancer and its impact on her life increases her willingness to learn preventive measures and seek early treatment.
"Breast self-examinations can help me find lumps in my breasts."	Breast self-examination is a helpful and important self-care tool.	Patient's perception of the procedure's benefit enhances her willingness to learn and perform it.
"I don't have to perform a self-examination each month. Besides, who has the time?"	Performing breast self-examination isn't important enough to make time for.	Patient's perception that the procedure isn't necessary and wouldn't fit her routine indicates a barrier that may compromise her willingness to learn it.

Does he still hold the values and customs of his ethnic group? If he doesn't, what changes has he made? Usually, the impact is less dramatic when several generations separate a patient from his family's country of origin.

Avoid stereotyping

If you're familiar with accepted behavior within your patient's sociocultural group, you can assess his learning needs with greater insight. At the same time, though, remember that each patient is an individual, not a stereotype.

RELIGIOUS BELIEFS

A patient's religion can also affect his willingness to learn by influencing his attitudes toward illness and traditional medicine. For example, a patient who regards his heart attack as a test of his faith or a divine punishment for wrongdoing may be unwilling to learn about cardiac rehabilitation.

Assess the nature and strength of your patient's religious beliefs. Does he have any religious beliefs about treating illness? For example, many Christian Scientists shun traditional medical treatment, believing that a person can cure illness by altering his thought processes.

What role does religion play in the patient's daily routine? If his religion prohibits certain foods, for instance, he may resist learning about dietary changes that conflict with his beliefs. Accommodating the patient's religious beliefs and practices in your teaching plan may increase his willingness to learn about and comply with treatment.

Assessing ability to learn

A patient's ability to learn hinges on his physical and mental status, preferred learning style, support system, and socioeconomic status. Explore the patient's current status, focusing on identifying problems.

PHYSICAL AND MENTAL STATUS
As a rule, a patient who's physically and mentally fit can master the skills and information necessary to manage his health problems, whereas a patient who has a physical or mental deficit, such as a disabling illness or severe stress, may be temporarily or permanently unable to do so.

PREFERRED LEARNING STYLE
How quickly and well a patient learns depends not only on his intelligence and education but also on his learning-style preference. *Visual* learners gain knowledge best by *seeing* or *reading* what you're trying to teach; *auditory* learners, by *listening*; and *tactile* or *psychomotor* learners, by *doing*.

You can improve your chances for teaching success if you assess your patient's preferred learning style, and

then plan teaching activities and use teaching tools appropriate to that style.

To assess learning style, you could, for example, ask the patient to describe what he likes at the seashore. If he talks mostly about images, such as the water's color or the sky's brilliance, he may be a visual learner. If he talks about the pounding of waves or seagulls' cries, he may be an auditory learner. If he describes primarily tactile sensations, such as the warmth of the sand or sun, he may be a tactile learner.

 TIPS AND TIMESAVERS: Another way to assess learning style is to experiment with different teaching tools, such as printed material, illustrations, videotapes, and actual equipment. Never assume, though, that your patient can read well—or even read at all.

SOCIOECONOMIC STATUS
External factors, such as socioeconomic status, may affect a patient's learning ability by causing or reducing stress. For instance, a patient who's financially secure tends to view illness more as a minor inconvenience than as a major disruption of his life and livelihood. This patient typically has job security, adequate health insurance coverage, and easy access to health care. For these reasons, he's less threatened by pain and illness than a patient with a lower income. This increases his sense of control over his condition and, as a result, improves his ability to learn.

Planning for teaching

Simply stated, a teaching plan is a carefully organized, written presentation of what the patient needs to learn and how you'll provide the instruction and evaluate the results. Broadly, it should be based on the patient's learning needs as he has identified them and as you and other health care team members have pinpointed them.

the response

A teaching plan should contain a statement of learning outcomes, a teaching content outline, selected teaching methods and tools, and some provision for evaluating teaching effectiveness. All aspects of the plan should be individualized to meet the patient's particular learning needs.

Be sure to state the patient's learning outcomes specifically so that anyone, including other health care members, can understand what will be taught, why it will be taught, and how it will be evaluated.

Keep in mind that your teaching plan should contain what you, the doctor, the nurse, and other members of the health care team determine the patient *needs* to know, blended with what the patient *wants* to know.

CHOOSE TEACHING METHODS
Most of your teaching will probably be done on a one-to-one basis, giving you the chance to learn about your patient, build a relationship with him, and tailor your teaching to his learning needs. But sometimes you'll need to teach a group of patients, give a demonstration, supervise practice and return demonstrations, or serve as part of a teaching team.

Individual teaching
Teaching patients one-on-one allows you to provide long- or short-term teaching and continually assess the patient's progress. It also gives you the chance to address individual needs. This teaching strategy promotes a personal relationship that helps the patient trust and confide in you, further enhancing the teaching-learning process.

The major disadvantage of individual teaching is that the patient can't exchange ideas with anyone but the teacher, forfeiting the opportunity to share experiences with others in similar situations. Also, this strategy demands more of your time as a teacher because patients can't be taught in groups, and it increases institutional expenses.

Group teaching
To maximize learning, members of a group should be similar in maturity, intelligence, and learning needs. Although many adults prefer small groups, most can learn in groups of almost any size. Teenagers typically require small groups because of their shorter attention spans and tendency to become distracted. Groups also should be restricted in size when the teaching topic requires hands-on participation or when personal sharing will enhance learning.

Group teaching may reduce patient and institutional expense and improve convenience (if classes are offered more frequently). Also, this method maximizes your time by providing services to multiple patients simultaneously. (See *Group teaching: Keys to success,* page 10.)

Discussion
Discussion encourages the open exchange of ideas and information between you and your patient. Rather than assuming that you have all the answers, the patient becomes involved in the problem-solving process. As he asks questions or makes comments, he begins to take some responsibility for his own learning.

Demonstration, practice, and return demonstration
You'll find this technique, like show-and-tell in a child's classroom, especially useful after a one-on-one discussion with your patient. In demonstration, you perform step-by-step so the patient can imitate what you do. Your demonstration can be impromptu at the patient's bedside or it can be given during a scheduled teaching session. Your choice depends on the circumstances.

A scheduled demonstration takes advance planning because you need to be knowledgeable and confident. Also, you must assemble required materials.

Team teaching
By interacting with several health care providers, the patient receives a

Group teaching: Keys to success

When you're teaching a group, you can enhance the learning process by helping patients develop a group identity and cohesiveness. Here are some tips.

Control the environment
● Hold the meeting at a round table, or arrange chairs in a circle. This increases interaction by making participants feel equal to one another and to the teacher.
● Limit the group size to five to seven patients. This allows maximum personal exchange and discussion.
● Adjust the temperature and lighting in the meeting room so that neither is uncomfortable nor distracting.
● Keep the atmosphere informal and relaxed.

Initiate discussion and maintain an overview
● Introduce yourself.
● Ask patients to introduce themselves and to share a bit of personal information.
● Explain the meeting's purpose.
● Invite the group to identify goals and ground rules.
● Suggest that the group develop learning outcomes.
● Encourage everyone to participate. Be gracious about allowing anyone to leave who isn't comfortable or doesn't want to participate.
● Keep the group focused on the agreed-upon discussion subjects.
● Act as a resource, providing information and clarification.
● Summarize and review at the end of the meeting; lead group members to agree on what they've learned.

range of viewpoints, expertise, and teaching styles. This versatility may prevent boredom and enhance learning.

The team teaching approach may be appropriate for groups or individuals. Team members may have similar qualifications and professions, or they may represent various disciplines.

SELECT TEACHING TOOLS
You can use various teaching tools to spur the patient's interest and reinforce learning. These tools, which may include printed pamphlets, audiocassettes, or closed-circuit television programs, help familiarize the patient with a topic.

Although some health care agencies and facilities prefer to develop their own teaching materials, others consider the process too expensive and time-consuming. Using existing materials may be more practical. When looking for materials, consult in-service instructors, librarians, and staff specialists. (Of course, the teaching aids you'll find in this book are designed for use in your practice.)

 TIPS AND TIMESAVERS: Other reliable sources for patient-teaching materials include local pharmaceutical and medical supply companies. And don't overlook national associations and foundations such as the American Heart Association. These organizations usually have large supplies of patient-education materials written with the layperson in mind. Many are free; some are offered at a nominal cost.

Obviously, prepackaged references can save you time. However, they're no substitute for your personal teaching; they only supplement it. Put your imprint on such auxiliary reference materials by marking significant passages for your patient and by reviewing the information with him.

Printed materials
Present background information and explain procedures with books, leaflets, and other printed materials.

Teaching the nonreader

To teach a patient who can't read, use teaching tools other than reading materials.

Illustrate the message
Make drawings of what you want the patient to do as you instruct him. Illustrate the most important points. For example, depict him taking his medicine rather than reading the label.

Your drawings needn't be works of art, but don't insult the patient's sensibilities with stick figures, either.

Tape the instructions
Making an audiotape of step-by-step procedures lets the patient play them back as often as necessary to memorize them.

Record the patient's words
If you have good rapport with the patient, try a variation of a technique used in basic reading classes. Start by telling him what you want him to know. Then have him repeat the instructions back to you.

Write down *exactly* what he says — grammatical mistakes, repetitions, sidetracks, and all. Correct any procedural mistakes immediately. Now have him repeat the instructions again. Prompt him if necessary, but he'll probably repeat almost verbatim because they're phrased in his own words.

Speak normally
Remind yourself to speak in a normal tone — don't shout. The patient can hear; he just can't read.

Remember, your responsibilities *don't* include conducting reading classes. But by individualizing the plan for this patient, you will have gone a long way in teaching him.

These allow the patient to read and reread information at his convenience.

When recommending printed materials, be sensitive to your patient's ability or inability to read and absorb information. Keep in mind that the printed word tends to work best with the patient who reads competently.

A patient who's not a skilled reader may be too embarrassed to admit it. He may even pretend that he can read and comprehend what you give him. (See *Teaching the nonreader*.) If the material proves too complex or difficult, he may quickly lose the motivation to learn.

Don't forget to observe whether the patient can see well enough to read. If he uses reading glasses, make sure he has them nearby. If he doesn't have them, suggest that he use a magnifying glass.

For the most part, the more pictures the printed materials contain, the better the patient will retain what he's learning. But take a minute to consider the best form. Although actual photographs of a step-by-step technique may seem to offer the most accurate illustrations, substituting abstract pictures, graphics, or diagrams can sometimes make a concept clearer by eliminating superfluous details. If your patient is a child, cartoons and pictures that use music, sports, or movie stars will create interest and help convey your message.

Audiocassette tapes
Use audiotapes for teaching auditory and performance skills. For instance, if you're teaching a parent how to care for an asthmatic child, you can play a tape of normal breath sounds and wheezing sounds. If you're teaching a patient who's uncomfortable with printed materials, you may want to tape-record the steps of the procedures he's to follow. He can listen to the tape with you; then, once

he understands it, he can go over it by himself.

Before using an audiocassette, consider whether the patient may have a hearing impairment — especially if he's older. For a hearing-impaired patient, auditory teaching tools may be a poor choice, unless he can hear the audiotape clearly with a hearing aid.

Working models

Convey visual and tactile information with anatomic models and actual equipment. Besides making your instruction seem more realistic than pictures, these materials can reduce the patient's anxiety by familiarizing him with equipment he'll be seeing or using later.

Posters and flip charts

You can use posters and flip charts to illustrate your teaching to a group of patients or to a single patient at his bedside. These materials can be supported by an easel or, if necessary, propped against the back of a chair. If you're planning to use these aids repeatedly, consider laminating them. This will make them easy to clean and will prevent them from becoming shabby and discolored with use.

Transparencies

You can augment a demonstration or lecture by using an overhead projector and transparencies to project images onto a screen or wall. Trans-parencies can be used in a normally lighted room and thus permit you to maintain eye contact with your audience.

Slides and filmstrips

Add color and drama to demonstrations, lectures, and individual teaching sessions with slides and filmstrips. You'll need a carousel projector and a screen. (If you can't obtain a screen, a wall or bedsheet will do.) Slides can be synchronized with an audiotape when a slide-tape projector is used.

Similar to a slide and tape show, filmstrips are merely slide frames connected in a continuous strip. They can prove awkward and difficult to change when you want to update your material or show only a portion of the strip. For this reason, they're used less often than slides.

Videotapes

If you work in a health care facility with a centralized hookup, you can show a videotape on the patient's television screen. He can wear earphones so that other patients won't be disturbed. If you're providing care in the patient's home, you can show a videotape on the patient's videocassette recorder or on one that you bring with you.

Closed-circuit television

You can plan to show prepared teaching programs on closed-circuit television if you work in a facility that has the necessary equipment. These programs provide important background teaching for patient groups with similar problems.

Computer-assisted instruction

Arrange for your patient to have access to a computer if the health care facility has computerized patient-teaching programs. If he needs instruction or orientation, arrange for that, too. Keep in mind, though, that some patients may feel threatened by a computer.

SIDESTEP OBSTACLES

You may have to become as creative as you can to sidestep typical teaching problems, such as insufficient teaching resources, lack of time, and lack of patient cooperation.

Overcome a resource shortage

If adequate resources (printed materials, working models, videotapes, and other tools) aren't available, you'll have to teach without them. But you still have the most important tool at hand: an active interchange between you and the patient.

Deal with time constraints

Another major obstacle to the best-laid teaching plans is time. A staff shortage can easily sabotage your planned time for teaching. Or you may have time for teaching, but your patient will be out of his room for tests. Or he'll be in too much discomfort to be receptive to teaching. Or he'll have visitors. And so on. At these times, try to share information with the patient's family, whose knowledgeable support can promote recovery.

Use any moment you're with the patient to do some teaching. You can incorporate teaching into your patient care in a number of ways. For instance, talk the patient through a new procedure as you're performing that part of his care. If the material to be taught is complicated, discuss one part at a time.

Explain what you're doing as you do it. If you're teaching a patient how to position himself for breathing ease and comfort, encourage him to ask questions and to repeat what you've just told him. Review the procedure with him the next time you see him. During subsequent visits, allow him to do more and more of the task by himself.

You can also give your patient written instructions that he can refer to between teaching sessions. When he's on his own, these instructions can help diminish his anxiety and remind him of the things you stressed in your teaching.

 TIPS AND TIMESAVERS: Because your time may be short, modify existing written instructions to your patient's specific needs. Cross out unnecessary or irrelevant information. Keep written instructions brief and close to the information and advice you gave the patient in person. Refer to things you talked about in teaching sessions. This will help refresh his memory and make the material more personal.

Cope with the unwilling learner

If your patient seems unmotivated to learn and you're convinced he's resistant to your teaching, document this and inform your supervisor or the doctor or nurse of the problem. Come back to this patient later to try again — perhaps with a fresh approach. His situation and attitude may change, making him a more willing learner.

Enhancing your teaching effectiveness

Although in some situations you work from a formal teaching plan, in others you'll be confronted with a "teachable moment" — a time when the patient is ready to learn and is asking pointed questions. Having a knowledge of basic learning principles will help you take advantage of these moments. Here are some principles proven to enhance teaching and learning.

SEIZE THE MOMENT

Teaching is most effective when it occurs in quick response to a need the learner feels. So even if you're in the middle of providing direct patient care, make every effort to teach the patient when he asks a question like, "What can I do to stop getting so many open sores?" In such situations, satisfy his immediate need for information now, and augment your teaching with more information later.

INVOLVE THE PATIENT IN PLANNING

Simply presenting information to the patient doesn't ensure learning or change. For learning to occur, you'll need to get the patient involved in identifying his learning needs and outcomes. Help him to develop attainable goals. As the teaching process continues, further engage him by selecting teaching strategies and materials that require his direct involvement, such as role playing and return demonstration. Regardless of the teaching strategy you choose, giving the patient the chance to test his ideas, take risks, and be creative will promote learning.

BEGIN WITH WHAT THE PATIENT KNOWS

You'll find that learning moves faster when it builds on what the patient knows. A patient who's been on peritoneal dialysis, for example, and now must undergo hemodialysis has some exposure to the concept of fluid exchange. Teaching that starts by comparing the old, known process and the new, unknown one allows the patient to grasp new information more quickly.

MOVE FROM SIMPLE TO COMPLEX

The patient will find learning more rewarding if he has the opportunity to master simple concepts first and then apply these concepts to more complex ones. Remember, though, that what one patient finds simple, another may find complex. A careful assessment takes these differences into account and helps you to plan the teaching starting point.

SORT GOALS BY LEARNING DOMAIN

You can combine your knowledge of the patient's preferred learning style with your knowledge of learning domains. Categorizing what the patient needs to learn into the proper domains helps identify and evaluate the behaviors you expect him to show.

Learning behaviors fall into three domains: cognitive, psychomotor, and affective.

• The *cognitive* domain deals with intellectual abilities.

• The *psychomotor* domain includes physical or motor skills.

• The *affective* domain involves expression of feelings about attitudes, interests, and values.

Most learning involves all three domains. For instance, when teaching a patient about subcutaneous injection sites, the cognitive domain has the essential task: identifying the sites. The psychomotor and affective domains have related tasks: finding the best site for the injection and expressing how the patient feels about giving

himself an injection. (See *Applying learning domains to patient teaching.*)

MAKE MATERIAL MEANINGFUL

Another way to promote learning is to relate material to the patient's lifestyle — and to recognize incompatibilities. For example, teaching a patient with hypertension how to take his blood pressure may be futile if he perceives this as something his spouse ought to do.

Similarly, discussing the need for a low-sodium diet with a traveling salesman may be futile if he often eats in fast-food restaurants and feels unable to control the ingredients in his diet. Instead, you may need to teach him about possible lifestyle adaptations.

ALLOW IMMEDIATE APPLICATION OF KNOWLEDGE

Promptly giving the patient the chance to apply his new knowledge and skills reinforces learning and builds confidence. For instance, a mother learning to perform postural drainage for her infant will learn better when she can quickly transfer what she's practiced on a doll to her own child (with supervision, of course). This immediate application translates learning to the "real world" and provides an opportunity for problem solving, feedback, and emotional support.

Similarly, providing sample menus to a diabetic patient helps reinforce his cognitive skills of food selection. This type of rehearsal reinforces his ability to select foods correctly on his own.

PLAN FOR PERIODIC RESTS

While you may want the patient to push ahead until he's learned everything on the teaching plan, remember that periodic plateaus occur normally in learning. When your instructions are especially complex or lengthy, the patient may feel overwhelmed and appear unreceptive to teaching. Be sure to recognize these

Applying learning domains to patient teaching

During the teaching process, you'll identify what the patient needs and wants to learn. You'll also evaluate what he has actually learned. Understanding learning domains — cognitive, psychomotor, and affective — can help with both steps.

Within each domain, learning can take place on several progressively complex levels. Understanding the degree of ability and comprehension each level demands helps you select the steps to take in guiding the patient toward appropriate outcomes. The chart below identifies the learning levels within each domain and gives an example of a patient outcome for each level.

COGNITIVE DOMAIN	PATIENT OUTCOME
Knowledge: Recalling information	Patient can identify signs and symptoms of hypoglycemia.
Comprehension: Understanding information and having the ability to draw conclusions	Patient can state the relationship between diet and blood sugar control.
Application: Adapting rules to specific behavior	Patient uses aseptic technique when giving himself a subcutaneous injection.
Analysis: Breaking down concepts into separate elements and identifying the relationships among them	Patient can distinguish between diabetes facts and myths.
Synthesis: Reassembling elements to create new concepts	Patient can use food exchange lists to develop weekly meal plans.
Evaluation: Appraising the value of material for a given purpose	Patient can judge the effectiveness of modifying activity to coincide with appropriate caloric intake.

PSYCHOMOTOR DOMAIN	PATIENT OUTCOME
Perception: Becoming aware of stimuli through the senses	Patient can recognize the difference between a fast and slow pulse.
Set: Being ready for a specific action or experience	Patient can place fingers correctly over wrist before taking pulse.
Guided response: Performing a procedure under supervision	After observing a demonstration, patient can perform the correct procedure for a monthly "teletrace" check of pacemaker.
Mechanism: Learning a behavior to the point of habit	Patient performs cardiac rehabilitation exercises at an established time daily.
Complex overt response: Performing a complex motor pattern	Patient can measure pulse accurately before and after exercising.

(continued)

Applying learning domains to patient teaching (continued)

PSYCHOMOTOR DOMAIN	PATIENT OUTCOME
Adaptation: Altering a motor response to solve new problems	Patient has adjusted activities of daily living (climbing stairs only twice a day) to avoid unnecessary fatigue.

AFFECTIVE DOMAIN	PATIENT OUTCOME
Receiving: Attending to and allowing continuation of a stimulus	Patient allows nasogastric tube placement.
Responding: Reacting voluntarily to a stimulus	Patient cooperates with urinary catheter insertion.
Valuing: Accepting the preferred value of a behavior to the point of acting it out	Patient accepts activity limits imposed by coronary artery disease.
Organization: Systematizing a behavioral framework based on values	Patient organizes schedule to include relaxation time.
Value characterization: Expressing feelings that portray health belief	Patient states, "I understand I have to adjust my activities and diet. I accept this and want to make every moment count."

signs of mental fatigue and let the patient relax. (You, too, can use these periods — to review your teaching plan and make any necessary adjustments.)

PROVIDE PROGRESS REPORTS

Learning is made easier when the patient is aware of his progress. Positive feedback can motivate him to greater effort because it makes his goal seem attainable.

Also remember to ask the patient how he feels he's doing. He probably wants to take part in assessing his own progress toward learning goals, and his input can guide your feedback. You'll find his reactions are usually based on what "feels right."

REWARD DESIRED LEARNING WITH PRAISE

Praising desired behavior improves the chances that the patient will repeat that behavior. For example, a child with cystic fibrosis may have difficulty learning how to perform breathing exercises. Praising his success associates the desired learning goal with a sense of growing and accepted competence. Reassuring him that he's learned the technique can help him refine it and motivate him to practice.

Evaluating your patient teaching

Evaluation refers to the continuous and systematic appraisal of the patient's learning progress during and after your teaching. Continuous evaluation provides the basis for feedback to the patient so that you can reinforce desirable behavior.

It can also help you correct undesirable behavior. For example, if your patient is injecting his insulin at the wrong site, your recognizing this will help him learn the correct sites to use. Ongoing evaluation also lets you measure the patient's progress in meeting learning outcomes by revealing how much progress he's making and how much he still has to learn.

 TIPS AND TIMESAVERS: Don't save your entire evaluation for the end of your teaching. Plan for brief, periodic evaluations throughout the teaching process. This serves a double purpose: It lets the patient immediately try out what he's learned, and it gives you immediate feedback for deciding the next step in your teaching — either reteaching the last step (possibly with new teaching strategies) or moving ahead. For instance, if you've just explained the sources of high-cholesterol foods and their risks, let the patient try selecting low-cholesterol foods from a menu.

To evaluate the patient's learning, use a mix of data-gathering techniques to obtain the broadest possible view. Techniques include direct observation, written tests, oral tests, interviews, rating scales, checklists, and simulation.

DIRECT OBSERVATION
In this method, often called *return demonstration,* you watch the patient demonstrate a skill or act out a simulated situation. This method works well in evaluating motor skills such as bathing a newborn. It doesn't work as well in evaluating attitudinal changes because these are more difficult to observe.

WRITTEN TESTS
You can use written tests before, during, and after teaching. Use them before teaching to measure what the patient already knows and what he needs to learn. Use them during

teaching to measure his progress and after teaching to measure what he's learned.

Although written tests can save time, they do have some disadvantages. They can work only with literate patients. They're also hard to construct — and that's a job best left to the patient-education specialists. In addition, written tests may intimidate some patients. Perhaps the biggest drawback is that written tests are indirect indicators of learning: A patient may say as you say, but not do as you do.

ORAL TESTS
Questioning the patient can evaluate his cognitive learning better than either direct observation or written tests. It lets you individualize evaluation for specific patients and situations.

This technique offers the advantage of providing instant feedback. Its main drawback is that it takes considerable time.

INTERVIEWS
Interviews are most effective when you ask sharply focused questions. Use a written outline to make your questions relate to each other, and use follow-up questions to elicit more information.

Interviews require creative listening. Try to restate each of your patient's answers. This assures him that you understand his answers and gives him the chance to change his answers if he feels they need clarification after he hears you restate them.

RATING SCALES
Rating scales are practical devices for gathering and evaluating data if they're thoughtfully conceived and constructed. They have two strong points: They save time and they don't require writing. You simply check the appropriate response.

Rating scales also have weaknesses. For instance, you may tend to choose the middle scale values because you don't like to use the extremes. Or you may rate patients higher or lower than is appropriate because of your feelings toward them. When you use a rating scale, try not to be swayed by your biases.

CHECKLISTS
The checklist enumerates specific characteristics or activities the patient should have mastered from the teaching session. With it, you can check off those the patient has mastered as you observe or interview him.

SIMULATION
In a simulation session, you present a typical problem for the patient to solve. For example, you might say to a diabetic patient, "Before taking a 2-week vacation in Hawaii, what plans would you make to manage your condition?"

Simulation has the advantage of actively involving the patient in applying knowledge and skills to realistic situations. It's also nonthreatening. In some situations, however, considerable time is needed for planning and execution.

Documenting your teaching

An essential part of successful patient teaching, documentation should reveal what teaching you've planned and accomplished, what the patient has learned, and what remains to be done.

WHY DOCUMENTATION IS CRUCIAL
Besides having important legal implications, documentation also helps ensure that the patient has learned the necessary skills. What's more, it saves time by preventing duplication of patient-teaching efforts by other health team members.

Documenting patient teaching also helps the other team members to start instruction where you left off, without reteaching or skipping essential information. This is especially important for patients with compli-

cated needs who may be cared for by multiple health care professionals. Documentation also can motivate your patient by helping him focus on skills to be learned and can bolster his confidence when you share documented success with him once he's learned these skills.

The Joint Commission on Accreditation of Healthcare Organizations (JCAHO) mandates that medical records include specific instructions to the patient and family about physical activity, medication, diet, and other follow-up care. The JCAHO also requires clear documentation that the patient and family not only received instruction in these areas but also understood it.

GENERAL DOCUMENTATION GUIDELINES
The JCAHO offers these general guidelines on how to document patient teaching:
● Record the patient's name on every page of your documentation.
● Record the time and date on all entries.
● Sign each entry.
● Write in black or blue ink.
● Write legibly.
● Be truthful and accurate.
● Be objective. Don't show personal bias or let others influence what you document.
● Be specific. Describe exactly what occurred.
● Be concise. Record information as succinctly as possible without compromising accuracy.
● Be comprehensive. Include all pertinent information.
● Record events in chronological order.

2

Cardiovascular conditions

Aneurysm

A ruptured aneurysm can quickly progress to shock and death without immediate treatment. To make matters worse, most patients don't know they're in danger because symptoms rarely occur. In fact, the diagnosis usually isn't made until the blood vessel ruptures or becomes apparent on an X-ray or studies performed for another health problem detect it.

Whether the patient requires immediate surgery or has time to consider treatment options, the primary goal of your teaching is to help relieve his anxiety. Then, if time permits, you'll cover other topics, such as aneurysm sites, types, and causes; tests to detect the disorder; and treatments, including surgery, drug therapy, and self-care.

Before teaching a patient about aneurysms, make sure you're familiar with the following topics:
• what an aneurysm is
• what causes an aneurysm
• signs and symptoms of an aneurysm
• diagnostic studies, such as X-rays, abdominal ultrasonography, magnetic resonance imaging (MRI), computed tomography (CT) scanning, angiography, echocardiography, and lumbar puncture
• required activity restrictions
• medications used to treat aneurysms
• surgery to repair the aneurysm, such as resection and bypass
• preoperative and postoperative care
• other care measures, including blood pressure monitoring
• sources of information and support.

ABOUT THE DISORDER
Inform the patient that an aneurysm is a localized, abnormal widening of a blood vessel. Explain that most aneurysms affect the aorta, the main trunk of the systemic circulation, although they can occur anywhere. If possible, show the patient on a diagram where his aneurysm is.

Explain that two factors — mural and mechanical — influence an aneurysm's development. Mural factors refer to the strength and integrity of the vessel wall. For example, in an atherosclerotic aneurysm, fibrin deposits clog the artery, causing the arterial wall to lose its elasticity and to stiffen. Meanwhile, plaques accumulate and mural thrombi form on the wall, obstructing the lumen (the artery's interior, hollow passageway for blood). Thrombi, which may break off and lodge in distal vessels, also narrow the lumen and critically impair blood flow. Over time, the artery weakens and bulges.

Mechanical factors, such as hypertension, trauma, infection, and congenital defects — even stress imposed on an artery by the pulse wave of each ventricular contraction — can also weaken vessel walls. Mechanical factors that can stress the arterial wall include rising blood pressure and increasing blood volume, which are normal during pregnancy. If the patient already has a risk factor, such as a congenital weakness in the vessel wall, an aneurysm may develop.

Finally, describe how signs and symptoms (if any) vary, depending on how quickly the aneurysm dilates and how it affects surrounding structures. Pain is the most common symptom; its location and nature depend on the aneurysm site. For example, a patient with a thoracic aortic aneurysm typically has constant, boring chest pain when he lies supine. A patient with an abdominal aortic aneurysm may suffer low back pain or persistent or intermittent abdominal pain when lying down.

Other symptoms stem from aneurysmal pressure on adjacent structures. For example, a thoracic aortic aneurysm may cause dyspnea from pressure on the trachea, main bronchus, or lung. Or it may cause difficulty swallowing if it presses on the esophagus.

Complications
Most patients don't realize they have an aneurysm until serious or even life-threatening complications occur from rupture or until the blood supply to the tissues fed by the affected vessel decreases enough to cause health problems.

DIAGNOSTIC WORKUP
Inform the patient that the doctor may order X-ray studies, abdominal ultrasonography, MRI, CT scans, angiography, echocardiography, and lumbar puncture to evaluate his condition. The specific tests ordered depend on the location of the suspected aneurysm. (For details on these tests, see *Teaching patients about cardiovascular tests,* pages 24 to 30.) For information on lumbar puncture, see *Teaching patients about neurologic tests,* pages 117 to 125.)

TREATMENTS
Inform the patient that surgery is the treatment of choice for an aneurysm, but that medications may reduce such symptoms as pressure, swelling, and pain. Tell the patient that he must restrict his activity and that he will have his blood pressure monitored closely and will be observed for signs and symptoms of aneurysm rupture.

Activity guidelines
Tell the patient that overexertion can trigger a sudden rise in blood pressure,

possibly leading to dissection, or tearing, of the aneurysm — a serious complication. For this reason, the doctor typically orders bed rest or other activity restrictions until after surgery.

Medication
Inform the patient that the doctor is likely to prescribe antihypertensive drugs to help control blood pressure and a beta-adrenergic blocker such as propranolol (Inderal) to reduce pulsatile blood flow and cardiac contractility. If the patient has a cerebral aneurysm, the doctor may order anticonvulsants to prevent seizures and corticosteroids to control edema.

Tell the patient that he may receive a sedative or narcotic to reduce anxiety, stress, or pain. If he does, he'll be monitored closely for a decrease in consciousness, a slow respiratory rate, and adverse effects.

 WARNING: Instruct the patient not to take aspirin, over-the-counter products containing aspirin, or foods or drugs containing caffeine. Aspirin impedes blood clot formation, which increases the patient's risk of bleeding should the aneurysm rupture. Caffeine is a stimulant that increases blood pressure.

Surgery
If the patient must undergo emergency surgery and if time allows, briefly explain the procedure. If surgery isn't immediately scheduled, take time to discuss the operation and possible complications. Be sure to include information on preoperative, postoperative, and home care.

Types of aneurysm repair
Inform the patient that to repair the aneurysm, the surgeon may perform surgical resection, bypass, clipping, or wrapping. The choice of surgery depends on the location, type, and size of the aneurysm; the patient's condition; and whether or not the aneurysm is intact.

To repair a thoracic aortic aneurysm, the surgeon may perform a thoracic aortic bypass; to repair a femoral-popliteal aneurysm, he may

Repairing an aortic aneurysm

If your patient has an aortic aneurysm — either abdominal or thoracic — and if he has time to learn about his impending operation, review the surgical procedure with him. If he's having emergency surgery, briefly describe aneurysmectomy to his family.

Inform them that the surgeon first resects the involved segment. Next, he replaces the diseased section with biologically neutral graft material, such as Dacron or a derivative (see illustration).

Then the surgeon cleans the diseased tissue of plaque or clotted blood and sutures this section around the graft. The section that once composed the aneurysm now covers the graft.

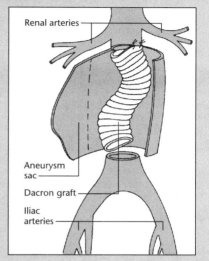

Renal arteries
Aneurysm sac
Dacron graft
Iliac arteries

perform a femoral-popliteal bypass. However, blood vessels may be repaired anywhere in the cardiovascular system.

If the patient is having bypass surgery, explain that the surgeon will graft an autologous or synthetic vessel above and below the aneurysm site to divert blood flow around the diseased tissue.

If the patient is scheduled for an aneurysmectomy (aneurysm resection), tell him that the surgeon will remove the aneurysm and reconnect the ends of the blood vessel or heart muscle. Or he may remove the diseased portion and graft a replacement vessel to the healthy ends of the blood vessel.

With a small aneurysm, the surgeon may clip or ligate the base of the aneurysm so blood can't flow into it. In wrapping, the surgeon wraps the arterial wall with a biologically neutral material, such as Dacron, to support it. (See *Repairing an aortic aneurysm*.)

Preoperative care
Tell the patient that he will bathe with a special antiseptic soap the day before surgery and may be shaved from neck to toes. If he has a cerebral aneurysm, his head will be shaved at least partially. Inform him that food and beverages are withheld after midnight before the surgery.

Mention that he may receive a sleeping pill to help him rest the night before surgery and a sedative to help him relax on the morning of surgery. Tell him that the peripheral pulses in his legs may be marked with an inklike substance; he should not wash off the markings when bathing with the antiseptic soap.

If the patient is scheduled for preoperative pulmonary artery catheterization or intracranial pressure monitoring, explain these procedures. Emphasize that the catheter will remain in place during and after surgery, but should cause little, if any, discomfort.

Postoperative care

Clarify what to expect after surgery. Tell the patient that immediately afterward, he will be transferred to a critical care unit. Then, after recovery, he will be moved to a regular hospital room. Describe the type of dressing and the various tubes and equipment he can expect after surgery. For example, if mechanical ventilation is used briefly, an endotracheal (ET) tube will be inserted through his nose or mouth into the lungs. If the aneurysm was in the chest, chest tubes connected to a suction apparatus will keep his lungs inflated properly and allow blood and fluid to drain from the thoracic cavity.

Inform the patient that he'll have a urinary catheter to measure fluid output and possibly a nasogastric (NG) tube to prevent vomiting, aspiration, and abdominal distention until his bowels resume normal function. The NG tube will be taped to his nose, connected to a suction machine, and irrigated every few hours. The tube may cause discomfort and dryness in the back of the throat. He'll receive I.V. fluids to help maintain hydration. Mention that when the ET and NG tubes are removed, he will be able to sit up and swallow liquids and will gradually start eating solid foods.

If the patient had a cerebral aneurysm, he will be positioned on his side after surgery, with the head of his bed raised 15 to 30 degrees to prevent increased intracranial pressure. Blood flow in his legs will be measured frequently with an ultrasound transducer.

Reassure him that coughing won't loosen or damage the graft or reopen the incision. However, if he has just had cerebral artery repair, warn him not to cough too vigorously because this may induce bleeding.

Active range-of-motion leg exercises help prevent clot formation. Tell the patient that a nurse will help him walk as soon as possible to improve his circulation and help prevent complications. Mention that he may wear antiembolism stockings to prevent complications. The stockings will be removed periodically to check his pulses and skin condition.

Home care

Tell the patient that when he starts to feel stronger, the doctor may revise his activity program to promote a gradual return to his previous activity levels.

If the patient underwent surgery for a ruptured cerebral artery, he may have some neurologic impairment and may need rehabilitation services. Advise him that the physical therapy and social service departments offer services that can help him and his family.

Make sure the patient understands which medications to take, how to take them, and what adverse reactions to watch for. Teach him how to recognize the warning signs of infection at the incision site, such as redness, swelling, tenderness, and drainage.

If the patient must wear antiembolism stockings at home, teach him how to check his pulses and examine his skin for signs of infection or decreased circulation. Tell him to immediately report cold, blue-tinged skin (which signals decreased circulation from a thromboembolism) as well as a fever, a skin color change, or pain in the area fed by the affected artery (which may indicate an anastomotic aneurysm).

Other care measures

If your patient is at home awaiting surgery for an aneurysm, discuss treatment measures with both him and his family. Emphasize that controlling blood pressure will decrease the risk of aneurysm rupture. Teach all family members how to take a blood pressure reading.

Until the aneurysm is surgically repaired, the patient's circulation will be decreased, increasing the risk of infection. Make sure all family members know the signs and symptoms of infection, and urge them to notify the doctor if these occur. Give them the address and phone number of the American Heart Association, which can provide more support and information. (See Appendix 2.)

Arrhythmias

Arrhythmias affect a broad section of the population. They range from mild, asymptomatic disturbances such as sinus arrhythmia to life-threatening emergencies such as ventricular fibrillation.

Such variation complicates teaching responsibilities. Not only must you teach about diverse degrees of illness, but you must also teach patients of diverse learning needs, ages, and health histories. Nonetheless, your goal is always the same: to inform the patient about his specific arrhythmia and its treatment.

Before teaching a patient about arrhythmias, make sure you are familiar with the following topics:
• normal cardiac conduction
• name and description of the patient's specific arrhythmia
• diagnostic tests, such as electrocardiography (ECG), serum electrolyte studies, and electrophysiologic studies
• appropriate activity guidelines and dietary restrictions
• name, purpose, and use of prescribed antiarrhythmic drugs
• prescribed treatments, such as carotid sinus massage, Valsalva's maneuver, temporary pacemaker implantation, and electrocardioversion
• preparation for placement of a permanent pacemaker or an automatic implantable cardioverter defibrillator (ICD), if necessary
• guidelines for pacemaker or ICD use and maintenance, if necessary
• how to measure the pulse rate
• sources of information and support.

ABOUT THE DISORDER
Inform the patient that arrhythmias are abnormal changes in heart rate, heart rhythm, or both. Tell him that normally the electrical impulses that cause the heart to contract originate in the sinoatrial node. The impulses travel across the atria through the atrioventricular node to the bundle of His. Then they disperse throughout the ventricles. Any disruption of this pathway can produce arrhythmias.

Complications
Explain that arrhythmias alter cardiac output, which can lead to a wide range of complications — from palpitations, dizziness, and fainting to life-threatening blood clots or cardiac arrest. Describe the causes of arrhythmias, including congenital abnormalities, lack of adequate blood to the heart, myocardial infarction (heart attack), heart disease, or drug toxicity.

DIAGNOSTIC WORKUP
Inform the patient that the doctor may order blood tests to measure levels of serum electrolytes such as potassium or certain drugs, such as quinidine and propranolol. If the doctor suspects an illicit or street drug as the underlying cause of the arrhythmia, he also may order tests for such drugs as heroin, amphetamines, and cocaine.

Other tests commonly used to identify the specific arrhythmia and to monitor antiarrhythmic therapy include ECG, ambulatory ECG, exercise ECG, and electrophysiologic studies. (See *Teaching patients about cardiovascular tests,* pages 24 to 30.)

TREATMENTS
Explain that treatment of an arrhythmia depends on the severity of the patient's symptoms. It may include medications, an artificial pacemaker, and other procedures.

Activity guidelines
Emphasize that the patient should not restrict his normal activities. In fact, a medically supervised exercise routine can improve his cardiovascular fitness.

However, remind the patient to avoid overexertion and to stop exercising immediately if he experiences dizziness, light-headedness, dyspnea, or chest pain. If his arrhythmia causes periodic dizziness or syncope, warn him not to drive a motor vehicle or operate heavy machinery.

(Text continues on page 31.)

Teaching patients about cardiovascular tests

TEST AND PURPOSE	TEACHING POINTS
Abdominal ultrasonography • To detect an abdominal aortic aneurysm	• Tell the patient that this painless 30-minute test can help detect an aneurysm in major blood vessels in the abdomen, such as the abdominal portion of the aorta. • Explain what happens during the test: The patient will lie on an examining table, and a technician will apply conductive jelly to his abdomen. Then the technician will move a transducer slowly over the abdominal area to scan the blood vessels. Tell the patient he will feel only mild pressure. Explain that sound waves bouncing off anatomic structures are translated into graphic images, which then are displayed on a monitor or printed as a sonogram.
Ambulatory electrocardiography (Holter monitoring, ambulatory monitoring) • To detect arrhythmias • To evaluate chest pain • To evaluate the effectiveness of antiarrhythmic therapy	• Inform the patient that this test records the heart's electrical activity as he carries out his normal activities over a prolonged period — usually 24 hours. Tell him the test takes 24 hours and causes no discomfort. • Describe physical preparation for the test: The technician will clean, dry, and possibly shave different sites on the patient's body and will apply a conductive jelly over them. Then the technician will attach electrodes at these sites. • If the patient will take the test at home, tell him he will wear a small, lightweight tape recorder with a belt or shoulder strap. He will be asked to log his usual activities (such as walking, sleeping, urinating), emotional upsets, physical symptoms (such as chest pain, palpitations, dizziness, or fatigue), and medication administration, in a diary. • Depending on the type of monitor being used, show him how to mark the tape at onset of symptoms or how to press the event button to activate the monitor if he experiences any unusual sensations. Remind the patient not to tamper with the monitor or disconnect leadwires or electrodes. Tell him to avoid magnets, metal detectors, high-voltage areas, and electric blankets. Demonstrate how to check the recorder for proper function. Light flashes, for example, may indicate a loose electrode. Make sure the patient receives a copy of an appropriate patient-teaching aid.

Teaching patients about cardiovascular tests *(continued)*

TEST AND PURPOSE	TEACHING POINTS
Angiography (arteriography) ●To examine arteries or veins for suspected abnormalities, such as aneurysms, thrombi, and atherosclerotic obstructions ●To detect vessel compression from an extravascular tumor ●To evaluate the patency of arterial grafting and reconstruction	●Explain that angiography is a type of X-ray study that examines arteries for blockages caused by atherosclerosis. Tell him that the test may take 30 minutes to 4 hours, depending on the vessels examined. ●Describe physical preparation for the test: An area of the patient's body will be shaved and cleaned. After a local anesthetic is injected, a catheter will be inserted into a vessel and advanced as necessary. ●Explain what happens during the test: A contrast dye will be injected into the vessels. Then a series of X-ray films will follow the dye's passage. Reassure the patient that any flushing sensation, nausea, or unusual taste will pass quickly. To avoid distorting the X-ray image, stress to the patient that he must stay perfectly still during the test. ●Discuss what happens after the test: When the catheter is removed, pressure is applied on the incision site for 15 to 30 minutes. After bandaging, additional pressure is applied by using sandbags on the affected limb. The patient must keep the arm or leg extended and immobile for 4 to 24 hours.
Cardiac blood pool imaging ●To assess left ventricular function ●To detect motion and structural abnormalities of the ventricular wall	●Tell the patient that this 30- to 45-minute test evaluates how well the main chamber of his heart (left ventricle) pumps. ●Explain that before the test begins, electrodes will be attached to various sites on the patient's body. ●Describe what happens during the test: The patient will lie on his back, and a mildly radioactive contrast dye will be injected into a vein. A scintillation camera will record the dye's passage through his heart, and then will be synchronized with an electrocardiogram (ECG) to correlate subsequent images with ECG waveforms. The patient must remain still during scanning.
Cardiac catheterization ●To assess valve and cardiac wall function ●To diagnose various abnormalities, such as valvular insufficiency or stenosis, septal defects, and congenital anomalies	●Inform the patient that this test evaluates the function of the heart and its vessels. Tell him that it usually takes 2 to 3 hours. Instruct the patient not to eat or drink anything after midnight before the procedure. ●Explain physical preparation for the test: The patient will be placed on a padded table, and his groin area will be shaved and cleaned. Mention that he will probably be strapped to the table to keep him from slipping when the table is tilted; this

(continued)

Teaching patients about cardiovascular tests *(continued)*

TEST AND PURPOSE	TEACHING POINTS
Cardiac catheterization *(continued)* • To evaluate coronary artery and bypass graft patency • To detect pulmonary artery hypertension • To evaluate the effectiveness of drug therapy	allows the doctor to view the heart from different angles. The technician will start a peripheral I.V. line and attach electrodes to various sites. The patient will receive a mild I.V. sedative to help him relax. • Describe what happens during the test: After a local anesthetic has been injected into the groin, a catheter will be inserted and threaded up through an artery to the left side of his heart or through a vein to the right side of his heart to his lungs. Next the doctor may inject a contrast dye through the catheter. This may cause flushing, nausea, or chest pain; reassure the patient that these sensations should pass quickly. Advise him to follow instructions to cough or breathe deeply to provide a better view of the heart. Inform him that he may receive nitroglycerin during the test to expand coronary vessels and aid visualization. • Discuss what happens after the test: The doctor will slowly remove the catheter and the site will be bandaged. The patient will be monitored closely. Caution him to keep the bandaged arm or leg straight and still for up to 24 hours. To help keep him from moving, the arm or leg may be splinted or weighed down with a sandbag. Once he's allowed to resume his diet, he should drink plenty of fluids.
Cardiac computed tomography scan • To perform rapid screening for aortic dissection • To detect and evaluate pericardial disease • To check bypass graft patency	• Inform the patient that this painless, noninvasive test produces X-ray images of the blood vessels in 30 to 60 minutes. If a contrast medium is ordered, the patient must not eat or drink anything for 4 hours before the test. • Describe what happens during the test: The patient will lie on a table in the appropriate position and a stabilizing strap will be placed across the body part to be scanned. Then the table will slide into the circular opening of the scanner. The scanner will revolve around the patient, taking radiographs at preselected intervals. Instruct the patient to remain still during the test. If the test calls for a contrast medium, it's infused I.V. over about 5 minutes. Tell the patient to report sensations of warmth, itching, or other discomfort immediately. Reassure him that he'll be able to communicate with the examiner throughout the procedure. • Explain what happens after the test: The patient can resume usual activities and diet. However, if he received a contrast medium, he'll need to increase his fluid intake for the rest of the day to help eliminate the contrast medium.

Teaching patients about cardiovascular tests *(continued)*

TEST AND PURPOSE	TEACHING POINTS
Cardiac magnetic resonance imaging (MRI) • To identify anatomic effects of a myocardial infarction (MI), such as ventricular aneurysm and mural thrombus • To detect and evaluate cardiomyopathy • To detect and evaluate pericardial disease • To identify and evaluate masses within or near the heart • To detect congenital heart disease • To identify vascular disease, such as thoracic aneurysm and thoracic dissection • To assess the structure of pulmonary blood vessels	• Inform the patient that this test assesses the heart's function and structure and that it takes up to 90 minutes. Explain that although MRI is painless, he may feel uncomfortable because he must remain still inside a small space (in most facilities). Ask if he suffers from claustrophobia; if he does, he might not be able to tolerate the procedure or may need sedation. • Describe preparation for the test: The patient must remove all jewelry and other metal objects. Ask if he has shrapnel, a pacemaker, or any surgically implanted joints, pins, clips, valves, or pumps containing metal that could be attracted to the strong MRI magnet. If he does, he won't be able to have this test. • Explain what happens during the test. The patient will be checked at the scanner room door one last time for metal objects. He may receive a sedative. Then he will lie supine on a narrow bed, which slides into a large cylinder housing the MRI magnets. Radiofrequency energy is directed at the chest; the resulting images are displayed on a monitor and recorded. Tell the patient that the scanner will make clicking, whirring, and thumping noises as it moves inside its housing to obtain different images and that he may receive earplugs. Reassure him that he'll be able to communicate with the technician at all times and that the procedure will be stopped if he feels claustrophobic. The patient must remain still during the procedure.
Doppler ultrasonography • To aid diagnosis of chronic venous insufficiency, superficial and deep vein thromboses, peripheral artery disease, and arterial occlusion • To detect abnormalities of carotid artery blood flow associated with such conditions as aortic stenosis • To monitor patency of arterial grafting and reconstruction	• Tell the patient that this painless test evaluates circulation in the blood vessels and that it takes about 20 minutes. • Describe physical preparation for the test: The patient will be asked to uncover his leg, arm, or neck and to loosen any restrictive clothing. • Explain what happens during the test: A transducer coated with conductive jelly will be placed on the patient's skin and moved along the vessel to be examined. Blood pressure will be checked at the calves, thighs, and arms. Mention that he may be asked to move his arms into different positions and to perform breathing exercises to vary blood flow while measurements are taken. *(continued)*

Teaching patients about cardiovascular tests (continued)

TEST AND PURPOSE	TEACHING POINTS
Echocardiography • To diagnose and evaluate valvular abnormalities • To identify aneurysms • To aid diagnosis of cardiomyopathy • To detect atrial tumors • To evaluate cardiac function after myocardial infarction • To detect pericardial effusion	• Inform the patient that this painless test evaluates the size, shape, and motion of various cardiovascular structures. Tell him that it takes 15 to 30 minutes. Mention that other tests such as electrocardiography may be performed at the same time. • Describe physical preparation for the test: Conductive jelly will be applied to the patient's chest. • Explain what happens during the test: A transducer will be angled over the patient's chest to observe different parts of the heart, and he may be repositioned on his left side. He may be asked to breathe in and out slowly, to hold his breath, or to inhale a gas with a slightly sweet odor (amyl nitrite) while changes in heart function are recorded. Tell him that amyl nitrite may cause dizziness, flushing, and tachycardia, but these effects quickly subside. Stress that he must remain still during the test because movement may distort results.
Electrocardiography (ECG) • To help identify primary conduction abnormalities, arrhythmias, cardiac hypertrophy, pericarditis, electrolyte imbalance, myocardial ischemia, and the site and extent of myocardial infarction • To evaluate the effectiveness of cardiac drugs • To monitor pacemaker performance	• Inform the patient that this 15-minute test evaluates heart function by recording electrical activity. Assure him that it is noninvasive and rarely causes discomfort. • Discuss physical preparation for the test: The technician will clean, dry, and possibly shave different sites on the patient's body, such as his chest and arms, and will apply conductive jelly over them. Then the technician will attach electrodes at these sites. • Explain what happens during the test: The patient will be asked to lie still, to relax and breathe normally, and to remain quiet. Explain that talking or limb movement will distort ECG recordings and require additional testing time.
Electrophysiologic studies • To diagnose arrhythmias • To evaluate the effects of antiarrhythmic drugs	• Inform the patient that these studies evaluate the heart's electrical activity and the effect of any medication he's taking to treat an irregular heart rhythm. Tell him that the tests may take 2 to 5 hours. Instruct him to avoid food, fluids, and nonprescription drugs for 6 hours before the test. • Discuss physical preparation for the test: A catheter insertion site on the groin will be shaved and cleaned. • Explain what happens during the test: After injection of a local anesthetic, a catheter will be inserted into the femoral vein and advanced into

Teaching patients about cardiovascular tests *(continued)*

TEST AND PURPOSE	TEACHING POINTS
Electrophysiologic studies *(continued)*	the right side of the heart. The patient will receive an I.V. sedative to help him relax. Tell him he may feel mild pressure at the groin site but that he should report any other discomfort. Explain that the doctor may try to induce extra heartbeats with the catheter. • Describe what happens after the test: The catheter will be removed, and pressure and then a heavy dressing will be applied to the site to control bleeding. The patient may need to lie with his leg straight for a few hours after the test.
Exercise ECG (stress test, treadmill test, graded exercise test) • To help diagnose the cause of chest pain or other possible cardiac pain • To identify arrhythmias that occur during exercise • To evaluate the effectiveness of antiarrhythmic or antianginal therapy	• Explain that this test records the heart's electrical activity while the patient walks a treadmill or pedals a stationary bicycle. Tell him that it takes about 30 minutes, and that a doctor or nurse will be present in the testing area at all times. Inform him that he mustn't eat, smoke, or drink alcohol for 3 hours before the test. However, he should continue any drug regimen, as ordered. • Advise the patient to wear comfortable shoes and loose, lightweight shorts or slacks; men usually don't wear a shirt during the test, and women usually wear a bra and a lightweight, short-sleeved top or a patient gown with front closure. Inform the patient that a technician will clean, shave (if necessary), and lightly rub sites on the chest and, possibly, back. Then he'll attach electrodes at these sites. • If the patient is scheduled for a multistage treadmill test, tell him that the treadmill speed and incline will increase at predetermined intervals and that he'll be told of each adjustment. If he's scheduled for a bicycle ergometer test, tell him that resistance to pedaling will increase gradually. • Inform the patient that he may receive an injection of thallium. Then the doctor will evaluate coronary blood flow on a scanner. Tell him that the injection involves negligible radiation exposure. • Tell the patient that he can stop the test if he experiences severe fatigue, chest pain, or leg pain. Typically, he'll feel tired, out of breath, and sweaty. However, he should report any feelings during the test. He'll have his blood pressure and heart rate checked periodically during the test. • Describe what happens after the test: The patient's blood pressure and ECG will be monitored for 10 to 15 minutes. Tell him to wait at least 1 hour after the test before showering and then to use warm water.

(continued)

Teaching patients about cardiovascular tests (continued)

TEST AND PURPOSE	TEACHING POINTS
Impedance plethysmography • To detect deep vein thrombosis in the legs	• Tell the patient that this reliable, noninvasive test helps detect blood clots in his leg veins. Tell him it takes 30 to 45 minutes to examine both legs. Assure him that it's safe and usually painless. • Describe what happens during the procedure: The patient will put on a hospital gown and then lie on his back on an examining table or bed. The technician will clean, dry, and possibly shave sites on his lower legs and then attach electrodes with conductive jelly. • Explain what happens during the test: The technician will wrap a pressure cuff around the patient's thigh, inflate the cuff for 1 or 2 minutes, and then quickly release the cuff. Usually, the test is repeated to confirm initial tracings. Stress that the patient should keep his leg muscles relaxed and breathe normally to ensure accurate test results.
Technetium scan • To confirm the presence, size, and location of an acute MI	• Tell the patient that this test detects any damaged areas of the heart muscle and that it takes 45 minutes. • Explain that the doctor will inject an I.V. tracer isotope called technetium pyrophosphate into an arm vein about 3 hours before the test. Reassure him that the injection causes only transient discomfort and involves negligible radiation exposure. • Describe what happens during the test: The patient will lie on his back and a series of scans will be taken at different angles. Instruct him to remain still.
Thallium scan (resting) • To assess myocardial perfusion • To locate and estimate the size of an acute or old MI • To evaluate the patency of a coronary artery bypass graft	• Explain that this test assesses the heart's blood supply, showing areas with poor blood flow as "cold spots" on a scan. Mention that it takes 45 to 90 minutes, although additional scans may be required. • Describe what happens during the procedure: Within the first few hours of MI symptoms, the patient will lie on a table and receive an injection of radioactive thallium. After 3 to 5 minutes, scanning will begin. The patient will be placed in various positions to produce multiple images. Reassure him that there is no known radiation danger from the thallium.

Dietary modifications

Instruct the patient to follow any special diet the doctor prescribes. Because a low serum potassium level sometimes contributes to arrhythmias, encourage him to eat potassium-rich foods, such as bananas, citrus fruits, figs, leafy green vegetables, meats, and seafood.

If dietary restrictions aren't required, advise the patient not to overeat or consume too much alcohol or caffeine. If he smokes, urge him to stop.

 WARNING: Caution the patient not to overindulge during the holidays. "Holiday heart syndrome" — a result of increased food and alcohol consumption, smoking, and emotional excitement associated with holiday get-togethers — can trigger or worsen arrhythmias.

Medication

Medications commonly used to treat arrhythmias include antiarrhythmics, such as digitalis glycosides, verapamil, propranolol, quinidine, or procainamide. These may be given in combination with other drugs to treat an underlying cardiovascular disorder.

Point out that medications can only control, not cure, the arrhythmia. Emphasize that the patient must take antiarrhythmics and other prescribed drugs on schedule, even when he has no symptoms. Warn him never to discontinue his medications without consulting the doctor.

Procedures

Depending on the patient's specific arrhythmia, the doctor may recommend carotid sinus massage, Valsalva's maneuver, or other procedures to help manage it. (See *Teaching patients about carotid sinus massage,* page 32.)

Valsalva's maneuver

Like carotid sinus massage, Valsalva's maneuver can restore normal heart rhythm in some arrhythmias. Tell the patient that to perform the maneuver, he inhales deeply, holds that breath, and strains hard for at least 10 seconds before exhaling. Explain that the maneuver increases chest pressure, which converts the arrhythmia to a normal rhythm.

Temporary pacemaker implantation

If the patient is scheduled for temporary pacemaker implantation, tell him that the doctor will insert a long, thin, electrode leadwire into a peripheral vein and, guided by fluoroscopy, will advance it through the vena cava into the right atrium and into the right ventricle. Once the electrode lead is in place, the doctor will attach its other end to a battery-powered pacemaker pulse generator, which will control the patient's heart rate.

Inform the patient that he may feel burning or stinging from the anesthetic used to numb his skin as well as transient pressure at the insertion site as the catheter is placed. He also may feel his heart flutter as the pacemaker is activated or adjusted but should otherwise have no discomfort.

Tell him that the pacemaker will remain in place for several days until the arrhythmia is controlled or until he undergoes other measures, such as permanent pacemaker insertion or cardiac surgery. Remind him that his activity will be limited and that he may require bed rest, depending on which vein was used.

Electrocardioversion

If the doctor orders electrocardioversion to control an unstable arrhythmia, tell the patient that cardioversion uses an electric current to restore the normal heart rate and relieve symptoms. Tell him he won't be allowed to consume food or fluids for at least 8 hours before the procedure.

Explain that just before the procedure, he'll receive an I.V. sedative to induce sleep. Then, while he's asleep, an electric current will be delivered to the heart through paddles placed on his chest. Reassure him that the procedure is painless.

Teaching patients about carotid sinus massage

If your patient has paroxysmal atrial tachycardia, the doctor may perform carotid sinus massage to quickly restore the heart's regular rhythm. Some patients may also be advised to self-administer this form of massage at home under certain circumstances.

Explain that this technique involves manual stimulation of blood pressure sensors in the carotid artery in the neck, slowing the heart rate and electrical conduction in the heart. Show the patient how to locate the carotid sinus on both the right and left sides of the neck (see the illustration).

Next, reinforce the doctor's or nurse's instructions on how to *firmly* massage the right sinus for no more than 5 seconds. *Caution the patient never to massage both sinuses at once.*

Emphasize that improper technique, such as using excessive pressure or massaging for too long, can block blood flow to the brain, which can cause a stroke. Improper technique also can trigger new, more dangerous arrhythmias.

Special precautions
The patient should not perform carotid sinus massage if he:
- has cholesterol-containing deposits in the carotid artery
- has a history of cerebrovascular disease (stroke)
- has had previous surgery on the carotid artery.

Also, the patient should make sure the doctor knows his complete medical history and all medications he's taking before performing carotid sinus massage.

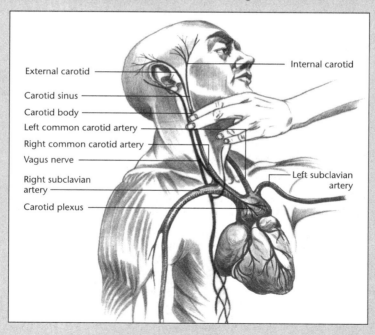

External carotid —
Carotid sinus —
Carotid body —
Left common carotid artery —
Right common carotid artery —
Vagus nerve —
Right subclavian artery —
Carotid plexus —
Internal carotid
Left subclavian artery

Inform the patient that he will be able to eat and move about once the sedative wears off. Tell him to expect a reddened area to appear where the paddles were placed as well as a feeling of tenderness and itching for a day or two.

Surgery

If the arrhythmia can't be controlled by medications or other conservative measures, the doctor may order surgery. The type of surgery selected depends on the specific arrhythmia and any underlying cardiovascular problems. It may involve complex open-heart surgery to correct structural defects, relatively uncomplicated permanent pacemaker implantation or, in recurrent life-threatening arrhythmias, ICD insertion.

Permanent pacemaker implantation

Explain the function of a pacemaker and the implantation procedure, and give preoperative and postoperative instructions. Tell the patient that he'll receive both a sedative and a local anesthetic before the procedure. During surgery, the pacemaker pulse generator will be implanted under the skin in an unobtrusive area, and electrodes will be threaded through a vein into the heart's right chamber.

Inform the patient that he'll be restricted to bed rest for the first 24 hours after surgery to allow the leads to seed, or attach well. If he previously had a temporary pacemaker, explain that it may be left in place for up to 24 hours after the permanent one is implanted, to serve as a backup. If a thoracotomy was done during implantation to attach electrodes directly to the epicardium, teach the patient proper postthoracotomy care.

ICD implantation

If the patient is scheduled to receive an ICD, explain that the device delivers an electrical shock to the heart to correct an abnormal heart rhythm.

Assure the patient that he'll receive both a sedative and an anesthetic be-

fore surgery. Tell him that the surgeon will make an incision down the center of the chest or on the left side between the ribs, and then will sew two small, rectangular patches onto the heart's surface. Attached to these patches are long, thin, insulated wires, which the surgeon will tunnel under the skin to a pocket he makes in the abdomen — where the ICD implant will be placed. Tell him that the implant is slightly larger than a deck of playing cards and weighs about ½ lb (227 g).

Inform him that he can expect to stay in the hospital about 1 week after ICD implantation. Before he is discharged, instruct him to check both the abdominal and chest incisions regularly for the first few weeks at home. Usually, the patient can see the ICD under the skin and feel its edges. Tell him that fluid accumulation in the implant area is normal, but that he should report any redness, swelling, drainage, warmth, or pain immediately.

Reassure the family that touching the patient when the ICD discharges a shock will not harm them, although they may feel a slight buzz on the patient's skin.

Finally, inform the patient that after about 2 years, he will require hospitalization to replace the ICD battery. Instruct him to always carry an ICD information card and to wear a medical identification tag.

Other care measures

Teach the patient — especially one with a pacemaker — how to take his pulse. Instruct him to keep an accurate record of daily pulse readings and to notify the doctor of any significant abnormalities — a rate 5 or more beats lower than the pacemaker's preset rate, a rate exceeding 100 beats/minute, or any unusually irregular rhythm. Tell the patient with atrial fibrillation to take a carotid pulse rather than a radial (wrist) pulse.

Also teach the patient ways to reduce long-term complications of arrhythmia. Suggest that at least one family member learn cardiopulmonary resuscitation — this training could make the difference between life and death if the patient develops sudden cardiac arrest or myocardial infarction.

Make the patient aware of other cardiovascular disorders that can contribute to or result from uncontrolled arrhythmias. Discuss general risk factors for these disorders — stress, obesity, smoking, and sedentary lifestyle, among others.

Finally, instruct the patient to contact the American Heart Association, Coronary Club, Heart Disease Research Foundation, or Heartlife for further information. (See Appendix 2.)

Arterial occlusive disease

Arterial occlusive disease often goes undetected until symptoms of arterial insufficiency force the patient to seek treatment. By the time symptoms appear, arterial damage is often extensive, limiting the effectiveness of treatment. Nevertheless, your teaching can help the patient cope with the demands of this chronic disorder.

Before teaching a patient about arterial occlusive disease, make sure you are familiar with the following topics:
• major causes of reduced arterial blood flow — atherosclerosis and arteriosclerosis
• how intermittent claudication and arterial ulcers develop
• diagnostic tests, such as arteriography, Doppler ultrasonography, blood clotting studies, and possibly serum lipid and lipoprotein measurements
• relief of intermittent claudication by resting or by placing the leg in a dependent position
• activity and dietary recommendations
• anticoagulants and other drugs and their proper use and precautions
• how to prevent infection and ulcers
• how to care for ulcers, including dressing changes

• preparation for treatment procedures, such as percutaneous transluminal angioplasty and laser-assisted angioplasty
• preparation for possible surgery: arterial bypass grafting, sympathectomy, or endarterectomy
• sources of information and support.

ABOUT THE DISORDER

Explain that in arterial occlusive disease, narrowing of the aorta and its major branches disrupts blood flow. This leads to interrupted blood flow, usually to the legs and feet, and prevents oxygen and nutrients from reaching the tissues. (See *Sites of arterial occlusion*.) Such occlusion, or blockage, can cause severe ischemia, skin ulceration, and gangrene.

Point out that changes in blood vessels — primarily arteriosclerotic and atherosclerotic changes — cause varying degrees of arterial occlusion and may appear in combination. In arteriosclerosis, calcification and blockage of arteries stem from a progressive loss of vessel elasticity associated with such factors as aging, hypertension, and diabetes. Explain that atherosclerosis — gradual buildup of fatty, fibrous plaques on the inner arterial walls — results from lipoprotein abnormalities, arterial wall injury, and platelet dysfunction.

Next, explain how these arterial changes lead to intermittent claudication: Insufficient blood flow through occluded arteries causes an oxygen deficiency in leg muscles — usually in the calves — resulting in a painful cramp. The patient usually feels no symptoms while resting, but pain and weakness develop in the calf muscles after he walks a certain distance without resting. When he does rest, his symptoms disappear as blood supply to the calf muscles is restored.

DIAGNOSTIC WORKUP

Explain that blood clotting studies will be done to check for blood clotting abnormalities or to evaluate the effectiveness of anticoagulant therapy. Inform the patient that the doctor also may order measurement of

Sites of arterial occlusion

Show the patient this anatomic diagram to help him understand the arterial system. Point out the location of the aorta, its major branching arteries, and the body areas affected by the blood flow from these arteries. Remember to pinpoint on the diagram the site of the patient's occlusion.

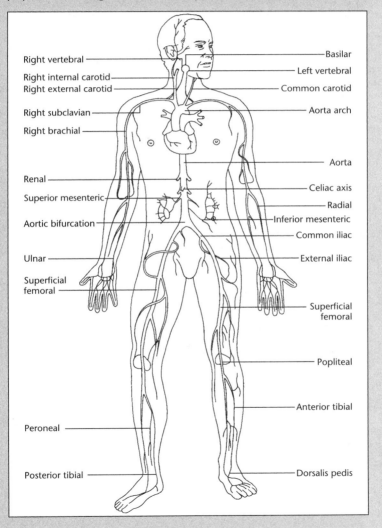

blood cholesterol, triglyceride, and fat levels to assess for atherosclerosis. Instruct him to abstain from alcohol for 24 hours and from exercise for 12 hours before these tests.

Teach the patient about other diagnostic tests he may undergo to evaluate the extent of arterial occlusive disease and collateral circulation, such as arteriography, Doppler ultrasonography, blood chemistry studies and, possibly, serum lipid and lipo-protein measurements. (See *Teaching patients about cardiovascular tests,* pages 24 to 30.)

TREATMENTS
Treatment of arterial occlusive disease may be medical, surgical, or a combination, depending on the cause, location, and size of the arterial blockage. Inform the patient that medical treatments may include risk-factor reduction (such as stopping smoking), exercise, dietary changes, foot and leg care, medications, and angioplasty. Surgery may involve such techniques as bypass grafting, sympathectomy, or endarterectomy.

Activity guidelines
Emphasize the importance of getting regular exercise to help prevent further arterial blockages. Point out that exercise also promotes development of collateral circulation, which reduces intermittent claudication and helps prevent leg ulcers. Depending on the patient's age and capabilities, the doctor may recommend daily walking, swimming, or bicycle riding.

Inform the patient that daily progressive exercise may gradually reduce the severity of claudication. Stress that in progressive exercise, the patient exercises until pain forces a halt; then he rests, and then he resumes the exercise. Instruct him to balance exercise and rest periods.

 WARNING: Caution the patient not to exercise too vigorously because this generates a great deal of heat in leg muscles, placing excessive demands on already compromised leg circulation. These demands, in turn, worsen leg pain and increase the risk of infection. For the same reasons, he should avoid crossing his legs and raising or applying heat to the affected leg.

Dietary modifications
Depending on the underlying cause of arterial occlusive disease, the doctor may restrict the patient's dietary intake of cholesterol, saturated fats, and salt. To help maintain skin integrity and reduce the chance of infection and ulcers, advise the patient to consume adequate protein, vitamin B_{12}, and vitamin C.

Medication
The patient may receive such drugs as anticoagulants, vasodilators, or pentoxifylline (Trental).

If the doctor prescribes anticoagulants, tell the patient that he must take certain precautions to prevent bleeding and must stay alert for adverse effects while on anticoagulant therapy. Make sure he is familiar with the purpose, adverse effects, and special instructions for all prescribed drugs. For instance, antiplatelet agents, such as aspirin and dipyridamole, reduce clot formation by interfering with platelet function.

If the patient is taking a vasodilator, such as isoxsuprine, tell him that the drug eases symptoms by expanding the arteries. Forewarn him that it may cause symptoms of low blood pressure, such as dizziness, flushing, and headache — especially when he gets up from a sitting or lying position. To help prevent dizziness, advise him to rise slowly.

If the patient is receiving pentoxifylline, explain that this drug aids blood flow through the blood vessels by making the blood less sticky. Tell him to report adverse effects — especially dizziness, tremors, agitation, palpitations, or fainting spells — to the doctor.

Procedures
Depending on the patient's condition, the doctor may recommend

percutaneous transluminal coronary angioplasty (PTCA) or laser-assisted angioplasty to open blocked arteries.

PTCA
Inform the patient that this technique (also called balloon angioplasty) allows the doctor to open a blocked or narrowed artery. Mention that he will be awake but sedated and must lie flat during the 1- to 4-hour procedure.

Preview the procedure for the patient: First, the catheter insertion site will be cleaned and anesthetized. Then the doctor will insert a thin, balloon-tipped catheter into a peripheral artery. With X-ray guidance, he will thread the catheter through the blocked artery and confirm the presence of the blockage by angiography (X-ray examination of blood vessels after a dye is injected). Tell the patient to expect a hot, flushing sensation or transient nausea when the dye is injected.

Next, the doctor will introduce a small, balloon-tipped catheter through the guide wire. After positioning the balloon tip in the blocked artery, the doctor will repeatedly inflate it. The inflated balloon compresses the cholesterol-containing deposits against the arterial wall, widening the diameter of the artery.

Tell the patient that angiography is repeated to confirm successful angioplasty. The catheter is left in the artery for up to 24 hours to provide emergency access in case arterial blockage develops. Tell the patient that he'll receive I.V. anticoagulants during this time.

The arterial catheter will be removed 6 to 24 hours after the procedure, and direct pressure will be applied to the insertion site for 30 minutes or until the bleeding stops. Then a pressure bandage will be applied.

Laser-assisted angioplasty
Explain that this alternative to standard angioplasty can be used to open vessels that are totally blocked or narrowed with dense plaque. The doctor makes a small incision to expose the artery or inserts a needle into the

artery. Next, he inserts a small catheter into the artery and advances it to the blockage site. A contrast dye is injected to outline the blocked area. Once the blocked area is identified, the doctor opens the blood vessel with a laser catheter alone. If some blockage remains, the doctor also may use a balloon-tipped catheter.

Tell the patient that he may feel a warm sensation in the affected limb from the laser. Assure him that this sensation lasts only seconds to minutes. Tell him the entire procedure usually takes 1 to 3 hours.

Surgery
Some patients with arterial occlusive disease require surgery, such as bypass grafting, sympathectomy, or carotid endarterectomy. Typically, surgery is done if claudication interferes with walking, if a blocked carotid artery causes neurologic problems, or if the procedure will improve blood supply to an ulcerated area.

Bypass graft surgery
If the doctor recommends this procedure, inform the patient that it uses a graft to divert blood flow around the blockage. Tell him that this procedure is the most effective surgical treatment for his condition. Depending on the blockage site, surgery may involve an aortofemoral bypass, an axillofemoral bypass, or a femoro-popliteal bypass graft.

If the patient is scheduled for an *aortofemoral* bypass, explain that he will receive a general anesthetic and will have two or three incisions — one midline abdominal and one groin site for each femoral graft done.

If he's scheduled for an *axillofemoral* bypass, tell him that he will receive a general anesthetic and have up to three incisions — one site under the arm and one or two at groin sites. Explain that after surgery, he won't be permitted to lie on the side of the graft. Advise him to avoid heavy lifting, carrying, sudden or forceful use of the arm on the affected side, and reaching high overhead.

Explain that passive range-of-motion exercises can help him regain use of the affected limb. These exercises involve alternately flexing and extending the legs, wiggling the toes, and rotating and flexing the feet. As his condition allows, the patient will be allowed to begin active exercises.

 WARNING: To prevent graft occlusion, caution the patient against sitting or standing for prolonged periods or wearing tight or constrictive garments (belts, girdles, or suspenders) over the graft.

Tell the patient undergoing *femoropopliteal* bypass that this procedure can be done under general or spinal anesthesia. The surgeon may make several incisions from the ankle to the groin, depending on the specific procedure.

Sympathectomy

Explain that this operation, which requires general anesthesia, usually is done in conjunction with other revascularization procedures. It involves the surgical removal of selected sympathetic nerve fibers. If successful, this surgery expands the arteries and increases blood flow to the limbs.

Carotid endarterectomy

Tell the patient scheduled for this procedure that it improves brain circulation by removing the atherosclerotic plaque that has built up in the carotid artery and blocked the blood flow. Mention that afterward, he will stay in the intensive care unit for at least 24 hours.

Instruct him to immediately report any changes in speech or level of consciousness, difficulty swallowing, hoarseness, paralysis or weakness in the arms or legs, or facial drooping. These symptoms could indicate neurologic damage.

Long-term management

Long-term management of arterial occlusive disease typically involves reducing cardiovascular risk factors and taking steps to prevent infection and skin ulcers.

Risk factor reduction

If the patient's job involves standing for prolonged periods or working outdoors in cold weather, suggest that he consider changing to an indoor, sedentary occupation or, if possible, retiring early.

Advise him to reduce cardiovascular risk factors by limiting his dietary salt and cholesterol intake, stopping smoking, losing weight, if necessary, and keeping hypertension or diabetes under control.

Infection and ulcer prevention

To help prevent infection and avoid skin ulcers, stress the importance of practicing meticulous skin care and avoiding any activity that could cause skin injury or irritation or that could apply pressure or heat to the skin.

To help safeguard the feet from injury and subsequent infection, instruct the patient to wash his feet daily with mild soap and warm water and to dry them carefully — especially between the toes.

If the patient has leg ulcers, explain that wet-to-dry dressings will help clean the ulcers and promote healing. Tell him to take prescribed pain medication about 30 minutes before changing dressings.

If the doctor prescribes an Unna's boot, inform the patient that this boot is a bandage that protects and medicates leg ulcers while preventing swelling.

Additional teaching points

Teach the patient to recognize and immediately report early warning signs and symptoms of an embolism or aneurysm — sudden onset of excruciating pain, abnormally pale skin or skin mottling (spotting with patches of color), difficulty breathing, loss of pulse, and paralysis in the affected extremity.

Refer the patient to the American Heart Association for more information and support. (See Appendix 2.)

Coronary artery disease

Coronary artery disease (CAD) claims more lives in the United States than any other disorder. Most patients lack symptoms until middle age or later, when the heart no longer receives an adequate blood supply for its needs.

Many patients with CAD first seek medical help after experiencing angina, which they may confuse with the chest pain of myocardial infarction (MI), or heart attack. Your teaching can help the patient prepare for diagnostic tests; understand prescribed drug therapy, surgery, or other necessary treatment; and identify and modify his risk factors for CAD.

Before teaching a patient about CAD, make sure you are familiar with the following topics:

• explanation of the disease mechanisms — atherosclerosis and coronary artery spasm
• cardiac physiology, with emphasis on coronary arteries
• how the patient's risk factors are evaluated
• how angina develops and how it can be treated and prevented
• importance of treating CAD to prevent such complications as MI
• diagnostic tests, such as cardiac catheterization, cardiac blood pool imaging, echocardiography, electrocardiography (ECG), exercise ECG, angiography, and serum lipid studies
• recommended exercise program
• dietary restrictions to lower blood cholesterol levels and control hypertension
• use of prescribed drugs
• preparation for percutaneous transluminal coronary angioplasty (PTCA) or coronary artery bypass grafting (CABG), if ordered
• modifying risk factors — reducing stress, controlling weight, and quitting smoking
• sources of information and support.

ABOUT THE DISORDER

Tell the patient that CAD is characterized by narrowing or blockage of one or more of the coronary arteries, leading to diminished blood flow to the heart. This deprives the heart of vital oxygen and nutrients, causing tissue damage.

Explain that atherosclerosis — buildup of fatty, fibrous plaques on inner arterial walls — usually causes CAD. These plaques narrow the vessels and reduce the amount of blood that can be pumped through them. (See *Atherosclerosis stages,* page 40.) Review the risk factors linked to atherosclerosis. Give the patient a copy of the teaching aid *Personalizing your exercise program,* pages 42 and 43.

Complications

Tell the patient that strict adherence to the treatment plan can reduce the risk of serious complications of CAD, such as heart attack, arrhythmias, heart failure, and even death.

DIAGNOSTIC WORKUP

Inform the patient that blood tests can detect and classify the type of hyperlipemia (high blood fat level) the patient has. (High blood fat level is a risk factor for CAD.) These tests include total cholesterol level, triglyceride level, lipoprotein phenotyping, and lipoprotein-cholesterol fractionation. Instruct the patient not to drink alcohol for 24 hours and not to eat for 12 to 14 hours before the tests. Stress the importance of getting periodic blood tests to help evaluate the effectiveness of drug and dietary therapy in reducing his blood fat levels.

Also explain other ordered diagnostic tests, which may include blood tests, cardiac angiography, cardiac blood pool imaging, cardiac catheterization, echocardiography, ECG, and exercise ECG. (For more information, see *Teaching patients about cardiovascular tests,* pages 24 to 30.)

TREATMENTS

Tell the patient that treatment for CAD typically includes increased exercise, dietary changes, and other risk factor–reduction measures along with drug therapy. If these treatments don't improve or eliminate angina, the doctor may recommend PTCA or CABG.

INSIGHT INTO ILLNESSES

Atherosclerosis stages

When explaining atherosclorosis to the patient, point out that the disorder doesn't happen all at once; it occurs in stages.

Intimal injury
Inform the patient that atherosclerosis starts with an injury to the intimal layer of the arterial wall. This makes the wall permeable to circulating lipoproteins.

Lesion formation
Next, lipoproteins invade smooth-muscle cells in the intimal layer, forming a fatty streak — a nonobstructive lesion.

Plaque development
Eventually, a fibrous plaque develops, impeding blood flow through the artery. Plaques contain lipoprotein-filled smooth-muscle cells, collagen, and muscle fibers.

Near-total occlusion
Explain that in the final stage of atherosclerosis, a complicated lesion develops, marked by calcification or rupture of the fibrous plaque. Thrombosis may occur, with near-total occlusion of the arterial lumen, as in the illustration below.

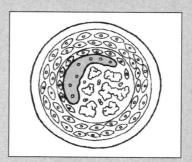

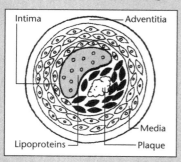

Activity guidelines
Emphasize that a sedentary lifestyle contributes to CAD, encourages overeating, leads to obesity and hypertension, and unfavorably alters the ratio of high-density lipoprotein (HDL) to low-density lipoprotein (LDL).

Point out that regular exercise has many benefits: It can increase the serum HDL level, promotes weight loss, lowers blood pressure, and tones the entire cardiovascular system. Encourage aerobic exercise, such as walking, jogging, bicycling, or swimming. Make sure the patient knows how to monitor his pulse during exercise.

 WARNING: Advise against isometric exercises such as weight lifting because they raise blood pressure and tax the heart and coronary arteries. Warn that occasional strenuous exercise may be more dangerous than no exercise. Tell the patient to take prescribed medication before engaging in any activity that normally provokes angina, including exercise and sex. If angina occurs, he should stop the activity immediately, sit or lie down with his head elevated, breathe deeply and slowly to relax, and take prescribed medication. Instruct him to have someone take him to the hospital emergency department if his angina persists longer than 10 minutes after he takes three spaced doses of his medication.

Dietary modifications

Explain how dietary adjustments can help modify three important CAD risk factors: high serum cholesterol level, high blood pressure, and obesity. Advise him to limit fat intake to no more than 30% of total daily calories, with saturated fats making up less than 10% of total calories. Also advise him to limit his cholesterol intake.

Instruct the patient to limit red meat, processed meat, lard, whole milk products, and saturated tropical oils (coconut, palm, and palm kernel), found mostly in processed foods. Tell him to trim visible fat from red meat, remove the skin from poultry before cooking, and substitute fish and margarine for meat and butter. Remind him that broiling, microwaving, grilling, or roasting meat on a rack is preferable to deep-frying. If he eats at fast-food restaurants, suggest he order food products cooked in unsaturated vegetable oils. Recommend that he eat no more than three egg yolks a week, including yolks in prepared foods.

 TIPS AND TIMESAVERS: Discuss the benefits of consuming fiber, fish oils, and olive oil. Explain that soluble fiber such as oat bran (but not wheat bran) may reduce the absorption of saturated fats in the intestines. Intake of fish oils, also known as omega-3 fatty acids or marine oils (found in salmon, mackerel, herring, and tuna), may improve the HDL:LDL ratio. But emphasize that the effectiveness of fish oil capsules hasn't yet been proven — only the eating of fish, especially as a substitute for red meat. If the patient drinks alcohol, advise him that up to two drinks a day can also improve the HDL:LDL ratio, but that more than this amount can adversely affect the heart.

To help the patient lower his blood pressure, advise him to eliminate caffeine and reduce sodium intake. If he's overweight, explain that obesity is closely linked to several other CAD risk factors. Explain how losing excess weight by itself affects CAD and also helps to lower hypertension. Inform him that the two best ways to lose weight are to limit caloric — especially fat — intake and to exercise (an activity that also corrects a sedentary lifestyle).

Medications

Reinforce the doctor's or nurse's explanation of the purpose of all prescribed medications, including antilipemics and antiplatelet drugs, beta blockers, calcium channel blockers, and nitrates. Explain, for instance, that antilipemics reduce the levels of certain protein and fat combinations in the blood. Antiplatelets, such as aspirin and dipyridamole, hinder blood clotting. Beta-adrenergic blockers lower blood pressure, reduce the frequency of anginal attacks, and control a rapid heart rate. Calcium channel blockers reduce the frequency and severity of chest pain and lower blood pressure. Nitrates prevent or alleviate anginal pain. Teach the patient to examine labels of nonprescription medications for sodium, caffeine, and aspirin content.

Procedures

If drug therapy fails to relieve angina, the doctor may order PTCA to repair a blocked artery. Explain that *percutaneous* means the procedure involves going through the skin; *transluminal* means that it's done inside the artery, *coronary* means the treated artery is one that involves the heart, and *angioplasty* signifies the technique of repairing the narrowed or blocked artery.

Tell the patient that before the procedure, he will receive a sedative to

(Text continues on page 44.)

Personalizing your exercise program

Dear Patient:
You can make your exercise program suit your individual needs by determining your aerobic training level, adjusting your pace accordingly, and allowing adequate time for warm up and cool down.

Finding your pace
How do you determine the aerobic training level that's best for you? Your target heart rate provides a guideline for achieving the greatest benefits during exercise while reducing risk.

First, find your maximum heart rate. To do this, subtract your age from 220. To determine your target heart rate, calculate 75% of your maximum rate (multiply your maximum rate times .75). For example, if your maximum rate is 180, your target rate is 135 beats per minute.

To determine your heart rate range, calculate the range between 70% and 80% of your maximum heart rate. By monitoring your pulse and staying in this range, you will achieve the greatest benefits from aerobic exercise. The chart below provides heart rate ranges according to age.

Keep in mind, however, that these numbers provide a measure of what a healthy heart can do. Gradually

slow down if you begin to experience any pain.

Warming up
Before starting any kind of demanding physical activity, you'll want to perform warm-up exercise to stretch muscles and loosen joints. This will lessen the risk of muscle strain or ligament damage. A good warm-up also offers psychological benefits. Use this time to focus on the activities ahead and to get rid of tension. First, take your pulse and then do 5 to 10 minutes of stretching exercises (such as those shown in the illustrations) and light calisthenics.

Adjusting the pace
Gradually work toward your optimal aerobic training level. During your exercise period, take your pulse two or three times as your doctor directs. Adjust your pace according to your pulse rate and how you feel. If you exceed your target

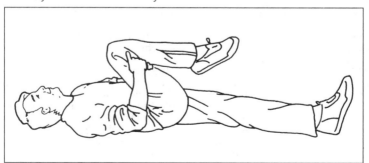

Personalizing your exercise program *(continued)*

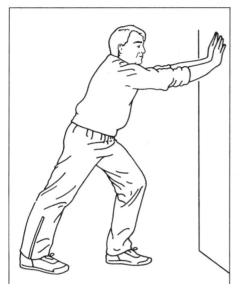

do, the amount of blood circulating back to the heart, which is still beating rapidly, won't be adequate to meet your body's needs. You need a cooldown period much as a horse needs to be walked after a race.

Gradually decrease the pace of your exercise for 5 to 10 minutes. Then do 5 minutes of light calisthenics and simple stretching exercises. At this point your pulse should be no more than 15 beats above your resting pulse. If you feel dizzy or faint after exercise, you may need a longer cooldown period.

rate, or if you have chest discomfort, breathlessness, or palpitations, slow down *gradually.* Don't stop suddenly unless symptoms persist or worsen.

Cooling down
Don't stop exercising abruptly. If you

Keeping records
Keep an exercise diary. List the date and time, the activity and its duration, your heart rate, and any symptoms you experience. Tracking your progress will help you keep up your motivation, and the record you develop will help you and your doctor.

Additional instructions

_____

_____

_____

_____

_____

_____

44 CARDIOVASCULAR CONDITIONS

promote relaxation. Explain that the
doctor may introduce the catheter
into either the arm or the groin. After
numbing the site with a local anesthetic, the doctor will insert a thin,
balloon-tipped catheter into a peripheral artery. Then he'll thread the
catheter through the blocked coronary artery to the obstruction site. To
verify catheter placement, the doctor
will instill contrast dye. Then he will
inflate the balloon tip. By compressing the obstruction against the arterial walls, balloon inflation expands
the vessel to increase blood flow.

Inform the patient that he will be
asked to cough several times during
the procedure to help clear contrast
dye from the heart. Advise him that
any flushing or angina he experiences when the contrast dye is instilled will pass quickly.

Mention that after PTCA, the patient will be on bed rest for 12 hours
and will require periodic blood tests
to evaluate blood coagulation and
cardiac enzyme and electrolyte levels.
He may receive I.V. nitroglycerin to
prevent coronary artery spasm and
anticoagulants to prevent clot formation. His blood pressure and pulses
will be checked frequently and he
may be connected to a cardiac monitor. Urge him to drink plenty of fluids
to help his kidneys excrete the contrast dye more readily.

Explain that mild chest pain is common immediately after PTCA but
should subside in 1 to 2 hours. Emphasize that the patient must report
worsening or returning chest pain immediately.

If the femoral approach was used,
tell the patient that short tubes or
sheaths may be left in the groin until
the next day. Urge him to keep the
affected leg straight to prevent the
tubes from kinking. Assure him that
he will be able to bend the leg and
then stand for a few hours after the
tubes are removed.

Surgery
If the doctor schedules CABG to re-
lieve angina (and possibly to prevent
MI), describe the surgery, including

preoperative and postoperative care
measures.

Tell the patient that CABG will restore normal blood flow to his heart.
Explain that the doctor will remove a
portion of a healthy vessel from another part of the body (usually a portion of a saphenous vein or a mammary artery) and then graft it above
and below the blocked coronary artery. Circulation will then be diverted
through the graft.

Preoperative care
Inform the patient that he'll be asked
to shower with a special antiseptic
soap and will be shaved from neck to
toes. Although he won't be allowed to
eat or drink anything after midnight,
he can ask for a sleeping pill to ensure
adequate rest. Tell him he may be giv-
en a sedative the morning of surgery
to promote relaxation.

If indicated, explain that the patient
may undergo preoperative pulmonary
artery catheterization. Tell him that
the catheter will remain in place after
surgery, but that the catheter, arterial
lines, and epicardial pacing wires will
cause minimal or no discomfort.

Postoperative care
Explain the complex, and often
frightening, equipment that will support the patient's vital functions after
surgery. For example, prepare him for
intubation and mechanical ventilation.

Explain that an intra-aortic balloon
pump may be inserted to provide circulatory support for several hours
postoperatively. A nasogastric tube, a
mediastinal chest tube, and an indwelling catheter will be in place for
the first day or two, and the patient
will be connected to a cardiac monitor.

Teach the patient about short-term
postoperative care measures. Start
with the expected course of the hospital stay — how many days he will
spend in the critical care area, step-
down unit, and regular room before
discharge.

Emphasize that his priority is to relax and rest; stress and anxiety will only hinder recovery. Encourage him to request pain medication to avoid discomfort. When the endotracheal and nasogastric tubes are removed, he will be able to sit up and swallow liquids. Tell him that solid foods will then gradually be reintroduced to his diet.

Discuss other self-care measures. For instance, tell him that about 6 days after surgery, he will probably be allowed to shower. Advise him to use warm, not hot, water and to wash all incision sites gently.

Explain that complete healing takes time. Assure him that although a scar will remain, it will fade. Recommend that he wear soft, loose clothing, such as cotton T-shirts, at first for maximum comfort.

To enhance circulation and reduce swelling in a leg from which a saphenous vein graft was taken, the patient also may need to wear support stockings, elevate the leg frequently, and avoid crossing the legs. Tell him to watch for and report any new tenderness, redness, swelling, or drainage from the chest and leg incisions.

Long-term care
Review the patient's prescribed exercise program. Stress the need to increase his activity gradually and to establish realistic goals. Advise him to alternate light and heavy tasks and to rest between tasks.

Address the patient's concerns about sex after surgery. Tell him that once the doctor has given approval, sex is no more dangerous to the heart than walking up a couple flights of stairs. Point out that a satisfying sex life can help speed recovery.

However, advise him to reduce strain on the heart by avoiding sex right after eating a big meal or drinking alcohol, when fatigued or emotionally upset, or when in an unfamiliar and stressful situation—in a strange environment or with a new partner, for example. Also suggest that he use positions that don't restrict breathing and avoid any position in which he must support his partner with his arms. Reassure him that impotence is fairly common but that it's almost always temporary and is no cause for concern.

Make sure the patient understands the administration schedules for all prescribed medications and is familiar with possible adverse effects. Also discuss dietary restrictions, emphasizing that a diet low in cholesterol and saturated fats can reduce his risk of arterial reocclusion. With the doctor's permission, he may have up to two alcoholic drinks a day beginning 2 to 3 weeks after surgery.

 WARNING: Counsel the patient to report warning signs and symptoms of reocclusion or other serious complications — angina, persistent fever, swelling or drainage at the incision site, dizziness, shortness of breath at rest, rapid or irregular pulse, and prolonged recovery time from exercise or sex.

If he has had surgery, prepare him for postoperative depression, which may not set in until he's home. Tell him that such depression is usually temporary.

Other care measures
Emphasize that smoking and stress are also CAD risk factors. Urge the patient to stop smoking because smoking reduces the serum HDL level, constricts the arteries (thereby elevating blood pressure), and reduces the blood's oxygen-carrying capacity. To help him reduce stress and other risk factors and obtain further information, provide him with the address and phone number of the American Heart Association. (See Appendix 2.)

Heart failure
Over 2 million Americans experience heart failure and thousands more are diagnosed each year. Although this disorder usually can't be cured, early intervention and comprehensive teaching can lessen its severity and improve the patient's outcome.

Heart failure can occur at any age, although its incidence rises with advancing age. *Note:* You and your patient may be more familiar with the term "congestive heart failure." However, "congestive" has been dropped because pulmonary and systemic congestion is only one aspect of the syndrome.

Before teaching a patient with heart failure, make sure you are familiar with the following topics:
• explanation of heart failure and the reasons for signs and symptoms
• causes of heart failure
• diagnostic tests, such as blood tests, chest X-ray, electrocardiography (ECG), echocardiography, radionuclide ventriculography, cardiac catheterization, angiography
• signs and symptoms of worsening heart failure
• what to do if symptoms worsen
• self-monitoring
• activity restrictions
• importance of smoking cessation
• activity guidelines
• dietary recommendations
• medications
• importance of complying with the treatment plan
• sources of information and support.

ABOUT THE DISORDER
Inform the patient that heart failure occurs when the heart can't provide sufficient cardiac output to meet the body's metabolic needs. Low cardiac output triggers a series of compensatory mechanisms, which may lead to pulmonary edema if they fail. (See *Understanding heart failure.*)

Review the possible causes of heart failure, such as myocardial infarction, angina, diabetes and uncontrolled hypertension. Also tell the patient about risk factors, such as cardiomyopathy, high cholesterol levels, smoking, chronic or excessive alcohol use, and a family history of the disease.

Explain that heart failure may reflect a systemic (left-sided) dysfunction, a diastolic (right-sided) dysfunction, or a combination. Point out that systolic heart failure (previously called left-sided heart failure) causes mostly pulmonary symptoms, whereas diastolic heart failure (previously

called right-sided heart failure) causes systemic symptoms. Diastolic failure, less common than systolic failure, occurs when the heart muscle loses its ability to relax after contractions.

DIAGNOSTIC WORKUP
Explain that no single diagnostic test confirms heart failure. Tell the patient that blood will be drawn for a complete blood count, serum albumin level, liver function tests, and arterial blood gas analysis. If the patient is over age 65 or has atrial fibrillation or evidence of thyroid disease, he'll also undergo a thyroid-stimulating hormone test. Mention that a urine specimen will be collected for urinalysis.

To determine the heart's size, evaluate the cardiac silhouette, and compare the sizes of major vessels, the patient will have a chest X-ray. This test will also reveal the extent of any pulmonary congestion. In addition, the doctor may order an ECG, echocardiography, cardiac catheterization, angiography, and radionuclide ventriculography (cardiac blood pool imaging). (For information on these tests, see *Teaching patients about cardiovascular tests,* pages 24 to 30.)

TREATMENTS
Treatment varies with the severity and cause of heart failure. However, its goals are always the same: to identify or prevent conditions that can bring on or worsen heart failure, to reduce the heart's workload, to improve pump performance, and to control sodium intake and fluid retention.

To help prevent complications, be sure to point out the importance of lifestyle changes and strict compliance with the prescribed treatment plan.

Activity guidelines
Tell the patient that, although in the past patients with heart failure were advised to limit physical activity, recent research indicates that the patient should stay as active as possible. However, urge him to pace himself to

INSIGHT INTO ILLNESSES

Understanding heart failure

Tell the patient that heart failure typically begins in the left ventricle when the heart fails to pump sufficient blood to meet the body's needs. Impaired pumping decreases cardiac output, elevates venous pressure, and reduces arterial pressure, triggering a series of *compensatory* mechanisms (shown here) to ensure perfusion of vital organs.

However, these mechanisms can't sustain themselves indefinitely. When they begin to fail (a phenomenon known as *decompensation*), heart failure progresses. Pulmonary edema then occurs if blood backs up and sodium and water enter the interstitial space.

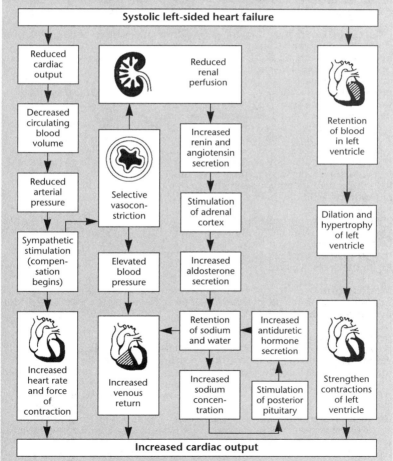

avoid fatigue, and stress the importance of following his doctor's recommendations on activity and exercise. Tell him to notify the doctor if activities seem to bring on or worsen shortness of breath, palpitations, or severe fatigue.

Dietary modifications
Teach the patient to adhere to the prescribed diet to diminish fluid retention and thus decrease the heart's workload. Point out that a low-sodium diet (2 to 3 g/day) promotes diuresis and inhibits further fluid accumulation. Advise him to follow his doctor's instructions on how much sodium he may consume daily.

Tell the patient that, although he should avoid excessive fluid intake, he need not restrict his fluid intake unless he develops a low serum sodium level (hyponatremia). To help monitor his fluid status, urge him to weigh himself daily, logging each measurement in a diary, and to report a weight gain of 3 to 5 lb (1.4 to 2.3 kg) or more in 1 week.

Depending on prescribed medication, the doctor may order a high- or low-potassium diet. As appropriate, help the patient identify foods high or low in potassium, or refer him to a dietitian.

 WARNING: Because alcohol decreases the heart's ability to contract, caution the patient to restrict his alcohol intake according to the doctor's guidelines.

Medication
In acute heart failure, drug therapy may include a rapid-acting I.V. diuretic such as furosemide. In chronic heart failure, long-term drug therapy is likely to include angiotensin-converting enzyme (ACE) inhibitors, diuretics, and digitalis glycosides.

ACE inhibitors
Tell the patient that an ACE inhibitor, such as captopril (Capoten), relaxes the blood vessels, making it easier for the heart to pump. Instruct him to report adverse effects such as cough, dizziness, and rash.

Diuretics
Inform the patient that a diuretic eases fluid overload by removing excess fluid and salt from the body. These effects reduce stress on the heart.

Encourage the patient taking a loop diuretic (bumetanide, ethacrynic acid, or furosemide) to increase his intake of high-potassium foods. If the patient takes a diuretic twice daily, advise him to take the second dose late in the afternoon rather than at night to prevent nighttime urination. To minimize postural hypotension, recommend rising slowly from a sitting or lying position.

 WARNING: Instruct the patient taking a diuretic to immediately report the following adverse effects: dizziness, light-headedness, blurred vision, muscle cramps, fatigue, mental confusion, rash, hives, weight gain or loss of more than 5 lb (2.3 kg), ankle swelling, or palpitations.

Digitalis glycosides
If the patient doesn't improve with ACE inhibitors or diuretics, the doctor may prescribe a digitalis glycoside such as digoxin (Lanoxin). Explain that digitalis glycosides strengthen cardiac contraction and regulate the heart rate by slowing the pulse. Instruct the patient to measure his pulse rate daily and to notify the doctor if it falls below 60 beats per minute.

 WARNING: Tell the patient taking a digitalis glycoside to report abdominal pain, dizziness, drowsiness, fatigue, headache, loss of appetite, malaise, nausea, visual disturbance, or vomiting to the doctor immediately.

Other care measures
Heart failure puts the patient at risk for pneumonia and other respiratory infections. To help prevent these complications, advise the patient to limit exposure to crowds and to people with infections, when possible. Urge him to get annual pneumonia and influenza vaccinations.

Encourage him to learn ways to reduce his anxiety level. Remind him that anxiety may raise his blood pressure, speed his heart rate, and decrease his urine output.

Stress the importance of calling the doctor if he notices early signs of pulmonary edema: cough, difficulty breathing, fatigue, restlessness, anxiety, increased pulse rate, weight gain, anorexia, dyspnea on exertion, persistent cough, frequent urination at night, and swelling of the ankles, feet, or abdomen.

To help the patient cope with his condition, refer him to the American Heart Association. (See Appendix 2.)

Hypertension

Hypertension is an insidious disorder affecting as many as 60 million Americans. Because many patients are asymptomatic, the disease may go undetected until it's revealed during a routine checkup.

The "silent" nature of hypertension can pose a challenge to your initial teaching efforts: The patient may need to be persuaded that he has a serious disorder that must be controlled — even though he feels fine. Your teaching must emphasize the importance of complying with long-term treatment.

Before teaching a patient about hypertension, make sure you are familiar with the following topics:
• explanation of hypertension, including normal and high blood pressure and factors that affect blood pressure
• type of hypertension the patient has (primary or secondary)
• importance of adhering to treatment to prevent complications
• diagnostic tests to rule out secondary hypertension, such as urinalysis, chest X-ray, angiography, electrocardiography (ECG), echocardiography, and cardiac catheterization
• exercise program and precautions
• dietary restrictions
• use of antihypertensives, diuretics, and other prescribed medications
• home blood pressure monitoring
• other measures to reduce long-term

complications, such as smoking cessation and stress reduction.
• sources of information and support.

ABOUT THE DISORDER
Explain that hypertension refers to abnormally high blood pressure. Blood exerts pressure against arterial walls as the heart pumps it through the body. In hypertension, this pressure is greater than it should be.

Tell the patient that a complex system involving the kidneys, brain, and nerves regulates blood pressure by making adjustments through hormone release into the bloodstream when pressure is too high or too low. Other factors governing blood pressure include the heart's strength and pumping ability, circulating blood volume, and arterial condition. Emphasize that blood pressure normally fluctuates with age, activity, and emotional stress and rises and falls many times daily.

Tell the patient that hypertension can be primary (essential hypertension) or secondary (resulting from another condition, such as kidney disease or an endocrine disorder).

Inform the patient that blood pressure is measured in millimeters of mercury (mm Hg) and that two values constitute a blood pressure reading. The first, or systolic, value measures maximum pressure, or that exerted when the heart is at work (contracting or beating). The second, or diastolic, value measures minimum pressure, or that exerted when the heart is at rest (relaxing between beats).

Complications
Point out that when sustained, hypertension eventually results in damage to blood vessels and reduced blood flow to tissues. This can lead to widespread organ damage, especially to the heart, brain, kidneys, and eyes. Cardiovascular damage increases the risk of potentially fatal heart failure, myocardial infarction, and cerebrovascular accident.

Classifying hypertension: Where does your patient fit in?

Inform your patient that hypertension classifications range from high normal to severe. Explain that the higher that the blood pressure reading is — especially the diastolic value — the greater and more imminent the health danger. Use this information to persuade your patient to schedule regular blood pressure evaluations.

Explain that normal systolic pressure ranges from 100 to 135 mm Hg; normal diastolic pressure, from 60 to 80 mm Hg. A blood pressure reading of 120/80 mm Hg is commonly accepted as normal for adults; a reading of 140/90 mm Hg or above is high and requires monitoring. At least three separate elevated blood pressure readings on different days are necessary to confirm a diagnosis of hypertension (unless a single reading is extremely high).

BLOOD PRESSURE RANGE (MM HG)	CLASSIFICATION	RECOMMENDED ACTION
DIASTOLIC		
85 to 89	High normal	Recheck blood pressure within 1 year.
90 to 104	Mild hypertension	Confirm blood pressure value within 2 months.
105 to 114	Moderate hypertension	Refer to doctor for evaluation within 2 weeks.
≥115	Severe hypertension	Refer to doctor for immediate evaluation.
SYSTOLIC (WHEN DIASTOLIC VALUE IS < 90)		
140 to 159	Borderline isolated systolic hypertension	Confirm blood pressure value within 2 months.
≥160	Isolated systolic hypertension	Confirm blood pressure value within 2 months.
≥200	Severe hypertension	Refer to doctor for evaluation within 2 weeks.

DIAGNOSTIC WORKUP

Tell the patient that consistently high blood pressure readings confirm hypertension. Explain that blood pressure is measured with a sphygmomanometer and that abnormally high pressure readings taken on at least three different days are necessary to confirm a diagnosis (unless a single reading is extremely high). In a patient under age 50, hypertension is diagnosed if the blood pressure exceeds 140/90 mm Hg; in a patient over age 50, it's diagnosed if pressure exceeds 150/95 mm Hg. (See *Classi-*

*fying hypertension: Where does your pa-
tient fit in?.*)

Discuss, if appropriate, which diagnostic studies the doctor has ordered
to rule out secondary causes of hypertension. These tests may include
urinalysis, chest X-ray, angiography,
ECG, echocardiography, and cardiac
catheterization. (See *Teaching patients
about cardiovascular tests,* pages 24 to
30.)

TREATMENTS
If the patient has newly diagnosed
mild hypertension, the doctor will
try to manage the condition by prescribing a low-salt diet, weight loss,
if appropriate, and a regular exercise
program. If these measures fail, he
will prescribe medications to lower
the blood pressure.

If the patient's hypertension results
from pheochromocytoma, discuss
the surgery he will undergo, if scheduled, to correct this disorder.

Activity guidelines
Encourage the patient to get regular
exercise to help lower his blood pressure. Explain that the doctor will recommend an exercise program based
on the patient's medical history, age,
and medication regimen. The program will emphasize aerobic exercise
to tone the cardiovascular system
and lower blood pressure. It won't include isometric exercise such as
weight lifting because such exercise
raises blood pressure.

Advise the patient to exercise frequently (at least three times a week),
vigorously (sufficient to raise the
heart rate to between 70% and 80%
of maximum capacity), and for a sustained time (gradually building up to
about 30 minutes a session).

 WARNING: Caution the patient not to overdo exercise,
because occasional bursts of
extreme activity can be worse than no
exercise at all. Emphasize that he must
stop exercising well before the point
of exhaustion. Instruct him to stop
exercising at once and call the doctor
right away if he becomes dizzy.

Dietary modifications
Explain that excessive sodium intake
contributes to hypertension. Recommend that the patient reduce the
sodium in his diet by avoiding or
limiting salty foods, such as most
and processed foods, luncheon
meats, and canned soups and vegetables as well as most snack foods and
condiments. Advise him to use alter-
natives to table salt, such as herbs,
spices, or sodium-free salt substitutes.

Also urge him to limit his intake of
caffeine and alcohol. Explain that
most alcoholic beverages are high in
calories, and beer contains considerable sodium.

If the patient is taking a potassium-
depleting diuretic, suggest that he ask
his doctor about following a potassium-rich diet. Name foods high in
potassium, such as bananas, dates,
salmon, carrots, and potatoes. Mention that many foods naturally high
in potassium are low in sodium.

Point out that obesity raises blood
pressure by increasing blood volume,
thus adding to the heart's workload.
Overweight people are three times
more likely to have hypertension
than people who maintain normal
weight. Under the doctor's supervision, encourage the patient to begin
a weight-reduction program that em-
phasizes a balanced diet, regular exercise, and gradual weight loss. When
teaching about diet, include the patient's family, especially if the patient
doesn't usually shop for groceries or
cook for the household.

Medication
If dietary restrictions and exercise fail
to lower blood pressure sufficiently,
drug therapy may be necessary.
Initial therapy usually consists of a
diuretic, a beta-adrenergic blocker, an
angiotensin-converting-enzyme inhibitor, or a calcium channel blocker.
Later, a combination of these drugs
or other antihypertensive agents may
be prescribed if the patient's blood
pressure is still not under control.
Explain that the doctor may "step
down" drug therapy, depending on
the patient's response.

Discuss the need for strict compliance with the prescribed drug regimen. Stress that drugs can only control, not cure, hypertension. Tell the patient that he may need to take antihypertensive drugs for the rest of his life.

 WARNING: Emphasize the importance of taking prescribed medication even if the patient feels well. Warn him that reducing or discontinuing medications without medical guidance may lead to severe rebound high blood pressure, possibly triggering a life-threatening hypertensive crisis.

Make sure the patient understands that many over-the-counter medications, especially cold and allergy remedies, contain ingredients that can make antihypertensives less effective. Also remind him that other over-the-counter drugs are high in sodium — particularly antacids, laxatives, diet pills, and cold and allergy medications.

Other care measures
Because stress and hypertension often go hand in hand, encourage the patient to use stress-reducing techniques, such as relaxation breathing or meditation. Advise him to practice these techniques twice a day for 10 or 20 minutes.

If the patient smokes, give him information to encourage him to quit. Explain how nicotine constricts blood vessels, further increasing blood pressure. As appropriate, refer him to community programs, agencies, or support groups that can help him stop smoking and provide follow-up services after he stops. For more information about hypertension, direct him to the American Heart Association. (See Appendix 2.)

Myocardial infarction

Few disorders arouse as much anxiety in a patient as myocardial infarction (MI) does. The patient who's had an MI worries not just about his immediate survival but about the quality of his life after recovery. When severe, anxiety can impair his ability to learn and cooperate. It can also increase his risk of complications. Fortunately, thorough patient education can reduce anxiety.

Before teaching a patient about MI, make sure you are familiar with the following topics:
• what happens during MI
• how such conditions as atherosclerosis and coronary artery spasm can occlude coronary blood flow and lead to MI
• diagnostic tests, such as blood enzyme studies, serial electrocardiograms (ECGs), resting thallium imaging, and technetium scan
• importance of following the prescribed treatment plan to aid recovery and prevent complications
• benefits of bed rest immediately after an MI
• prescribed exercise program and precautions
• dietary restrictions
• drug therapy for acute MI and for long-term care
• percutaneous transluminal coronary angioplasty (PTCA), pulmonary artery catheterization, or other treatment procedures
• coronary artery bypass surgery, if scheduled
• measures to reduce long-term complications, such as controlling weight, quitting smoking, and reducing stress
• sources of information and support.

ABOUT THE DISORDER
Tell the patient that MI results from reduced blood flow through one of the coronary arteries. The reduced flow, in turn, decreases blood supply to a portion of the heart. Explain that the chest pain of MI results from myocardial ischemia (reduced oxygen supply to the heart). The pain may range from a mild discomfort to a burning or crushing sensation that may radiate to the arm, jaw, neck, or shoulder blades.

Point out that if blood flow isn't restored, tissue in the affected area of the heart is destroyed, becoming necrotic. Later, scar tissue forms but isn't able to contract. This reduces the heart's ability to pump blood, placing the patient at risk for another MI.

Discuss the causes of MI. By far, the most common cause is atherosclerosis in one or more coronary arteries. Inform the patient that atherosclerosis is characterized by buildup of fatty, fibrous plaques that narrow or occlude the artery. Thrombosis, or clot formation, commonly occurs in atherosclerotic arteries and is a contributing factor in many MIs.

Tell the patient that some MIs result not from atherosclerosis or thrombosis but from a sudden spasm, or smooth-muscle contraction, in a coronary artery, which then blocks blood flow to part of the heart. Such spasms can occur in both normal and atherosclerotic arteries.

DIAGNOSTIC WORKUP
Inform the patient with an acute MI that his condition will be confirmed on the basis of symptoms, serial blood studies, an ECG, and thallium and technetium scans. Tell him that blood samples will be collected regularly to detect fluctuations in cardiac enzyme levels, reflecting evidence of MI.

After the patient's condition stabilizes, explain that the doctor may order an exercise ECG (possibly with a thallium scan), an ambulatory ECG, or electrophysiologic studies. (See *Teaching patients about cardiovascular tests,* pages 24 to 30.)

TREATMENTS
Initial treatment focuses on reducing pain and preventing further myocardial damage through activity restrictions, diet, and medication. The doctor also may recommend certain treatment procedures.

Activity guidelines
Explain to the patient that bed rest for the first 24 to 48 hours after an MI greatly reduces the demands on his heart and improves his chance of recovery. Encourage him to wiggle

his toes regularly while in bed to reduce the risk of blood clots.

 WARNING: Caution the patient not to press his feet against the footboard, raise his legs off the bed, or perform any other activity that strains the heart.

Review the patient's prescribed activity program. Emphasize the need to resume activities gradually. Help him plan activities so that he alternates light and heavy tasks, takes frequent rest breaks, and shares the workload with a friend or family member.

Dietary modifications
For the first few days after an MI, the patient receives only clear fluids because digesting solid foods places a greater strain on the heart. Tell him he must avoid caffeine, which stimulates the heart.

Medications
If the doctor discovers a coronary artery thrombus, he may attempt to dissolve it by administering a thrombolytic drug — either I.V. or directly into the heart through a catheter.

If it's too late to administer thrombolytic therapy (it should be given in the first few hours after an MI) or if such therapy is contraindicated, emergency surgery may be required.

Supplemental oxygen is administered through a nasal cannula for the first 24 to 48 hours and as needed thereafter. Inform the patient that this therapy keeps the heart and other tissues well oxygenated.

If the doctor orders nitroglycerin or morphine, explain that these drugs relieve chest pain by increasing oxygen supply to the heart. Also describe the purpose of other prescribed medications, such as nitroprusside (which lowers blood pressure, thereby reducing demands on the heart), lidocaine (which controls arrhythmias), and dopamine or dobutamine (which strengthens cardiac contractions).

Discuss other prescribed drugs. For instance, the doctor may order a stool softener to prevent straining during defecation, sedatives to decrease anxiety, and hypnotics to promote rest. Later, he may prescribe such drugs as calcium channel blockers, beta-adrenergic blockers, digoxin, antiarrhythmics, diuretics, antilipemics, antihypertensives, and even aspirin to help regulate cardiovascular function and prevent complications. Stress the importance of taking all drugs exactly as prescribed.

Procedures

Before any ordered procedure, provide clear, simple explanations of patient preparation, how the procedure is done, and postprocedure care. Even if the patient or family members don't absorb all the details, your concern and reassurance can improve the patient's prospects for recovery.

PTCA or percutaneous transluminal atherectomy

To reexpand coronary arteries narrowed by coronary artery disease, the doctor may recommend PTCA or percutaneous transluminal atherectomy. If the patient will undergo PTCA (also known as balloon angioplasty), tell him that this procedure uses a tiny balloon catheter to widen the narrowed coronary artery, thus improving blood flow. Explain that the catheter serves as an alternative to coronary artery bypass grafting (CABG).

Inform the patient that he'll receive a local anesthetic and a sedative and that during the procedure, he must lie flat on a hard table. Tell him that after the catheter site is cleaned and anesthetized, the doctor inserts a guide wire through the skin into an artery in the arm or groin. With fluoroscopic guidance, he threads the catheter into the coronary artery, confirms the presence of the blockage by angiography, and introduces a small, balloon-tipped catheter through the guide wire. After positioning the balloon tip in the blocked artery, the doctor repeatedly inflates it. The inflated balloon compresses the cholesterol-containing deposits against the wall of the artery, widening the diameter of the artery. Be sure to tell the

patient that he'll be asked to take deep breaths so the balloon catheter can be clearly seen.

Explain that the catheter is left in the artery for up to 24 hours to provide emergency access in case coronary blockage develops. Assure the patient that he'll be monitored closely after the procedure.

If percutaneous transluminal atherectomy will be done in addition to PTCA, tell the patient he'll receive a local anesthetic and a sedative and that during the procedure, he must lie flat on a hard table. Tell him that the catheter site is cleaned and anesthetized, and then the doctor inserts a catheter into the groin. Next, a guide wire is passed and advanced until it extends past the area to be treated. At this point, the patient may hear the Rotablator device as the small diamond crystal tip is advanced across the blocked area several times. Tell the patient that after the artery is opened and the guide wire is removed, the catheter will be left in the artery for up to 24 hours. Reassure him that he'll be monitored closely after the procedure.

If another form of atherectomy, laser-enhanced angioplasty, will be done in addtion to PTCA, describe the procedure. Tell the patient that the doctor threads a laser-containing catheter into the diseased artery. When the catheter nears the blockage in the artery, the doctor triggers the laser to emit rapid bursts. Between bursts, he rotates the catheter, advancing it until the occlusion is destroyed. The procedure takes about 1 hour and requires only a local anesthetic. Clearing a completely occluded artery requires ten 1-second bursts of laser energy, followed by PTCA.

Pulmonary artery catheterization

The doctor may perform this procedure if the patient develops heart failure, hypotension, hypertension, or oliguria. Or he may use it to assess cardiac function or monitor the effects of drug therapy.

Tell the patient that a sheath will be inserted into the subclavian, jugu-

Resuming sex after a heart attack

Once the patient is discharged from the hospital, he can expect to gradually resume most, if not all, of his usual activities, including sex. Inform him that most patients can resume having sex 3 to 4 weeks after a heart attack. Explain that in terms of physical demands, sex is a moderate form of exercise — no more stressful than a brisk walk. However, point out that sex can place a strain on the heart if it's accompanied by emotional stress.

Review the following guidelines with the patient to help him have a satisfying sex life. Tell him to discuss any related concerns with his doctor or nurse.

Choosing the right setting

Advise the patient to choose a quiet, familiar setting for sex. A strange environment may cause stress. Tell him that a comfortable room temperature is important because excessive heat or cold makes the heart work harder.

When to have sex

Recommend having sex when the patient feels rested and relaxed. A good time is in the morning, after he has had a good night's sleep.

When not to have sex

Caution the patient not to have sex when he's tired or upset or after drinking a lot of alcohol. Alcohol expands the blood vessels, which makes the heart work harder. Also tell him not to have sex right after a big meal but to wait a few hours.

Positioning for comfort

Advise the patient to choose positions that are relaxing, permit unrestricted breathing, and don't require him to use his arms to support himself or his partner. Encourage him to experiment. At first, he may be more comfortable if his partner assumes a dominant role.

A few precautions

Instruct the patient to ask the doctor if he should take nitroglycerin before having sex. This medication can prevent angina attacks during or after sex.

Point out that it's normal for the pulse and breathing rates to rise during sex, but that they should return to normal within 15 minutes. Instruct the patient to call the doctor at once if he has any of these symptoms after sex:

● sweating or palpitations for 15 minutes or longer
● breathlessness or increased heart rate for 15 minutes or longer
● chest pain that's not relieved by two or three nitroglycerin tablets (taken 5 minutes apart), a rest period, or both
● sleeplessness after sex or extreme fatigue the next day.

---

lar, or femoral vein under local anesthesia and will then be sutured in place. The doctor will introduce a thin, balloon-tipped catheter through the sheath. The catheter will be carried by the circulation through the right atrium and right ventricle into the pulmonary artery. There, the catheter will allow measurement of certain pressures until the patient's condition stabilizes.

Intra-aortic balloon pump (IABP)
The doctor may insert an intra-aortic balloon pump (IABP) to increase the supply of oxygen-rich blood to the heart and decrease the heart's oxygen demand. Tell the patient that the IABP displaces blood within the aorta by means of a balloon attached to an external pump console. Explain that the balloon catheter will temporarily reduce the heart's workload to promote rapid healing of the ventricular

muscle. Assure him that it will be removed after his heart can resume an adequate workload.

Briefly explain the insertion procedure. The patient will be attached to an ECG machine and will have several lines (arterial, pulmonary artery, and peripheral I.V.) in place, as well as an indwelling urinary catheter.

Explain that the doctor may insert the balloon surgically or through the femoral artery into the aorta. With the femoral approach, the doctor advances the balloon catheter into the correct position in the vessel, and then attaches the balloon to the control system to initiate counterpulsation. The balloon catheter then unfurls.

Tell the patient that crucial pressures will be measured while the IABP is in use, and that he will gradually be weaned from the intra-aortic balloon — usually about 24 hours after balloon insertion. For approximately 24 hours after balloon removal, the patient is restricted to bed rest and is monitored closely.

Surgery

If the patient will undergo CABG to treat acute MI or complications associated with cardiac catheterization or PTCA, explain that CABG will restore normal blood flow to his heart.

Mention that before surgery, the patient will shower with a special antiseptic soap and may be shaved from neck to toes. Tell him he won't be allowed to eat or drink anything after midnight before the surgery, although he can request a sleeping pill. Inform him that he may receive a sedative the morning of surgery to help him relax.

Discuss what will happen during surgery: The doctor will excise a portion of a healthy vessel from another part of the body, then graft it above and below the blocked coronary artery. Tell the patient that his circulation will then be diverted through the graft.

Other care measures

Reassure the patient that he'll be able to resume regular sexual activity after discharge. Emphasize that a satisfying sex life can help speed his recovery. (See *Resuming sex after a heart attack,* page 55.)

Educate the patient about the importance of correcting or reducing risk factors for MI, such as obesity, excessive stress, and smoking.

Mention that to aid his recuperation, the doctor may recommend a cardiac rehabilitation program and prescribe medications. Urge him to follow the treatment regimen closely. Also refer him to such sources of information as the American Heart Association. (See Appendix 2.)

3

Respiratory conditions

Asthma

Teaching for this chronic respiratory disorder focuses on helping the patient to prevent and control asthma attacks. Because the patient usually lacks symptoms between attacks, he may stop taking prescribed medications. So teaching should stress the need to comply with drug therapy.

Other goals include helping the patient identify and avoid asthma triggers — which can range from eggs and aspirin to infection and emotional stress — and helping him achieve some control over it. Thorough teaching also can help ensure that asthma doesn't prevent him from leading a normal life.

Before teaching a patient about asthma, make sure you are familiar with the following topics:
• how asthma triggers bronchospasm, airway edema, and mucus production
• diagnostic studies, such as arterial blood gas (ABG) analysis and pulmonary function tests
• importance of diet and adequate hydration
• warning signs of an acute asthma attack
• ways to prevent respiratory infection
• how to identify and avoid asthma triggers
• how to control an asthma attack
• sources of information and support.

ABOUT THE DISORDER

Inform the patient that asthma is a chronic respiratory disorder marked by recurrent episodes of respiratory distress, shortness of breath, wheezing, difficulty breathing, and coughing. These episodes are triggered by exposure to an allergy-producing substance (allergen), infection, emotional stress, or other factors.

Explain that an asthma attack may begin dramatically, with severe, multiple symptoms occurring all at once, or it may come on gradually, causing respiratory distress that grows more and more severe. An acute attack can cause difficulty breathing, wheezing, chest pressure or tightness, and a productive cough with thick, clear sputum. The attack may last from minutes to hours and may subside spontaneously or in response to drug therapy.

Tell the patient that during an asthma attack, the muscles of the smaller bronchi and bronchioles contract, causing bronchospasm (narrowing of the airways), which makes it difficult for air to pass in and out of the lungs. The airway linings become congested and swollen and secrete excess mucus, further obstructing airflow. Some patients can't speak more than a few words without pausing for breath.

Complications

Warn the patient that if he doesn't adhere strictly to his treatment plan, he may experience a prolonged severe attack called status asthmaticus. Explain that this condition may lead to respiratory arrest.

DIAGNOSTIC WORKUP

Before the doctor diagnoses asthma, he must rule out other causes of airway obstruction and wheezing. In children, such conditions may include cystic fibrosis, aspiration, congenital abnormalities, acute viral bronchitis, and benign or cancerous tumors of the bronchi, thyroid gland, thymus, or mediastinum. In adults, other causes of airway obstruction and wheezing include obstructive pulmonary disease and heart failure.

Tell the patient that no single test conclusively diagnoses asthma. Therefore, the doctor may order numerous tests, such as blood tests, ABG analysis, allergy tests, bronchial challenge testing, chest X-ray to diagnose asthma or monitor its progress, and pulmonary function tests to evaluate lung function and the effectiveness of therapy. (For information on ABG analysis, chest X-ray, and pulmonary function tests, see *Teaching patients about respiratory tests,* pages 70 to 80.)

Blood tests
Blood tests can help confirm a diagnosis of asthma and monitor its treatment. Tell the patient that blood samples typically detect increased levels of immunoglobulin E, an antibody that rises during an allergic reaction.

If the doctor prescribes theophylline, inform the patient that he may require daily blood studies to monitor the effectiveness of this drug.

Allergy tests
If the patient has asthma symptoms but no history of allergy, he may undergo skin tests to identify specific allergens. Inform him that the suspected allergen is either applied to the forearm (using paper backed by a layer of material that the allergen can't penetrate) or is injected in small doses, usually into the forearm. Test results are read after 1 or 2 days to detect an early reaction and again after 4 or 5 days to detect a late reaction.

Bronchial challenge testing
Depending on the results of allergy tests, the doctor may order bronchial challenge testing. Tell the patient that the doctor will ask him to breathe in an identified allergen such as pollen through a handheld inhaler. His reaction to this test helps determine drug therapy and required lifestyle changes, if any.

TREATMENTS
Make sure the patient understands that asthma can be controlled but not cured. Explain that treatment consists mainly of drug therapy. Other measures include appropriate exercise, a well-balanced diet, and avoidance of asthma triggers.

Activity guidelines
Inform the patient that exercise generally promotes good health, but that he may need to avoid or curtail certain forms of exercise — especially if they trigger an asthma attack (from heat and moisture loss in the upper airways).

Encourage him to use trial and error to find the exercise that's right for him. For instance, if he starts wheezing when he jogs, suggest that he slow his pace or try a different exercise, such as bicycling. Advise him to consult the doctor about taking prescribed medication before exercise to prevent an attack.

Dietary modifications
Emphasize the importance of a well-balanced diet to help prevent respiratory infection and fatigue. Encourage the patient to try to associate what he eats with his asthma attacks. Foods known to trigger asthma in some persons include egg yolks, chocolate, and shellfish. Instruct him to avoid the foods that trigger his attacks. (See *Avoiding asthma triggers.)*

 TIPS AND TIMESAVERS: Tell the patient to drink plenty of fluids (1½ to 2 qt [1.4 to 2 L] daily). Explain that this will help him to maintain adequate hydration and keep the mucus thin, which may ease bronchospasm.

Medication
Drugs used to treat or prevent asthma come in inhalable and oral forms. Inhalable forms include adrenergics, some corticosteroids, and cromolyn sodium.

Cromolyn sodium
Inform the patient taking cromolyn sodium (Intal) that this drug is used to prevent airway spasm — not to reverse spasm. Tell him not to increase the dose to treat acute airway spasm.

Avoiding asthma triggers

To make it easier for your patient to live with asthma, teach him to avoid the following common asthma triggers.

At home
- Such foods as nuts, chocolate, eggs, shellfish, and peanut butter
- Such beverages as orange juice, wine, beer, and milk
- Mold spores, pollens from flowers, trees, grasses, hay, and ragweed; if pollen is the offender, advise the patient to install a bedroom air conditioner with a filter and to avoid long walks when pollen counts are high
- Dander from rabbits, cats, dogs, hamsters, gerbils, and chickens; suggest that the patient consider finding a new home for the family pet, if necessary
- Feather or hair-stuffed pillows, down comforters, wool clothing, and stuffed toys; advise patient to use smooth (not fuzzy), washable blankets on his bed
- Insect parts, such as those from dead cockroaches
- Medicines such as aspirin
- Vapors from cleaning solvents, paint, paint thinners, and liquid chlorine bleach
- Fluorocarbon spray products, such as furniture polish, starch, cleaners, and room deodorizers
- Scents from spray deodorants, perfumes, hair sprays, talcum powder, and cosmetics
- Cloth-upholstered furniture, carpets, and draperies that collect dust; tell patient to hang lightweight, washable cotton or synthetic-fiber curtains and to use washable, cotton throw rugs on bare floors
- Brooms and dusters that raise dust; instead, advise patient to clean bedroom daily by damp dusting and damp mopping and instruct him to keep door closed
- Dirty filters on hot-air furnaces and air conditioners that blow dust into the air
- Dust from vacuum cleaner exhaust

In the workplace
- Dust, vapors, or fumes from wood products (western red cedar, some pine and birch woods, mahogany); flour, cereals, and other grains; coffee, tea, or papain; metals (platinum, chromium, nickel sulfate, soldering fumes); and cotton, flax, and hemp
- Mold from decaying hay

Outdoors
- Cold air, hot air, or sudden temperature changes (when going in and out of air-conditioned stores in the summer)
- Excessive humidity or dryness
- Changes in seasons
- Smog
- Automobile exhaust

Anywhere
- Overexertion, which may cause wheezing
- Common cold, flu, and other viruses
- Fear, anger, frustration, laughing too hard, crying, or any emotionally upsetting situation
- Smoke from cigarettes, cigars, and pipes; advise patient not to smoke and not to stay in a room where people are smoking

Preventive measures
To help prevent asthma attacks, instruct the patient to:
- drink six to eight glasses of fluid daily
- take all prescribed medications exactly as directed
- tell his doctor about any and all medications he takes — even nonprescription ones
- avoid taking sleeping pills or sedatives to promote sleep during a mild

(continued)

Avoiding asthma triggers *(continued)*

asthma attack. (Explain that these medications may slow down his breathing and make it more difficult. Instead, suggest that he try propping himself up on extra pillows while waiting for antianxiety medication to work.)

• schedule only as much activity as he can tolerate and to take frequent rests on busy days.

If the patient is also taking an inhaled bronchodilator, advise him to take the bronchodilator before cromolyn sodium. Suggest that he rinse his mouth after taking the drug to minimize its taste.

Bronchodilators

If the patient is using a bronchodilator, such as albuterol (Proventil), explain that this drug should reverse or control wheezing and airway spasm. Warn him not to increase the prescribed dosage because this could cause potentially lethal complications. Also instruct him not to take the drug more frequently than ordered.

Methylxanthines

If the doctor prescribes a methylxanthine (such as aminophylline or theophylline), tell the patient that this drug will control his wheezing and prevent airway spasm. Mention that it may cause mild GI upset or a bitter taste. If he experiences GI upset, advise him to take the drug with food.

Instruct the patient to report adverse reactions — such as appetite loss, diarrhea, dizziness, headache, irritability, insomnia, nausea, palpitations, restlessness, seizures, and vomiting — to the doctor. Tell him to take his pulse daily and to notify the doctor if the rhythm changes or the pulse rate rises or falls 20 or more beats per minute.

Oral prednisone

Instruct the patient taking oral prednisone (Deltasone) to report abdominal pain, acne, back or rib pain, bloody or tarry stools, easy bruising, fever, leg swelling, extreme personality changes, sore throat, vomiting, weakness, weight gain, and wounds that don't heal.

Emphasize that he must strictly follow the doctor's orders when starting, ending, or tapering the use of prednisone in conjunction with inhalable steroids. Warn him that sudden withdrawal of prednisone may be fatal.

Instruct the patient to eat a salt-restricted diet high in protein and potassium. If the drug causes stomach irritation, suggest that he take it with food.

Desensitization treatment

If the patient can't avoid a particular airborne allergen, the doctor may try desensitization treatment. Explain that in this therapy, tiny amounts of the offending substance are injected under the skin at regular intervals — but only as much as the patient can tolerate without experiencing symptoms. Over several years, doses are increased until his body learns not to react to the substance with bronchospasm.

Chest physiotherapy

Teach the patient to perform chest physiotherapy at least twice daily to clear mucus from the lungs. He may find it easier to comply with this regimen if other family members learn how to perform the technique and can assist him.

Preventive measures

If stress or emotional upset is a known asthma trigger, the doctor may advise the patient to take additional medication during a prolonged

How to control an asthma attack

Inform your patient that an asthma attack usually is preceded by warning signs that give him time to take action. Instruct him to stay alert for:
● chest tightness
● coughing
● awareness of breathing
● wheezing.

Taking action

Once the patient has had a few asthma attacks, he'll have no trouble recognizing these early warning signs. Emphasize that he *must not ignore them.* Instead, tell him to follow these steps:

1. Take prescribed medicine with an oral inhaler, if directed, to prevent the attack from getting worse.

2. Try to relax as the medicine goes to work. Although you may understandably be nervous or afraid, keep in mind that these feelings only worsen your shortness of breath.

To help relax, sit upright in a chair, close your eyes, and breathe slowly and evenly. Then relax your muscles. Begin by consciously tight-

ening and relaxing the muscles in your body. First tighten the muscles in your face and count to yourself: one-1,000; two-1,000. Don't hold your breath. Then, relax these muscles and repeat with the muscles in your arms and hands, legs and feet. Finally, let your body go limp.

3. Perform the pursed-lip breathing exercises you've been taught to regain control of your breathing. Don't gasp for air. Continue pursed-lip breathing until you no longer feel breathless.

4. If the attack triggers a coughing spell, control your cough so that it effectively brings up mucus and helps clear the airways. To do so, lean forward slightly, keeping your feet on the floor. Then breathe in deeply and hold that breath for a second or two. Cough twice, first to loosen mucus and then to bring it up. Be sure to cough into a tissue.

5. Call the doctor right away if the attack gets worse even after you have followed these steps.

---

period of upset. To further reduce the risk of an asthma attack, advise the patient to practice breathing exercises and relaxation techniques when he becomes fearful, angry, sad, or excited. (See *How to control an asthma attack.*)

 WARNING: Instruct the patient and family to report the following danger signs and symptoms to the doctor right away: respiratory infection (a common asthma trigger), temperature over 100° F (37.8° C) during an asthma attack, chest pain, uncontrollable cough, and shortness of breath when not coughing or exercising. Finally, encourage the patient to contact the American Lung Association for further information and support. (See Appendix 2.)

Chronic obstructive pulmonary disease

Chronic obstructive pulmonary disease (COPD) is the second leading cause of disability in the United States. Although COPD can't be cured, thorough teaching can make a tremendous difference in the patient's quality of life.

Before teaching a patient about COPD, make sure you are familiar with the following topics:
● explanation of COPD, including the patient's specific type
● diagnostic studies, such as pulmonary function tests, chest X-ray, computed tomography (CT) scan of the chest, magnetic resonance imaging (MRI), and exercise electrocardiography (ECG)

- exercise program, activity tips, and breathing exercises to avoid dyspnea
- importance of diet, adequate hydration, and combating obesity
- drugs and their administration
- how to use an oral inhaler, perform chest physiotherapy, and use home oxygen therapy
- importance of avoiding bronchial irritants, such as cigarette smoke, allergens, and adverse weather conditions
- sources of information and support.

ABOUT THE DISORDER

Tell the patient that COPD is the name given to a group of progressive, irreversible respiratory conditions in which the airways are blocked, causing chronic breathing difficulty and exhaustion. Review the patient's particular type of COPD, such as chronic bronchitis, emphysema, or asthma. (For a discussion of asthma, see pages 57 to 61.)

If the patient has chronic bronchitis, explain that repeated exposure to irritants inflames the airways, causing them to swell and clog with mucus.

Tell the patient with emphysema that this condition is marked by airway inflammation, which eventually destroys air sacs (alveoli) in the lungs and small airways (bronchioles). Mention that he may experience ruptured blebs and bullae, leading to spontaneous pneumothorax or pneumonia. Emphasize the importance of calling the doctor immediately if he experiences sudden, sharp chest pain made worse by chest movement, breathing, or coughing. Such pain is a sign of spontaneous pneumothorax.

Complications

No matter which form of COPD the patient has, be sure to explain that an untreated respiratory infection can lead to life-threatening respiratory failure. Also mention that COPD increases the risk of lung collapse from mucus plugs that block the bronchi.

If COPD involves the pulmonary blood vessels, tell the patient that pressure in these vessels may rise too high and the heart's right side may fail. When this happens, breathing

becomes more difficult; the ankles, lower back, and scrotum become swollen; and the skin becomes bluish or mottled.

DIAGNOSTIC WORKUP

Inform the patient that the doctor typically relies on pulmonary function tests and chest X-rays to assess respiratory impairment or detect possible complications. However, he also may order a CT scan of the chest, MRI, or exercise ECG. If the doctor suspects a coexisting respiratory infection, tell the patient he will undergo a complete blood count and sputum analysis. (See *Teaching patients about respiratory tests,* pages 70 to 80.)

TREATMENTS

Inform the patient that the goal of COPD treatments is to relieve symptoms and prevent complications. Treatment may include daily exercise, limits on activity, dietary changes, drug and oxygen therapy, chest physiotherapy, and other measures.

Activity guidelines

After evaluating the results of the patient's exercise ECG, the doctor may prescribe an exercise program to boost endurance and strength without causing severe breathing difficulty.

Encourage regular participation in such exercises as walking or riding a stationary bicycle. Advise the patient to perform several minutes of warm-up exercises (slow walking, bending, stretching) and to finish with cool-down exercises. He should start slowly and gradually increase the pace and duration of activity. If he needs low-flow oxygen during exercise, instruct him and his family on how to use oxygen at home. Also show him how to take an accurate radial pulse to monitor exercise effects. Tell him that the doctor will reevaluate his exercise tolerance from time to time and modify the program as necessary.

 WARNING: Tell the patient to stop exercising and notify the doctor immediately if he experiences increased difficulty breathing, heart fluttering, extreme fatigue, nausea, dizziness, or muscle cramps or if his skin becomes pale, mottled, or clammy.

Counsel the patient to plan daily activities to conserve his energy and best cope with breathing difficulty. Advise him to alternate light and heavy tasks, rest frequently, practice pursed-lip breathing, minimize body movements, and use labor-saving devices as appropriate. (See *Overcoming shortness of breath*, page 64.)

Dietary modifications
Point out that a well-balanced, nutritious diet helps compensate for the extra calories the patient expends in breathing. Because difficulty breathing and increased sputum production can discourage eating and lead to weight loss, help the patient maintain caloric intake.

 TIPS AND TIMESAVERS: To stimulate the patient's appetite and enjoyment of food, advise him to maintain good oral hygiene, chew food slowly, and eat small and more frequent meals to reduce fatigue and air swallowing. Also recommend that he perform breathing exercises 1 hour before meals (so secretions won't interfere with eating) and that he rest before eating.

Encourage the patient to drink plenty of water — at least eight glasses daily — to thin secretions and make expectoration easier. Explain that adequate fluid intake also helps prevent constipation and avoid breathlessness caused by straining during defecation.

Obesity interferes with the movement of the diaphragm and adds to the heart's workload. This, in turn, can increase the work of breathing. If the patient is overweight, urge him to follow a medically supervised weight-loss diet.

Medication
Drugs used to treat COPD include inhalers, oral bronchodilators, corticosteroids, and antibiotics. Teach the patient about prescribed drugs as appropriate.

Inhalers
Inhaled bronchodilators such as metaproterenol (an adrenergic agonist also known as Alupent) are fast-acting, well tolerated, and highly effective in treating bronchospasm. Make sure the patient understands correct use of an inhaler, which requires a certain degree of mind-muscle coordination.

Tell the patient to notify the doctor if the inhaled drug seems to have lost its effectiveness or if he experiences tremors, nausea, vomiting, or a rapid or irregular pulse. Instruct him to store the medication away from heat. Tell him not to take nonprescription medications such as cold preparations because of potential interactions with the inhaler.

After assessing the patient's technique for inhaler use, the doctor may suggest the use of a spacer device, such as InspirEase or Aerochamber, with the inhaler. Make sure the patient knows how to used the spacer device correctly.

Oral bronchodilators
Oral bronchodilators such as theophylline (Theo-Dur) are sometimes used when inhalers alone don't effectively control bronchospasm. They are rarely a first-line treatment because they're associated with such adverse effects as tremors, fast pulse, and palpitations. Also, they're slower-acting than inhalers.

Tell the patient to take a xanthine-derivative bronchodilator (such as aminophylline [Aminophyllin] or theophylline) with a full glass of water at mealtimes if GI upset occurs. Also instruct him to take the medication at regularly scheduled intervals. Warn him not to combine the drug with over-the-counter products such as cold preparations because of possible interactions. Instruct him to avoid foods and beverages high in caffeine, such as coffee, tea, cola, and chocolate. Explain that they may increase adverse effects of bronchodilators and cause tremors and palpitations.

Overcoming shortness of breath

The patient who's having trouble breathing can feel better by performing special exercises. Provide instructions on performing these exercises, and tell the patient to practice them twice a day for 5 to 10 minutes until she is used to doing them.

Abdominal breathing

Instruct the patient to lie comfortably on her back and place a pillow beneath her head. Tell her to bend her knees to relax her stomach.

Next, tell her to press one hand on her stomach lightly — but with enough force to create slight pressure. Her other hand rests on her chest.

Then instruct her to breathe slowly through her nose, using her stomach muscles. The hand on her stomach should rise during inspiration and fall during expiration. The hand on her chest should remain almost still.

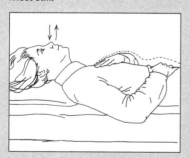

Pursed-lip breathing

Instruct the patient to breathe in slowly through her nose to avoid gulping air. Tell her to hold her breath as she counts to herself: one-1,000; two-1,000; three-1,000.

Next, tell her to purse her lips as if she's going to whistle. Then have her breathe out slowly through pursed lips as she counts to herself: one-1,000; two-1,000; three-1,000; four-1,000; five-1,000; six-1,000.

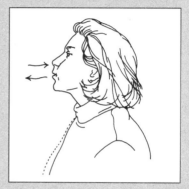

Tell her that she should make a soft, whistling sound while she breathes out. Explain that exhaling through pursed lips slows her breathing and helps get rid of the stale air trapped in her lungs.

Describe how to perform pursed-lip breathing during activity: The patient inhales before exerting herself and then exhales while performing the activity.

If the recommended counting rhythm feels awkward to the patient, tell her to find one that feels more comfortable. Remind her to breathe out longer than she breathes in.

Corticosteroids

Corticosteroids are anti-inflammatory drugs that have become a mainstay in the treatment of asthma and other airway diseases. When administered by inhalation, the drug is delivered directly to the bronchial wall.

Aerosol administration causes fewer overall adverse effects, but it may lead to thrush, a yeast infection in the mouth.

Warn the patient using an inhaled corticosteroid (such as beclomethasone dipropionate [Beclovent] or flunisolide [AeroBid Inhaler]) to stay alert for signs and symptoms of systemic absorption, including Cush-ing's syndrome and hyperglycemia, and to notify the doctor if these occur. If the patient also uses inhaled bronchodilators, advise him to inhale the bron–chodilator 15 minutes before he inhales the corticosteroid. Tell him to rinse his mouth after using the inhaler to reduce the risk of oral fungal infections. Instruct him to call the doctor if he notices a decreased response to the drug. If fever or local irritation develops, advise the patient to discontinue corticosteroid use and report the effect to the doctor promptly.

In more severe cases, the doctor may prescribe an oral corticosteroid such as prednisone (Deltasone). Instruct the patient on long-term oral corticosteroid therapy to watch for adverse effects, including weight gain, fluid retention, and stomach ulcers. To minimize these effects, the doctor may prescribe alternate-day therapy. Caution the patient not to stop taking the drug abruptly because serious complications could result. Suggest that he take the drug with food or milk to decrease the risk of stomach irritation. Advise him to wear a medical identification tag or carry a wallet card and to notify any health care provider about his corticosteroid therapy. Explain that this therapy suppresses the immune system.

Antibiotics
If infection complicates COPD, explain that the patient will require antibiotic therapy and may have to undergo culture and sensitivity testing to ensure effective treatment.

 WARNING: Instruct the patient to avoid cough suppressants, sedatives, and sleep aids because they can cause respiratory depression. Point out that coughing is an important reflex that helps clear secretions from the airway and that suppressing a productive cough can worsen the patient's oxygen deficiency.

Procedures
Other treatments for COPD include chest physiotherapy and supplemental oxygen.

Chest physiotherapy
Teach both the patient and a family member (or another caregiver) how to perform chest physiotherapy. Explain that this technique helps mobilize and remove mucus from the lungs. If the patient's caregiver has limited arm strength, recommend use of a mechanical percussor.

Oxygen therapy
If the doctor prescribes home oxygen therapy, provide instructions to the patient and caregiver. Acquaint them with the types of oxygen delivery devices available. The doctor will write a prescription for oxygen therapy specifying the type of system, liter flow rate, and hours of use.

Advise the patient to investigate different oxygen suppliers before choosing one. Encourage him to ask about the costs of initial setup, delivery, monthly supplies, service calls, and insurance coverage.

Make sure the patient understands that oxygen should be treated as a medication. Advise him to use it exactly as prescribed. Give him a copy of the teaching aids *Learning to use breathing devices,* page 66, and *Using oxygen safely and effectively*, page 67.

Self-care
Review self-care measures, such as watching for complications, preventing infection, avoiding irritants, and developing effective coping techniques. Point out that these measures can improve the patient's quality of life and prevent a long, severe attack of COPD. Add that they may also eliminate the need for hospitalization.

 WARNING: Urge the patient to report early signs and symptoms of COPD complications: increasing difficulty breathing, wheezing, fatigue, or a change in cough or sputum production.

Learning to use breathing devices

Dear Patient:

Your doctor has prescribed a nasal cannula or an oxygen face mask so you can breathe in extra oxygen. Follow these steps for using your breathing device.

Attaching the tubing

Whether you use a nasal cannula or mask, attach one end of the oxygen tubing to the device. Attach the other end to the humidifier nipple.

Setting the flow rate

Next, turn on the oxygen and set the flow rate to the prescribed level. If you're receiving oxygen at a rate of 2 liters per minute or more, you should feel it flowing from the prongs. If you can't, briefly turn up the flow rate. Then turn it back to the prescribed level.

Positioning the device

If you use a nasal cannula, insert the two prongs in your nostrils. Make sure the prongs face upward and follow the curve of your nostrils. Also make sure the flat surface of the tab rests above your upper lip. Position the tubing for the nasal cannula behind each ear and adjust it below your chin for a comfortable fit.

If you use an oxygen mask, place

the device over your face. Position the elastic strap over your head so that it rests above your ears and the mask fits snugly against your face.

Preventing skin irritation

To keep the cannula or mask strap from irritating your skin, pad it with 2-inch-square gauze pads, moleskin, foam rollers, or cotton balls. Place them against your cheeks and behind your ears.

Every 2 hours, check for reddened areas around your nose and ears. If you see redness, rub the area gently; then wash your face and dry it well. Call your doctor if redness continues.

You may moisten your lips and nose with a water-soluble lubricating jelly (such as K-Y Jelly), but take care not to get any in the cannula or mask.

Every 8 hours, remove the cannula or mask and wipe it clean with a wet cloth.

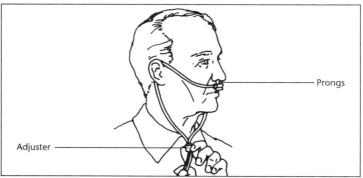

Prongs

Adjuster

Using oxygen safely and effectively

Dear Patient:

To help you breathe easier, the doctor wants you to receive extra oxygen. You'll use an oxygen concentrator, a liquid oxygen unit, or an oxygen tank. Your prescribed oxygen flow rate is _____ liters a minute for _____ hours a day.

Obtaining equipment

When you obtain your home oxygen system from your medical equipment supplier, you'll learn how to set it up, check for problems, and clean it. Your system will include a humidifier to warm and add moisture to the oxygen and a nasal cannula or a face mask through which you'll breathe the oxygen. Keep the supplier's phone number handy in case of problems and get a backup system to use in an emergency.

General guidelines

When using oxygen, be sure to follow these important guidelines:
• Check the water level in the humidifier bottle often. If it's near or below the refill line, pour out any remaining water and refill it with sterile or distilled water.
• If your nose dries up, use a water-soluble lubricant like K-Y Jelly.
• If the tubing irritates your skin, use cotton balls or moleskin to protect your skin from the tubing.
• If you'll need a new supply of oxygen, order it 2 or 3 days in advance or when the register reads one-quarter full.
• Maintain the oxygen flow at the prescribed rate. If you're not sure whether oxygen is flowing, check the tubing for kinks, blockages, or disconnection. Then make sure the system is on. If you're still unsure, invert the nasal cannula in a glass of water. If bubbles appear, oxygen is flowing through the system. Shake off extra water before reinserting the cannula.

Safety tips

• Oxygen is highly combustible. Don't use it near electrical equipment or while using an electric razor. Alert your local fire department that oxygen is in the house, and keep an all-purpose fire extinguisher on hand.
• If a fire does occur, turn off the oxygen immediately and leave the house.
• Don't smoke — and don't allow others to smoke — near the oxygen system. Keep the system away from direct sunlight, space heaters and other sources of heat, and open flames, such as a gas stove.
• Don't run oxygen tubing under clothing, bed covers, furniture, or carpets.
• Keep the oxygen system upright.
• Make sure the oxygen is turned off when it's not in use.
• Keep oxygen concentrators away from the wall to allow air to circulate.

When to call the doctor

You may not be getting enough oxygen if you have these symptoms: difficult, irregular breathing; restlessness, anxiety, tiredness, or drowsiness; blue nail beds or lips; confusion; or distractibility.

You may be getting too much oxygen if you notice these symptoms: headaches, slurred speech, sleepiness or difficulty waking up, or shallow, slow breathing.

If any of these symptoms develops, call your doctor immediately. And — above all — *never change the oxygen flow rate* without checking with the doctor first.

Infection prevention
Point out that the patient's limited pulmonary reserve makes him susceptible to respiratory infection. To reduce his risk of infection, encourage him to get prompt treatment for infection, to use proper hand-washing technique, and to avoid people with infections.

Avoiding irritants
Tell the patient that pollutants can worsen his symptoms. Whenever possible, he should try to avoid heavy traffic and smog. Also counsel him to refrain from using aerosol sprays and to keep his home as dust-free as possible.

Advise the patient to carefully assess his home and workplace for pollutants that may cause excessive irritation and to make changes to reduce or remove these pollutants or to limit his exposure to these areas.

Inform the patient that exposure to blasts of cold or dry air can trigger bronchospasm and that dry air can also thicken mucus. Whenever possible, he should avoid cold winds or cover his mouth with a scarf or mask when outdoors in cold weather.

Point out that heat can also be dangerous. Urge him to stay indoors, keep the windows closed, and use an air conditioner on hot days when the air quality is poor. Instruct him to maintain environmental humidity at levels between 40% and 50% whenever possible.

If the patient smokes, emphasize that smoking has harmful effects on respiratory function. If he has chronic bronchitis, tell him that his respiratory function may gradually improve if he stops smoking. (Unfortunately, the same rarely holds true for the patient with emphysema.)

Coping techniques
To help the patient deal with chronic anxiety and depression related to COPD, tell him about such techniques as relaxation exercises and biofeedback. Encourage him to join a support group. Also help family members deal with the added emotional strain in their lives.

 TIPS AND TIMESAVERS: If breathing difficulty interferes with the patient's sexual activity, suggest that he use pursed-lip breathing during intercourse, assume a comfortable position that won't restrict breathing such as lying on one side, have his partner take a more active role, rest before and after sexual activity, and keep oxygen nearby to relieve any breathing difficulty.

To help the patient cope with his condition, give him the address and phone number of the American Lung Association; for help in quitting smoking, refer him to the American Cancer Society. (See Appendix 2.)

Pleural disorders
When pleural effusion, pleurisy, or empyema causes sharp, stabbing chest pain and impairs breathing, the patient will certainly feel apprehensive. And when diagnostic tests such as pleural biopsy and treatments such as thoracentesis are ordered, he's likely to feel increasingly frightened. Clearly, one of your major teaching goals is to relieve his anxiety by helping him understand his disorder.

Before teaching the patient about pleural disorders, make sure you are familiar with the following topics:
• how the pleural system functions
• an explanation of the patient's specific pleural disorder — pleural effusion, empyema, pleurisy, or chylothorax
• diagnostic studies, such as chest X-rays, computed tomography (CT) scans, pleural biopsy, and thoracentesis
• importance of balancing rest and activity
• dietary guidelines
• drug therapy, including antibiotic and anticancer drugs via chest tube, I.V. or I.M. antibiotics, and oral drugs for symptomatic relief
• oxygen therapy to relieve dyspnea and thoracentesis to remove fluid
• comfort measures, such as the or-

thopneic position to ease breathing and chest binding for support and pain relief
• sources of information and support.

ABOUT THE DISORDER
Define a pleural disorder as a lung problem. Then describe how normal pleural function promotes smooth and efficient respiration.

Review the causes of the patient's disorder. If he has *pleural effusion,* explain that excess fluid in the pleural space causes his signs and symptoms. Add that the causes of pleural effusion may be classified as transudative (most often associated with heart failure) or exudative (associated with cancer or lung infections such as tuberculosis).

If the patient has *empyema,* explain that pus or necrotic tissue is found in the pleural space. The infection is typically associated with cancer, pneumonitis, esophageal perforation or rupture, tuberculosis, chest trauma, or chest surgery.

If the patient has *pleurisy,* explain that this disorder is marked by inflammation of the pleural linings (the parietal pleura and the visceral pleura). Pleurisy may complicate such disorders as cancer, chest trauma, pneumonia, systemic lupus erythematosus, and rheumatoid arthritis.

If the patient has *chylothorax,* explain that this rare disorder occurs when chyle, a milky fluid produced during digestion, accumulates in the pleural space.

Complications
Tell the patient that poorly treated pleural effusion or pleurisy may lead to respiratory failure and systemic sepsis.

DIAGNOSTIC WORKUP
Tell the patient with a suspected pleural disorder that the doctor confirms the diagnosis by obtaining a health history, performing a complete physical examination, and ordering such diagnostic studies as chest

X-rays, CT scan, pleural biopsy, and pleural fluid aspiration (thoracentesis) and analysis. (See *Teaching patients about respiratory tests,* pages 70 to 80.)

TREATMENTS
Depending on the patient's disorder, treatments include medication, thoracentesis, oxygen therapy, coughing and deep breathing, adequate rest and nutrition and, as a last resort, surgery.

Activity guidelines
Most patients with pleural disorders experience fatigue and breathlessness because the disorder deprives the body of adequate oxygen. The lower the patient's oxygen level, the greater his fatigue. Emphasize that he'll need to find the right balance between rest (for healing) and activity (to prevent complications such as pneumonia). Suggest that he take short naps (long ones may interfere with a good night's sleep), alternate exercise and rest periods, and schedule treatments and medications when they won't interrupt rest periods.

If he has trouble breathing when lying down, recommend the orthopneic position. Instruct the patient to prop several pillows behind his back to keep him upright and to place several more on his lap (or on the overbed table). They will help support and cushion the weight of his arms, shoulders, and head.

Dietary modifications
Nutrition problems are common in patients with pleural disorders. The patient may complain of impaired taste and smell (from nasal congestion), coughing attacks that make eating difficult, and a bad taste in the mouth (from sputum and accompanying nausea). Encourage him to brush and floss his teeth; rinse with mouthwash frequently; eat small, protein-rich meals or snacks to conserve energy and ease digestion; and drink plenty of fluids, unless directed otherwise.

(Text continues on page 80.)

Teaching patients about respiratory tests

TEST AND PURPOSE	TEACHING POINTS
Arterial blood gas analysis • To evaluate the efficiency of gas exchange in the lungs • To assess integrity of the ventilatory control system • To determine the acid-base level of the blood • To monitor respiratory therapy	• Inform the patient that this test evaluates how well the lungs are delivering oxygen to the blood and eliminating carbon dioxide. Tell him which puncture site will be used (radial, brachial, or femoral artery) and, if appropriate, whether he should continue oxygen therapy during the test. • Describe what happens during the test: The patient will be instructed to breathe normally while an arterial puncture is performed to collect a blood sample. Forewarn him that he may experience a brief cramping or throbbing pain at the puncture site.
Bronchoscopy • To help identify the cause of dyspnea and other respiratory symptoms • To visually examine a possible tumor, secretions, or other obstruction demonstrated on X-ray • To help diagnose bronchogenic carcinoma, tuberculosis, interstitial pulmonary disease, or fungal or parasitic pulmonary infection by obtaining a tissue or mucus specimen for examination • To locate a bleeding site in the tracheobronchial tree • To remove foreign bodies, mucus plugs, or excessive secretions from the airways	• Explain that this test allows direct examination of the patient's airways and takes 45 to 60 minutes. • Describe pretest restrictions: The patient must not eat or drink for 6 hours before the test. However, he should continue taking prescribed drugs unless the doctor orders otherwise. • Explain what happens during the test: If the test will be done with a local anesthetic, the patient may receive a sedative to help him relax. Prepare him for the unpleasant taste and coolness of the anesthetic throat spray used to suppress the gag reflex and ease bronchoscope passage. • Inform the patient that he'll probably be positioned supine on a table or bed, although he may be asked to sit upright in a chair. Tell him to remain relaxed, with his arms at his sides, and to breathe through his nose during the test. Mention that the doctor will insert the bronchoscope tube through the patient's nose or mouth into the airway. Then he'll flush small amounts of anesthetic through the tube to suppress coughing and wheezing. Reassure him that although he may experience dyspnea during the test, he won't suffocate. Also tell him that oxygen will be given through the bronchoscope. • Describe what will happen after the test: The patient's blood pressure, heart rate, and breathing will be monitored for about 15 minutes. He should lie on his side or sit with his head elevated at least 30 degrees until his gag reflex returns. Food, fluid, and oral drugs will be withheld for about 2 hours or until his gag reflex returns. Reassure him that hoarseness or a sore throat is

Teaching patients about respiratory tests *(continued)*

TEST AND PURPOSE	TEACHING POINTS
Bronchoscopy *(continued)*	temporary. He can have throat lozenges or liquid gargle when his gag reflex returns. ●Advise the patient to report bloody mucus, dyspnea, wheezing, or chest pain immediately.
Chest X-ray (chest radiography) ●To detect respiratory disorders, such as pneumonia, atelectasis, pneumothorax, pulmonary bullae, and tumors ●To detect mediastinal abnormalities (such as tumors) and cardiac disease ●To evaluate the effectiveness of therapy	●Tell the patient that this test detects or monitors the progress of his illness. Mention that it takes only minutes, but that the technician or doctor will need additional time to check the quality of the films. ●Describe what will happen before the test: The patient must put on a gown without snaps but may keep on his pants, socks, and shoes. Instruct him to remove all jewelry from his neck and chest. ●Explain what will happen during the test: The patient will stand or sit in front of the X-ray machine (if the X-ray is performed in the radiology department) or will be helped to a sitting position (if it's performed at bedside). He must take a deep breath and then hold it for a few seconds while the X-ray is taken. Make it clear that he must remain still for those few seconds. Reassure him that he'll be exposed to only slight amounts of radiation.
Computed tomography scan (CT scan, thoracic computed tomography) ●To locate or monitor lesions in the lungs, mediastinum, thoracic lymph nodes, blood vessels, or other tissues	●Inform the patient that this test uses multiple computed X-ray images to help diagnose or evaluate respiratory disorders. Mention that it takes 30 to 60 minutes and causes little discomfort. Reassure him that the technician will be able to see and hear him from an adjacent room. ●Describe pretest preparations: If a contrast dye will be used, he must fast for 4 hours before the test. Just before the test, he should remove all jewelry. ●Explain what will happen during the test: The patient will lie supine on an X-ray table. To restrict movement, a strap will be placed across the body part to be scanned. The table will then slide into the large, tunnel-shaped machine. When the dye is injected, the patient may experience transient nausea, flushing, warmth, and a salty taste. Stress that he must not move during the test but should relax and breathe normally. Movement may invalidate test results and require repeat testing. Reassure him that radiation exposure during the test is minimal. ●Tell the patient that he can resume his usual activities and diet immediately after the test.

(continued)

Teaching patients about respiratory tests *(continued)*

TEST AND PURPOSE	TEACHING POINTS
Doppler ultrasonography • To aid diagnosis of chronic venous insufficiency, superficial and deep vein thromboses, peripheral artery disease, and arterial occlusion • To detect abnormalities of carotid artery blood flow associated with such conditions as aortic stenosis • To monitor patency of arterial grafting and reconstruction	• Tell the patient that this painless test evaluates circulation in the blood vessels and that it takes about 20 minutes. • Describe physical preparation for the test: The patient will be asked to uncover his leg, arm, or neck and to loosen any restrictive clothing. • Explain what happens during the test: A transducer coated with conductive jelly will be placed on the patient's skin and moved along the vessel to be examined. Blood pressure will be checked at the calves, thighs, and arms. Mention that he may be asked to move his arms into different positions and to perform breathing exercises to vary blood flow while measurements are taken.
Electrocardiography (ECG) • To help identify changes in heart activity that may suggest pulmonary embolism	• Inform the patient that this 15-minute test evaluates heart function by recording electrical activity. Assure him that it is noninvasive and rarely causes discomfort. • Discuss physical preparation for the test: The technician will clean, dry, and possibly shave different sites on the patient's body, such as the chest and arms, and apply conductive jelly over them. Then the technician will attach electrodes at these sites. • Explain what happens during the test: The patient will be asked to lie still, to relax and breathe normally, and to remain quiet. Explain that talk or limb movement will distort ECG recordings and require additional testing time.
Exercise ECG (stress test, treadmill test, graded exercise test) • To help diagnose the cause of breathing problems • To help evaluate the effectiveness of bronchodilator therapy • To assess the degree of pulmonary dysfunction	• Explain that this test evaluates cardiopulmonary function while the patient walks a treadmill or pedals a stationary bicycle. Tell him that it takes about 30 minutes, and that a doctor or nurse will be present in the testing area at all times. Inform him that he mustn't eat, smoke, or drink alcohol for 3 hours before the test. However, he should continue any drug regimen, as ordered. • Advise the patient to wear comfortable shoes and loose, lightweight shorts or slacks; men usually don't wear a shirt during the test, and women usually wear a bra and a lightweight, short-sleeved top or a patient gown with front closure. Inform the patient that a technician will clean,

Teaching patients about respiratory tests (continued)

TEST AND PURPOSE	TEACHING POINTS
Exercise ECG (stress test, treadmill test, graded exercise test) (continued) • To help plan or evaluate an exercise program	shave (if necessary), and lightly rub sites on the chest and, possibly, the back. Then he'll attach electrodes at these sites. • If the patient is scheduled for a multistage treadmill test, tell him that the treadmill speed and incline will increase at predetermined intervals and that he'll be told of each adjustment. If he's scheduled for a bicycle ergometer test, tell him that resistance to pedaling will increase gradually as he tries to maintain a specific speed. He'll be asked to breathe in and out of a mouthpiece during the test and may need to wear a noseclip. • Tell the patient that he can stop the test if he experiences severe fatigue or dyspnea. Typically, he'll feel tired, out of breath, and sweaty. However, he should report any feelings during the test. Tell him that he may receive low-flow nasal oxygen during the test to see whether this therapy improves his cardiopulmonary function. • Describe what will happen after the test: The patient's blood pressure and ECG will be monitored for 10 to 15 minutes.
Impedance plethysmography • To detect deep vein thrombosis • To evaluate for suspected pulmonary embolism	• Tell the patient that this reliable, noninvasive test helps detect blood clots in leg veins. Tell him it takes 30 to 45 minutes to examine both legs. Assure him that it's safe and usually painless. • Describe what happens during the procedure: The patient will put on a hospital gown and then lie on his back on an examining table or bed. The technician will clean, dry, and possibly shave sites on the patient's lower legs and then attach electrodes with conductive jelly. • Explain what will happen during the test: The technician will wrap a pressure cuff around the patient's thigh, inflate the cuff for 1 or 2 minutes, and then quickly release the cuff. Usually, the test is repeated to confirm initial tracings. Stress that the patient should keep his leg muscles relaxed and breathe normally to ensure accurate test results.
Lung perfusion scan (lung scan, lung scintigraphy) • To detect and assess pulmonary vascular obstruction, such as a pulmonary embolism	• Explain that this test evaluates blood flow in the lungs and that it takes about 30 minutes. • Describe what will happen during the test: The patient will lie supine on a table as a radioactive protein substance is injected into an arm vein. This substance will flow through the bloodstream

(continued)

Teaching patients about respiratory tests (continued)

TEST AND PURPOSE	TEACHING POINTS
Lung perfusion scan (lung scan, lung scintigraphy) (continued)	to the lungs, where it will be detected by a large scanning camera. Pictures will be taken while the patient is supine, lying on one side, prone, and sitting. More dye will be injected when the patient is positioned on his stomach. Reassure him that the radioactive substance exposes him to minimal radioactivity. However, he may experience some discomfort from the venipuncture and from lying on a cold, hard table.
Magnetic resonance imaging (MRI) • To help diagnose respiratory disorders by providing high-resolution, cross-sectional images of lung structures and by tracing blood flow	• Inform the patient that this painless, noninvasive test relies on a powerful magnet, radiowaves, and a computer to produce clear cross-sectional images of the chest. Tell him that the test doesn't expose him to radiation but does involve exposure to a strong magnetic field. • Explain that although MRI is painless, the patient may feel uncomfortable because he must remain still inside a small space (in most facilities). Ask if he suffers from claustrophobia; if he does, he might not be able to tolerate the procedure or may need sedation. • Describe preparation for the test: The patient must remove all jewelry and other metal objects. Ask if he has shrapnel, a pacemaker, or any surgically implanted joints, pins, clips, valves, or pumps containing metal that could be attracted to the strong MRI magnet. If he does, he won't be able to have this test. • Explain what happens during the test. The patient will be checked at the scanner room door one last time for metal objects. He may receive a sedative. Then he will lie supine on a narrow bed, which slides into a large cylinder housing the MRI magnets. Radiofrequency energy is directed at the chest; the resulting images are displayed on a monitor and recorded. Tell the patient that the scanner will make clicking, whirring, and thumping noises as it moves inside its housing to obtain different images, and that he may receive earplugs. Reassure him that he'll be able to communicate with the technician at all times, and that the procedure will be stopped if he feels claustrophobic. The patient must remain still during the procedure; advise him to relax and try to concentrate on a favorite subject or image or on his breathing.

Teaching patients about respiratory tests *(continued)*

TEST AND PURPOSE	TEACHING POINTS
Mediastinoscopy • To visualize and obtain a biopsy of the mediastinal area to confirm an occupational respiratory disorder • To detect bronchogenic carcinoma, lymphoma, or sarcoidosis • To determine staging of lung cancer	• Tell the patient that this test allows the doctor to visualize and biopsy the mediastinal area and thereby confirm the diagnosis. • Describe physical preparation for the test: The patient must not eat or drink for 8 hours before the test. He'll receive an I.V. sedative before the test and then a general anesthetic. • Explain what will happen during the test: After inserting an endotracheal tube, the surgeon will make a small transverse suprasternal incision. Then he'll insert a mediastinoscope through this incision and obtain tissue specimens for analysis. • Discuss what will happen after the test: The patient may remain intubated for several hours or overnight. He may experience pain or tenderness at the incision site, a sore throat, and hoarseness. He also may experience nausea and vomiting and a sense of unreality from the anesthetic. Reassure him that these effects soon pass. Advise him to request analgesics for pain.
Pleural biopsy • To differentiate between nonmalignant and malignant disease • To diagnose viral, fungal, or parasitic disease and collagen vascular disease of the pleura	• Inform the patient that this test allows the doctor to biopsy the pleural tissue, which is then analyzed to determine the cause of his pleural disorder. Tell him that the test takes 30 to 45 minutes, although the needle remains in the pleura less than 1 minute. Reassure him that he should experience little pain. • Explain pretest preparation: Blood will be drawn for various studies, and chest X-rays will be taken. The biopsy site will be cleaned and a local anesthetic will be injected. • Describe what will happen during the test: The patient may sit on the edge of the bed and lean forward on the overbed table with arms resting on a pillow and feet resting on a stool; he may straddle a chair; or he may sit in bed in the semi-Fowler position. The doctor will probably use an ultrasound device to guide a needle (an Abrams' or a Cope's needle) through the chest wall to obtain a sample of pleural tissue. Tell the patient that he may feel some pressure as the needle enters the chest cavity. Caution him not to move, breathe deeply, or cough while the needle is in place. Instruct him to let the doctor know if he feels short of breath, dizzy, weak, or sweaty or as if his heart is racing.

(continued)

Teaching patients about respiratory tests *(continued)*

TEST AND PURPOSE	TEACHING POINTS
Pleural biopsy *(continued)*	• Discuss what will happen after the test: The doctor will apply pressure and a bandage to the site. The patient will have a chest X-ray to check for complications. Instruct the patient to tell the doctor if he feels faint or experiences increased breathing difficulty, chest pain, or uncontrollable coughing. Mention that the biopsy sample will be sent to the laboratory for analysis to identify the cause of his disorder. • If the doctor decides to make a chest incision to obtain a tissue sample, the biopsy will be done in the operating room.
Pulmonary angiography (pulmonary arteriography) • To confirm diagnosis of a pulmonary embolism	• Tell the patient that this test allows confirmation of pulmonary embolism. Mention that it takes about 1 hour. • Describe pretest restrictions: The patient must fast for 6 hours before the test, or as ordered. He may continue taking prescribed drugs unless the doctor orders otherwise. • Describe preparation for the test: The patient should remove his clothing, except for socks, and don a gown that fastens in the front. He will be asked to void just before the test. • Explain what will happen during the test: The patient will need to remove the gown, but will be covered with sheets and sterile drapes. Tell him that he'll lie supine on a table and that ECG electrodes will be attached to his arms and legs to monitor his heart. A blood pressure cuff will be wrapped around his arm and an I.V. line started. After injecting a local anesthetic, the doctor will make a small incision or a percutaneous needle puncture in an antecubital, femoral, jugular, or subclavian vein. Warn the patient that he may feel pressure. Next, the doctor will insert and advance a catheter through the vein to the right side of the heart and the pulmonary artery, where he'll measure pressures and withdraw blood samples. Inform the patient that a radiopaque dye will be injected into the catheter. Forewarn him that he may experience a flushed feeling, nausea, or a salty taste for a few minutes after dye injection. X-ray films will be taken as the dye circulates through the pulmonary vessels. When the test is completed, the doctor will withdraw the catheter and ap-

Teaching patients about respiratory tests *(continued)*

TEST AND PURPOSE	TEACHING POINTS
Pulmonary angiography (pulmonary arteriography) *(continued)*	ply a pressure dressing to the insertion site. Instruct the patient to tell the doctor if he experiences shortness of breath, palpitations, chest pain, persistent nausea, numbness or tingling, or wheezing during the test. ● Describe what will happen after the test: The patient's vital signs will be monitored during the first 1 or 2 hours, and the catheter insertion site will be checked. If a femoral or antecubital vein was used, he may need to restrict activity in the affected limb for 4 to 6 hours. Instruct him to report wheezing, palpitations, chest pain, itching, nausea, vomiting, irritability, or euphoria after the test. Also tell him to report redness, swelling, or bleeding at the insertion site.

Pulmonary function tests
● To determine the cause of breathing problems
● To determine whether a functional abnormality is obstructive or restrictive
● To estimate the degree of pulmonary dysfunction in obstructive and restrictive diseases
● To evaluate the effectiveness of therapy, such as use of bronchodilators or steroids
	● Explain that these tests evaluate lung function. If the patient has asthma, tell him that the tests can help determine whether prescribed drugs are effective in treating asthma.
	● Describe pretest restrictions: The patient must not smoke for 4 hours before testing and must avoid eating a large meal or drinking a large amount of fluid before the test.
	● Discuss preparation for the test: The patient should put on loose, comfortable clothing. If he wears dentures, advise him to keep them in to help form a tight seal around the mouthpiece. Just before the test, he will be asked to void.
	● Explain what will happen during the test: The patient will sit upright and wear a nose clip. Or he may sit in a small airtight box called a *body plethysmograph* and will not need the nose clip. Forewarn him that inside the plethysmograph, he may experience claustrophobia. Reassure him that he won't suffocate and that he will be able to communicate with the technician through the window in the box.
	  Tell him that he will be asked to breathe in a certain way for each test; for example, to inhale deeply and exhale completely or to inhale quickly. Explain that he may receive an aerosolized bronchodilator and may then repeat one or two tests to evaluate the drug's effectiveness. An arterial puncture may also be performed during the test for ABG analysis.
	  Emphasize that the test will proceed quickly if the patient follows directions, tries hard, and

(continued)

Teaching patients about respiratory tests *(continued)*

TEST AND PURPOSE	TEACHING POINTS
Pulmonary function tests *(continued)*	keeps a tight seal around the mouthpiece or tube to ensure accurate results. Tell the patient that he may experience dyspnea and fatigue during the test but will be allowed to rest periodically. Instruct him to tell the technician if he experiences dizziness, chest pain, palpitations, nausea, severe difficulty breathing, or wheezing.

Sputum analysis
• To identify the cause of pulmonary infection, thus aiding diagnosis of respiratory diseases (most frequently bronchitis, tuberculosis, lung abscess, and pneumonia)
	• Tell the patient that this test isolates and identifies the cause of his infection. Inform him that the best time to collect the specimen is early morning after secretions have accumulated overnight.
	• Discuss preparation for the test: The patient should drink plenty of fluids the night before and avoid brushing his teeth before collection. If the specimen will be collected by bronchoscopy, instruct him to fast for 6 hours before the procedure.
	• Describe what will happen during the test: If the specimen will be collected by expectoration, the patient will be instructed to take several deep abdominal breaths. When he's ready to cough, he should take one more deep abdominal breath, bend forward, and make a soft, staged, shortened cough into the provided sterile container.
	  If the specimen will be collected by tracheal suctioning, tell the patient that he'll receive oxygen before and after the procedure, if necessary. The doctor will pass a suction catheter through the patient's nostril and advance it into the trachea. Then he'll apply suction briefly to obtain the specimen. Warn him that he'll experience some discomfort as the catheter passes into the trachea.
	  If the specimen will be collected by bronchoscopy, inform the patient that a local anesthetic will be sprayed into his throat or that he will gargle with a local anesthetic. Next, the bronchoscope will be inserted into the bronchus. Secretions are then collected, and the bronchoscope is removed.
	• Explain what will happen after the test: After tracheal suctioning, the patient will be given a drink of water. After bronchoscopy, he will be observed for possible complications. Tell him that he can have liquids once his gag reflex returns.

Teaching patients about respiratory tests *(continued)*

TEST AND PURPOSE	TEACHING POINTS
Thoracentesis (pleural fluid aspiration) • To obtain a specimen of pleural fluid for analysis • To relieve lung compression caused by pleural fluid, blood, or air • To obtain a lung tissue biopsy specimen	• Inform the patient that thoracentesis provides samples of tissue or fluid from around the lungs to help diagnose his respiratory disorder. It may also be done therapeutically to relieve respiratory distress. • Describe preparation for the test: The patient will put on a hospital gown, and the area around the needle insertion site will be shaved. • Explain what will happen during the test: The patient will be comfortably positioned — either sitting with his arms on pillows or lying partially on his side in bed. The doctor will clean the needle insertion site with a cold antiseptic solution, then inject a local anesthetic. Tell the patient that he may feel a burning sensation as the doctor injects the anesthetic. After the patient's skin is numb, the doctor will insert the needle, obtain the necessary sample, and withdraw the needle. Warn the patient that he will feel pressure during needle insertion and withdrawal. Instruct him to remain still and to avoid coughing, breathing deeply, or moving. Tell him to inform the doctor right away if he experiences dyspnea, palpitations, wheezing, dizziness, weakness, or diaphoresis, which may indicate respiratory distress. After withdrawing the needle, the doctor will apply slight pressure and then an adhesive bandage. • Describe what will happen after the test: The patient's vital signs will be monitored frequently for the first few hours. Instruct him to report any fluid or blood leakage from the needle insertion site and any signs of respiratory distress. Explain that a chest X-ray will be taken to detect any posttest complications.
Ventilation scan • To assess general and regional lung ventilation • To help diagnose respiratory disorders, such as pulmonary embolism and chronic obstructive pulmonary disease	• Inform the patient that this 30-minute test evaluates lung ventilation during respiration. • Describe pretest restrictions: The patient must avoid large meals, drinking a large volume of fluid, and smoking for 3 hours before the test. He may continue to take his medications unless the doctor orders otherwise. Before the test, he will be asked to remove all jewelry and metal objects. • Explain what will happen during the test: The patient will be asked to sit down and breathe a radioactive gas through a mouthpiece or a tightly fitted face mask. A nuclear scanner will monitor

(continued)

Teaching patients about respiratory tests *(continued)*

TEST AND PURPOSE	TEACHING POINTS
Ventilation scan *(continued)*	gas distribution in his lungs. Tell the patient that he'll be instructed to breathe deeply, hold his breath, breathe out, and then breathe normally. Instruct him to remain still when he's asked to hold his breath. Assure him that the amount of radioactive gas used is minimized and that it's mixed with air. Tell him to report any dyspnea or wheezing during the test.

Medication

Tell the patient that medications are the primary treatment for pleural disorders. Discuss the drugs prescribed for the patient's particular disorder, explaining that they may be discontinued once the disorder is controlled.

Pleurodesis

If the patient has pleural effusion, explain that he may receive a solution of tetracycline hydrochloride (Achromycin) or bleomycin sulfate (Blenoxane) through a chest tube to produce inflammation and adhesions. Called pleurodesis, this condition may deter pleural fluid from reaccumulating. Explain that the inflammation and adhesions in the pleural space eliminate areas for further effusion. Reassure the patient that adverse effects are usually mild.

Antibiotics

If the patient has empyema, inform him that high doses of antibiotic drugs may destroy the organism causing this infection. The drugs may be administered through a chest tube or parenterally (I.V. or I.M.). Before starting antibiotic therapy, the patient will undergo culture and sensitivity tests.

Symptomatic therapy

Tell the patient with pleurisy that drug treatment aims to relieve his symptoms. If the doctor recommends antitussive therapy to control coughing,

tell the patient he can obtain some antitussives without a prescription.

 WARNING: Caution the patient about adverse effects of antitussives, including insomnia, nervousness, irritability, unusual excitement, dizziness, drowsiness, and stomach upset. Warn him to avoid alcohol when taking an antitussive because alcohol may increase central nervous system depression. Also caution him to avoid activities that require alertness if the medication makes him feel drowsy.

If the doctor prescribes a nonsteroidal anti-inflammatory drug such as ibuprofen, inform the patient that this drug reduces inflammation. Clarify the prescribed dosage, and caution him that this drug may cause behavioral changes, confusion, dizziness, edema, GI upset, headache, insomnia, and nausea and vomiting. Reassure him, however, that adverse effects are usually mild with short-term therapy.

If the patient needs a narcotic analgesic for severe pleuritic pain, the doctor may prescribe morphine (Duramorph), codeine, or meperidine (Demerol). Mention that most narcotic analgesics have antitussive (anticough) properties. Point out the adverse effects of these controlled substances, including possible breathing problems, confusion, constipation, dry mouth, drowsiness, and nausea and vomiting.

WARNING: Advise the patient to avoid alcohol when taking a narcotic because alcohol may increase central nervous system depression, worsening such symptoms as drowsiness and confusion. Also warn him that prolonged use can lead to physical and psychological dependence and tolerance.

Procedures

Inform the patient that oxygen therapy is usually necessary to treat pleural effusion or empyema. The flow rate, type of delivery system, and duration of therapy depend on the patient's disorder and the severity of his dyspnea.

Tell the patient with pleural effusion, empyema, or pleurisy with pleural effusion that thoracentesis may be performed to drain the pleural space and relieve breathing difficulties. Add that thoracentesis may be followed by insertion of a chest tube (to remove fluid or air) and closed drainage. Describe the chest tube insertion and drainage procedure, as appropriate.

Surgery

If the patient has severe empyema, explain that decortication (removal of the visceral pleura) may be performed. Rib resection may also be necessary to allow for open drainage and lung expansion.

Other care measures

If the doctor recommends chest support for the patient with pleurisy, show the patient how to tape his chest to provide support and firm pressure at the pain site. Even without chest binding, he can apply pressure to relieve discomfort, especially during coughing and deep breathing. Demonstrate how to use a folded blanket or pillow as a splinting device.

For information and support, refer the patient to an appropriate organization, such as the American Lung Association, the National Jewish Center for Immunology and Respiratory Medicine, or the Respiratory Health Association. (See Appendix 2.)

Pneumonia

Despite the availability of vaccines and anti-infective drugs, pneumonia remains a leading cause of death and disability, especially among already debilitated patients. For this reason, your teaching should underscore the need to comply with prescribed treatment. However, if breathing difficulty, fever, coughing, and fatigue impede the patient's ability to learn, you'll need to provide simple explanations and brief instructions about diagnostic tests and treatment.

As the patient's condition improves, you should discuss the cause of pneumonia and how the disease develops. Remember, though, that the patient may lose his motivation to comply with treatment as he starts to feel better. Therefore, you must be sure to caution him about risk factors for recurrent pneumonia. To prevent a relapse, urge him to take all prescribed medications as directed and stress the importance of adequate rest.

Before teaching a patient about pneumonia, make sure you are familiar with the following topics:
• respiratory defense mechanisms and how pneumonia develops
• signs and symptoms of pneumonia
• diagnostic studies, such as chest X-rays, sputum analysis, and blood tests
• how pneumonia is classified — by cause, location, and type
• risk factors, including chronic health conditions and smoking
• treatment, such as activity restrictions, drug therapy, breathing and coughing exercises, chest physiotherapy, hydration, and oxygen therapy
• preventive measures, including pneumococcal and influenza vaccinations for high-risk patients and methods to prevent the spread of infection, such as proper hand washing and tissue disposal
• sources of information and support.

ABOUT THE DISORDER

Inform the patient that pneumonia is a lung infection that interferes with oxygen and carbon dioxide exchange. Explain that it develops when pathogens overwhelm the body's respiratory defenses. Normally, the upper and lower airways stop most pathogens from reaching the air sacs in the lungs, or alveoli, where gas exchange takes place. The immune system backs up failed airway defenses by destroying any remaining pathogens. If all natural defenses fail, pneumonia can develop. (See *How the body fights respiratory infection.*)

Point out the cardinal signs and symptoms of pneumonia: fever, pleuritic chest pain, shaking chills, dyspnea, tachypnea, and coughing. Explain that sputum color may vary, depending on the causative organism. Colorless sputum implies a noninfectious process; creamy yellow sputum suggests staphylococcal pneumonia; green sputum denotes pneumonia caused by *Pseudomonas* organisms; and sputum that looks like currant jelly indicates pneumonia caused by *Klebsiella.*

Inform the patient that pneumonia may be classified by causative organism, location, or type. Causative organisms include bacteria, viruses, fungi, and protozoa. Pneumonia may be located in the distal airways and alveoli (bronchopneumonia), part of a lobe (lobular pneumonia), or an entire lobe (lobar pneumonia). By type, pneumonia may be primary (usually a result of inhaling or aspirating a pathogen), or secondary (following initial lung damage from a noxious chemical or other insult or caused by the spread of bacteria to the lung from elsewhere in the body).

Discuss predisposing factors for pneumonia. Point out that viral infections, such as a cold or influenza, may weaken the body's defenses against the viruses that cause pneumonia. Age is also a factor. Individuals under age 1 and over age 65 have the fewest natural immune factors. With aging, too, chronic disease and less efficient lung function are more likely, predisposing the body to lung infection. Other risk factors for pneumonia are smoking and alcohol consumption.

Inform the patient that chronic lung disease, such as emphysema, asthma, or cystic fibrosis, heightens the risk for pneumonia. So does a depressed immune system associated with such conditions as cancer, chemotherapy, organ or bone marrow transplant, and acquired immunodeficiency syndrome. List the other risk factors for pneumonia, including prolonged bed rest, use of general anesthetics or narcotics, chest or abdominal surgery, neuromuscular disease, chronic illness, and exposure to contaminated air or water.

Complications

Emphasize that untreated or inadequately treated pneumonia can lead to life-threatening complications, such as septic shock, hypoxemia, and respiratory failure. With inadequate treatment, the infection can spread within the lung, or it may spread by the bloodstream or by cross-contamination to other parts of the body, causing bacteremia, endocarditis, pericarditis, or meningitis.

DIAGNOSTIC WORKUP

Tell the patient about tests used to diagnose pneumonia and evaluate his condition. Standard tests include sputum analysis, blood studies, and a chest X-ray to detect and monitor the progression of pneumonia. (For more information on chest X-rays, see *Teaching patients about respiratory tests,* pages 70 to 80.)

Sputum analysis and blood studies

Explain that a sputum analysis, including a Gram stain and culture and sensitivity studies, isolates and identifies the cause of infection and can guide the selection of antimicrobial therapy. If the patient is seriously ill, blood cultures may also be ordered.

If sputum analysis and blood culture results don't identify the causa-

INSIGHT INTO ILLNESSES

How the body fights respiratory infection

As you explain the pathophysiology of pneumonia to your patient, point out how the upper airway structures form a front-line defense against infection. Add that lower airway structures stand ready to expel pathogens that escape upper airway defenses. Finally, explain how the immune system backs up failed airway defenses by destroying any remaining pathogens.

Upper airway defenses
Inform the patient that nasal hairs trap inhaled dust and grit. Mucus then traps finer particles such as bacteria, which the cilia move to the oropharynx (mouth area).

At the same time, turbinates — bony structures that project into the nasal cavity — humidify and warm the air, which keeps secretions warm and moist.

In the pharynx, the soft palate and epiglottis separate air and food, preventing choking. Gag and cough reflexes also prevent choking, and the cough reflex clears secretions that might harbor bacteria.

Lower airway defenses
Tell the patient that the lower airways — containing the larynx, trachea, bronchi, and lungs — form a second line of defense against infec-

tion. Upon entering the trachea, particles small enough to pass through the upper airway defenses fall into a blanket of cilia and mucus that carries these invaders away from the lungs. In this process, known as the *mucociliary escalator,* continuously undulating cilia move contaminated mucus to the pharynx (where it's swallowed), to the larynx (where coughing expectorates it), or to the nose (where sneezing and blowing expel it).

Macrophages: Last line of defense
Inform the patient that specialized reticuloendothelial cells called macrophages greet any bacteria and foreign particles that escape airway defenses and reach the pulmonary alveoli. Explain that macrophages carry out phagocytosis.

First, bacteria attach to the cell surfaces, initiating opsonization — an antibody coating that enables phagocytosis. Then the macrophages surround the bacteria by forming pseudopods — footlike extensions. Phagosomes digest the bacteria and merge with lysosomes to form phagolysosomes, which help destroy the bacteria. Finally, the macrophages release digestive debris and continue to fight infection.

tive organism and the patient remains ill despite conventional therapy, the doctor may order more invasive studies, such as bronchoscopy, transtracheal aspiration, and needle or open-lung biopsy. Provide information about these tests as necessary.

TREATMENTS
Explain that treatment includes rest, medication, and procedures to re-

move excess secretions, such as deep-breathing exercises, therapeutic coughing, hydration therapy, and chest physiotherapy.

Activity guidelines
Urge the patient to get adequate rest, emphasizing that rest promotes a full recovery and helps to prevent a relapse. Mention that the doctor will

advise him when he can resume normal activities and return to work.

Explain that convalescent time depends on the patient's age, health history, and the severity of the infection. For example, a young, usually healthy patient can resume typical activities within a week of recovery, whereas a middle-aged or chronically ill patient may need several weeks before regaining his usual strength, vigor, and feeling of well-being. Caution such a patient that he may tire easily, and encourage him to alternate activity with rest to conserve his energy.

Medication
Inform the patient that the doctor usually prescribes a broad-spectrum antibiotic, such as penicillin or erythromycin, based on results of the Gram stain of the sputum. Once culture and sensitivity tests identify pneumonia's cause, the doctor may prescribe an antibiotic specific to the infecting organism. Discuss the prescribed medication and reinforce the doctor's or nurse's instructions for taking it.

 WARNING: Although the patient's condition may improve dramatically after only a few days of treatment, stress that he must take prescribed medication for the entire course of therapy (7 to 10 days) to prevent a relapse. Warn him that recurrent pneumonia can be far more serious than the initial illness.

Procedures
Teach the patient procedures to clear lung secretions, such as breathing and coughing exercises, hydration therapy, chest physiotherapy, and home oxygen administration.

Breathing and coughing exercises
Show the patient how to perform deep breathing and pursed-lip breathing. Begin by demonstrating the proper position for maximum effectiveness. Instruct him to sit upright, placing both feet on the floor. If he must remain in bed, have him assume a high Fowler position. Then demonstrate prolonged deep inspiration through the nose and slow exhalation through pursed lips.

Tell the patient that effective coughing can help expel lung secretions. He should use the same position he uses for deep breathing. Show him how to flex his body at the waist if he's sitting or how to bend his knees if he's in a high Fowler position. If he must lie flat, direct him to lie on one side and bend his knees. Then instruct him to breathe deeply through his nose, hold his breath for a few seconds, and cough twice to bring up any sputum. Finally, tell him to inhale by sniffing gently and then expectorate into a strong tissue. (Swallowed mucus can upset the stomach.)

Hydration therapy
Encourage the patient to drink 2 to 3 quarts of fluid a day to promote adequate hydration and keep mucus secretions thin for easier removal. Without adequate hydration, infected secretions become thick and tenacious. Fever and tachypnea also increase mucoid thickening, thereby providing an excellent medium for growth of the infecting organism.

Chest physiotherapy
Include the patient's family when you discuss chest physiotherapy. Explain that postural drainage, percussion, and vibration help to mobilize and remove mucus from the lungs. Show the patient how to position himself for gravity drainage of the affected lung segment or lobe. Ambulatory and upright positions naturally drain the upper lobes. The lower lobes (except for the superior segments) are best drained with the patient in the prone Trendelenburg position.

Oxygen therapy
If the patient will be receiving oxygen at home, teach him how to use the equipment. Give him copies of the teaching aids *Learning how to use breathing devices,* page 66, and *Using oxygen safely and effectively,* page 67.

Other care measures

Urge the patient to avoid irritants that stimulate secretions, such as cigarette smoke, dust, and significant environmental pollution. Refer him to community programs that can help him stop smoking.

To avoid spreading infection to others, remind the patient to sneeze and cough into tissues and to dispose of the tissues in a waxed or plastic bag. Advise him to wash his hands thoroughly after handling contaminated tissues.

Because pneumonia caused by influenza usually carries a poor prognosis — even with treatment — encourage the patient to obtain yearly flu immunization, unless he has a demonstrated allergy to eggs or to a previous flu vaccine. Encourage the high-risk patient (over age 65, with chronic heart, renal, or lung disease, sickle cell anemia, or diabetes) to ask the doctor about the pneumococcal pneumonia (Pneumovax) vaccination.

To promote a full recovery, advise the patient to contact the American Lung Association or the Coalition on Smoking or Health. (See Appendix 2.)

Pulmonary embolism

More than any other respiratory disorder, pulmonary embolism is likely to complicate the recovery of a hospitalized patient. As a result, many patients need to learn about risk factors and warning signs of pulmonary embolism. And once an embolus resolves, some patients may not comply fully with prolonged anticoagulant therapy. These problems can pose a challenge to patient education.

Before teaching a patient about pulmonary embolism, make sure you are familiar with the following topics:

• how emboli obstruct pulmonary blood flow

• risks and causes associated with emboli

• diagnostic tests, such as perfusion and ventilation scans, arterial blood gas (ABG) analysis, pulmonary angiography, electrocardiography (ECG), ultrasonography, impedance plethysmography, chest X-ray, and blood tests

• patient preparation for clotting studies to monitor anticoagulant therapy

• importance of exercise and proper positioning to prevent venous stasis

• anticoagulant therapy

• how to use a sequential compression device and apply antiembolism stockings

• signs and symptoms of recurrent pulmonary embolism and of complications, such as thrombophlebitis, ventricular failure, and arrhythmias

• sources of information and support.

ABOUT THE DISORDER

Tell the patient that pulmonary embolism occurs when a mass, such as a dislodged thrombus or a blood clot, lodges in an artery of the lung. (See *How a clot travels from the leg to the lung,* page 86.) The clot obstructs perfusion, or blood flow, to a portion of the lung. As a result, the air in this lung portion can't participate in gas exchange. To compensate for the mismatch between ventilation and perfusion, the patient must breathe faster and with more effort to avoid hypoxemia. He may also wheeze in response to distal airway constriction — the body's attempt to shunt ventilation from nonperfused to perfused areas of the lung.

Briefly discuss the most common cause of pulmonary embolism — dislodged thrombi, usually originating in the deep leg veins, which form as the result of vascular wall damage, venous stasis, or hypercoagulability of the blood. The thrombi may have embolized spontaneously during clot dissolution or may have become dislodged during trauma, sudden muscle action, or a change in peripheral blood flow.

Complications

Emphasize that the patient can avoid or minimize lung tissue collapse (atelectasis) by strictly adhering to the

INSIGHT INTO ILLNESSES

How a clot travels from the leg to the lung

Inform the patient that a blood clot may develop in a leg vein if a blood vessel is torn, if blood accumulates in his legs, or if his blood clots more easily than normal.

Perilous path

Explain that if the clot breaks free, it will travel from the legs through progressively larger veins to the heart. Point out that the clot flows freely until it reaches the lungs, where the blood vessels again become small. Here it can cause a blockage, stopping blood flow to the lungs.

treatment plan. Explain how atelectasis may worsen breathing distress. Note that the patient is at risk for atelectasis until the embolus resolves.

DIAGNOSTIC WORKUP

Discuss the studies used to detect pulmonary embolism and to evaluate the patient's response to anticoagulant therapy. To help confirm pulmonary embolism, the doctor may order a lung perfusion scan, a ventilation scan, ABG measurements, pulmonary angiography, and an ECG. To detect peripheral venous thrombosis, he may schedule Doppler ultrasonography or impedance plethysmography. (See *Teaching patients about respiratory tests,* pages 70 to 80.)

To rule out other disorders, the doctor may order blood tests to determine the white blood cell count, erythrocyte sedimentation rate, fibrin split products, and serum lactate dehydrogenase, aspartate aminotransferase, and bilirubin levels. He may also order a chest X-ray.

Coagulation tests

If the patient has acute pulmonary embolism, tell him that the doctor will monitor his clotting time, thrombin time, or activated partial thromboplastin time. Inform him that test results help evaluate his response to heparin therapy. Mention that once he begins oral anticoagulants, the doctor will monitor pro-

thrombin time (PT) until the desired anticoagulant level is reached.

Remind the patient that after discharge on anticoagulant therapy, he must return for periodic blood tests to monitor PT. Usually, blood is drawn once a week until PT stabilizes, then every 2 weeks and, eventually, once a month.

TREATMENTS

Inform the patient that the goal of treatment is to maintain adequate heart and lung function until the obstruction resolves — and to prevent recurrence of the embolism. (Most emboli resolve within 10 to 14 days.)

If the patient's embolism was caused by a thrombus, explain that treatment generally consists of oxygen therapy as needed and anticoagulation with heparin. Inform the patient who's on heparin therapy that he needs daily coagulation studies. He may also receive warfarin for 3 to 6 months, depending on his risk factors.

If the patient has a massive pulmonary embolism and shock, the doctor may prescribe fibrinolytic therapy with thrombolytic agents (such as streptokinase or urokinase). Explain that when given early, thrombolytic agents dissolve clots within 12 to 14 hours. If the embolus causes hypotension, the patient may need a vasopressor such as dopamine.

Tell the patient who has a septic embolus that he will require antibiotic therapy specific to the causative agent, not anticoagulants, and that he will be evaluated for the infection source (most likely endocarditis).

Activity guidelines
Inform the patient that prolonged standing, sitting, or inactivity can cause venous stasis, which sets the stage for blood clots in the legs. Encourage him to exercise his legs frequently to promote blood flow. Demonstrate exercises that can be easily done such as rocking on the heels or toes. If the patient is disabled or restricted to bed rest, instruct family members or other caregivers to perform passive leg exercises by flexing and extending his feet at the ankles.

Instruct the patient to elevate his legs 30 degrees or more whenever possible — without bending his knees — to prevent blood from pooling in the legs.

 WARNING: Caution the patient to avoid standing or sitting with legs dangling or crossed.

Also advise the patient to stop frequently for short walks if he takes long car rides and to periodically stroll up and down the aisle on airplane trips.

Medication
Make sure the patient understands that prescribed anticoagulants — warfarin or heparin — aim to prevent recurrent emboli. Teach the patient how to detect signs of drug toxicity, such as bleeding gums, nosebleeds, bleeding hemorrhoids, red or purple skin spots, or excessive menstrual flow (in females). Instruct him to report these signs immediately.

If the patient is taking warfarin, stress the importance of continuing this medication at home and returning for periodic blood tests. If he can't tolerate anticoagulants, the doctor may order aspirin or dipyridamole instead. Tell the patient to take these medications exactly as ordered.

Procedures
A patient who can't take anticoagulants or who develops recurrent emboli during anticoagulant therapy requires surgery to interrupt the inferior vena cava. Explain that this surgery consists of vena caval ligation, plication, or insertion of a device (an umbrella filter) that filters blood returning to the heart and lungs. Tell the patient that he may receive heparin or other medications to prevent blood clots after surgery.

To prevent postoperative venous thromboembolism or in patients who can't take anticoagulants, pneumatic boots, sequential compression devices, or antiembolism stockings will be required.

Other care measures
Stress the importance of coughing and deep-breathing exercises to prevent atelectasis. Then teach the patient how to apply antiembolism stockings or elastic bandage wraps, if ordered, to improve circulation in the legs. (See *Applying antiembolism stockings,* page 88.) Emphasize that the stockings must fit properly and be applied smoothly.

To ensure safety, advise the patient to remove throw rugs and small objects from floors to help prevent falls. If the patient does fall, tell him to call the doctor, who may want to examine him to rule out internal bleeding.

 WARNING: Instruct the patient to immediately report signs of thrombophlebitis — calf pain and swelling — especially if pulling the toes backward toward the head makes the calf hurt more. Also tell him to report signs of postphlebitis syndrome — lower leg and ankle swelling, hyperpigmentation, and ulceration.

Teach the patient how to recognize signs and symptoms of recurrent pulmonary embolism, including dyspnea; tachypnea; chest pain (especially when trying to take a deep breath); coughing up of blood; a dry, annoy-

Applying antiembolism stockings

To improve circulation in the lower legs, the doctor may want your patient to apply antiembolism stockings. Be sure to cover the following points when teaching him about these stockings.

Applying the stockings

Emphasize that the patient should put the stockings on in the morning before getting out of bed and remove them at night once he's in bed.

To put the stockings on, tell him to lightly dust his ankles with powder to make them easier to apply. Then instruct him to insert his hand into the stocking from the top, and grab the heel pocket from the inside. He should turn the stocking inside out so that the foot section is inside the stocking leg.

Next, tell him to hook the index and middle fingers of both hands into the foot section and then ease the stocking over his toes, stretching it sideways as he moves it up his foot. Advise him to point his toes to help ease on the stocking.

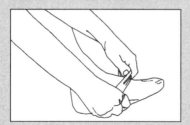

Then, instruct the patient to center his heel in the heel pocket. Tell him to gather the loose material at his ankle and slide the rest of the stocking up over his heel with short pulls, alternating front and back.

Tell him to insert his index and middle fingers into the gathered stocking at his ankle, and then ease the stocking up his leg to the knee.

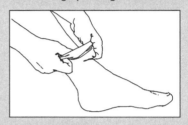

To distribute the material evenly, instruct the patient to stretch the stocking toward the knee, front and back. The stocking should fit snugly, with no wrinkles.

Precautions

• Stress that the top of the stocking must be below the crease at the back of the knee. Explain that if the top of the stocking sits in the crease, it can put pressure on the vein and decrease circulation to the legs.
• Caution the patient never to let the stockings be rolled part way down his leg or bunched up in any way. This can create too much pressure on the leg veins.

ing cough; or apprehension or a feeling that "something isn't right."

If the patient has underlying cardiopulmonary disease, instruct him to immediately report fatigue, swelling of the feet or ankles, unexplained steady weight gain, and chest tightness. And because pulmonary embolism can also trigger arrhyth-

mias, such as atrial fibrillation or atrial flutter, tell the patient to report palpitations.

If the patient is at high risk for recurrence of pulmonary embolism, refer him to the American Lung Association for information and support. (See Appendix 2.)

4

Gastrointestinal conditions

Gallbladder disease

Diseases of the gallbladder are painful conditions commonly associated with deposition of calculi and inflammation. About 25 million Americans (mostly women) have cholelithiasis, or gallstones, making it the most common biliary tract disorder in the United States.

Despite its prevalence, few patients know much about the causes of gallbladder disease or its treatments. Even fewer understand how the gallbladder functions. Most express surprise that untreated gallstones can be life-threatening. Therefore, patient education should start with the basics.

Before teaching a patient about gallbladder disease, make sure you are familiar with the following topics:
• biliary system anatomy and physiology
• how gallstones develop
• risk factors for cholelithiasis, including obesity, age, and multiple pregnancies
• signs and symptoms of biliary colic, such as pain, belching, and nausea
• cholecystitis and other complications
• diagnostic tests, such as biliary ultrasonography, oral cholecystography, endoscopic retrograde cholangiopancreatography (ERCP), and percutaneous transhepatic cholangiography
• drug therapy, including analgesic and antibiotic agents, oral dissolution drugs, and topical solvents
• procedures to remove gallstones, including ERCP, endoscopic sphincterotomy, and extracorporeal shock-wave lithotripsy (ESWL)
• surgery, such as cholecystectomy,

cholecystotomy, choledochostomy, and laparoscopic cholecystectomy
• the importance of follow-up care to detect recurrent gallstones.

ABOUT THE DISORDER

Inform the patient that cholelithiasis refers to stones, or calculi, in the gallbladder. Gallstones reflect a change in bile components. They signal that the gallbladder has become sluggish, giving cholesterol, calcium bilirubinate, or a mixture of cholesterol and bilirubin pigment a chance to settle and crystallize. Usually pea-sized, the resultant stone can be as tiny as a pinhead or as large as a hen's egg. To better explain how and where gallstones occur, review biliary structures and functions. (See *How the biliary system works,* page 90.)

Point out that although no one knows for sure what causes gallstones, certain contributing factors set the stage for stone formation. At highest risk for cholelithiasis are women — especially obese women over age 40 who have had several pregnancies. Pregnancy causes increased abdominal pressure, which leads to bile flow stasis and subsequent stone formation. In addition, hormonal changes during pregnancy may delay gallbladder emptying, which may also promote stasis. Increased cholesterol levels during the third trimester contribute as well.

Mention other risk factors associated with a sluggish gallbladder: oral contraceptive use, diabetes mellitus, celiac disease, cirrhosis of the liver, pancreatitis, and heredity.

How the biliary system works

To help your patient understand how and why gallstones interfere with her digestion, describe the biliary system and its functions. Use this illustration to point out common gallstone sites and to reinforce your discussion.

The role of bile

Inform your patient that bile is a greenish-yellow fluid that forms in the liver, helping the digestive system to break down fats and absorb fats and fat-soluble vitamins. Tell her that bile is concentrated and stored in the gallbladder, a muscular, membranous, pear-sized sac situated just under the liver.

Where bile travels

To reach the gallbladder, bile flows from the liver through the hepatic and cystic ducts. Point out that these ducts join to form the common bile duct, which connects the gallbladder and the liver.

Explain that the common bile duct joins the pancreatic duct, which opens into the duodenum (the beginning of the small intestine). Bile flow into the duodenum is controlled by sphincter muscles. When these sphincters close, bile returns to the gallbladder for storage.

How gallstones impede bile flow

Tell the patient that when food enters the duodenum, a hormone stimulates the gallbladder to contract and release stored bile into the common bile duct. At the same time, the pancreas secretes juices, which join the bile as it flows to the duodenum. Both substances aid digestion. Gallstones that form and lodge in biliary structures (either ducts or organs) block bile flow and interfere with digestion.

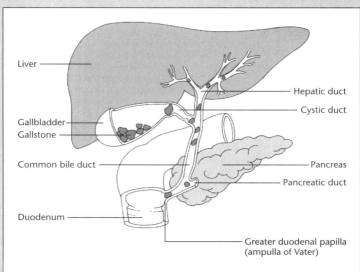

Explain that about half of patients lack symptoms and may not realize they have gallstones until an X-ray or ultrasonography performed for other reasons detects them. The other half suffer the severe, episodic pain of acute cholelithiasis (also called gallbladder attack or biliary colic). Severe pain in the middle of the abdomen or the right upper quadrant commonly spreads to the back and shoulders and lasts up to several hours. Walking or changing position offers no relief. Inform the patient that the pain results from a stone lodged in the gallbladder's neck or in the cystic duct. The pain diminishes when the stone dislodges and either slips back into the gallbladder or passes into the intestine.

Complications

Emphasize that untreated gallstones can cause life-threatening complications, such as prolonged obstruction, infection, and gallstones in the common bile duct (possibly leading to obstruction of bile flow into the duodenum, with subsequent abscess, necrosis, perforation, and peritonitis.)

DIAGNOSTIC WORKUP

Tell the patient that several diagnostic studies can detect gallstones. The most commonly performed tests are biliary ultrasonography and oral cholecystography. If these tests fail to reveal gallstones, despite symptoms, the doctor may order ERCP or percutaneous transhepatic cholangiography. (For information on these tests, see *Teaching patients about gastrointestinal tests,* pages 101 to 109.)

Routine laboratory tests also may be done to support the diagnosis. Inform the patient that blood samples and urine specimens will be studied to assess serum and urine bilirubin, total serum cholesterol, cholesterol ester, plasma phospholipid, and serum alkaline phosphatase levels; activated partial thromboplastin time; and white blood cell count.

TREATMENTS

Explain that treatment for cholelithiasis depends on signs and symptoms. If the patient is asymptomatic, she won't require treatment. If she has had at least one gallbladder attack and test results confirm cholelithiasis, the doctor may recommend gallstone removal. The removal procedure depends on the gallstones' location, their size and number, and potential or confirmed complications, such as acute cholecystitis or choledocholithiasis.

Also tell the patient that medications may be prescribed. If she asks whether a special diet (such as a fat-free diet) can relieve her symptoms, tell her that clinical findings no longer validate diet therapy.

Medications

Review medications prescribed to treat gallstones. These medications may include analgesics to relieve pain, antibiotics to prevent infection, and drugs to dissolve the stones.

Analgesics

A narcotic analgesic such as meperidine (Demerol) may be prescribed for the patient with episodic biliary colic or for the hospitalized patient with gallstones complicated by acute cholecystitis. Reassure the patient that pain and inflammation usually subside in 2 to 7 days.

Antibiotics

For the patient with gallstones and acute cholecystitis, the doctor may prescribe a broad-spectrum antibiotic such as tetracycline to prevent infection — especially if the patient is elderly, has gallstones in the common bile duct, or has diabetes mellitus or another serious disorder.

Oral dissolution agents

If the patient's gallstones are noncalcified and contain mainly cholesterol, the doctor may recommend oral dissolution therapy. Explain that the bile salts chenodiol (Chenix) and ursodiol (Actigall), alone or in combination, can shrink or dissolve existing gall-stones and prevent new formations. Inform the patient that this therapy will continue for about 2 years and that the patient's progress will be monitored by ultrasonography.

Teach the patient how to take these drugs. Because the dosage is based on weight, tell her to alert the doctor to significant weight loss. Urge her to keep scheduled appointments for laboratory tests to monitor how the therapy affects her liver function. Tell her to report these adverse reactions immediately: diarrhea, severe abdominal pain, nausea, and vomiting.

Topical solvents
If the doctor prescribes the topical solvent methyl *tert*-butyl ether (MTBE) to dissolve cholesterol stones, explain that this drug can dissolve any size or number of cholesterol stones within hours; however, the stones may recur later. Point out that the solvent is instilled through a catheter inserted either into the abdomen or through the nose to the hepatic duct, depending on the gallstones' location. Explain that the procedure usually requires a local anesthetic and takes place in the hospital outpatient department.

For gallstones in the gallbladder, the doctor may insert a small catheter through the right upper abdomen. Inform the patient that after guiding the catheter into the gallbladder and using X-rays to verify its placement, the doctor will pump the solvent in and out of the gallbladder until fluoroscopy shows that the stones are completely dissolved. The process may take several hours.

For gallstones in the hepatic duct, the doctor may insert an endoscope nasally, thread a nasobiliary catheter through it, and verify its placement in the hepatic duct with X-rays. Then he'll instill MTBE through the catheter. Every 30 minutes, he'll aspirate the drug with a syringe, gradually increasing the dose. After 4 hours of this treatment, a second X-ray will confirm whether MTBE has dissolved

the stones. When the stones have dissolved, the doctor will remove the endoscope and catheter.

If the doctor instills the topical solvent monooctanoin (Moctanin) immediately after a cholecystectomy to dissolve retained stones, he'll infuse the drug by nasobiliary tube or through a small T tube inserted through an abdominal incision into the common bile duct. The solvent may infuse continuously up to 3 weeks until the stones dissolve. Tell the patient she will remain hospitalized during this time. When an X-ray shows that the gallstones have dissolved, the doctor will remove the tube.

Procedures
Besides drug therapy to dissolve gallbladder stones, any of several nonsurgical procedures, such as ERCP, endoscopic sphincterotomy, and ESWL, may be used to remove them.

Therapeutic ERCP
If gallstones are detected during diagnostic ERCP, the doctor may attempt to remove them at the same time. He'll insert a basketlike device via the endoscope to secure and retrieve them.

Endoscopic sphincterotomy
If the doctor schedules this procedure, tell the patient that an endoscope and special devices will be used to remove gallstones in the common bile duct. Tell her to fast after midnight the day before the procedure. She can expect to receive medications to relax her and insertion of an I.V. line in her hand or arm to administer medication. A local anesthetic will be given to ease endoscope insertion. During the procedure, she'll assume various positions to help advance the endoscope for proper placement.

Tell the patient that afterward, her vital signs will be monitored until they're stable. She can eat and drink when the gag reflex returns, but will remain in bed for 6 to 8 hours (or overnight in the hospital). Warn her that she may have abdominal discomfort for 1 to 2 weeks.

ESWL

Explain that ESWL is a noninvasive, painless procedure that uses high-energy shock waves to shatter gallstones, thereby allowing them to be eliminated naturally. The 30- to 60-minute procedure works best for patients with mild to moderate symptoms and only a few small-diameter stones consisting mainly of cholesterol.

Inform the patient that immediately before ESWL, the doctor will locate the stones precisely by ultrasonography, which might be augmented by use of a contrast medium. The patient may receive I.V. narcotics or, occasionally, a general anesthetic.

Tell the patient that she will be placed in a semireclining position on the machine's hydraulic stretcher. Then she'll be lowered into the water tank and her position adjusted so that the shock-wave generator focuses directly on the gallstones. Next, the lithotriptor will discharge serial shock waves through the water to shatter the stones without damaging surrounding tissue. The doctor will synchronize the shock waves with the patient's heart rhythm to prevent arrhythmias. Ultrasonic or fluoroscopic devices will monitor the process until the gallstones disintegrate — usually in 1 to 2 hours.

Reassure the patient that she won't feel pain but may feel a fluttering sensation or mild blows. If a catheter has been inserted, the doctor may also inject monooctanoin through the catheter to decrease the stones' size.

After ESWL, instruct the patient to report posttreatment abdominal pain, fever, nausea, or vomiting without delay. The doctor may order narcotic analgesics to relieve pain if stone fragments congest the bile ducts and cause biliary colic. The patient also may require oral bile salt therapy for several months to ensure gallbladder and bile duct patency. However, in the days immediately after ESWL, most of the stones should

travel from the gallbladder to the intestine and are excreted naturally.

 WARNING: Because incompletely pulverized stones can lodge in the biliary tract or pancreas or develop into new calculi, urge the patient to keep scheduled follow-up appointments.

Surgery

When nonsurgical treatments fail or if a complication such as cholecystitis develops, surgery may be necessary. Standard gallbladder surgeries include cholecystectomy (the most common), cholecystotomy, and choledochostomy. Or laparoscopic cholecystectomy, a relatively new procedure, may be performed.

Standard gallbladder surgery

Tell the patient that most gallbladder operations require a general anesthetic before surgery and 1 week recovery time in the hospital. Advise her to consume only clear liquids the day before surgery and nothing after midnight before the operation.

Forewarn the patient that she'll have a nasogastric (NG) tube in place for 1 to 2 days after surgery and a drain at the incision site for 3 to 5 days. She may also have a T tube inserted in the common bile duct to drain excess bile and allow removal of retained stones. If appropriate, explain that the T tube may remain in place for up to 2 weeks, depending on the type of surgery, and that she may be discharged with the tube. Teach her how to perform coughing and deep-breathing exercises to help prevent postoperative atelectasis, which can lead to pneumonia.

Prepare the patient for self-care after discharge. If she's going home with a T tube in place, make sure she knows how to perform tube care. Instruct her in caring for her incision, and direct her to report signs or symptoms of infection, such as redness, tenderness, or drainage at the incision site. Also advise her to report signs or symptoms of biliary obstruction: fever, jaundice, itching, pain, dark urine, and clay-colored stools.

Laparoscopic cholecystectomy

Inform the patient that the surgeon may remove her gallbladder through one of four small, slitlike abdominal incisions. The surgery takes about 90 minutes and requires a general anesthetic. Usually, fewer complications follow this operation than traditionally follow gallbladder surgery.

Tell the patient that she'll probably be admitted to the hospital on the day of surgery and discharged the next day. Instruct her to fast after midnight the day before surgery. Inform her that a urinary catheter and an NG tube will be inserted just before surgery.

Describe how the surgeon will begin the operation with a small incision above the navel. He'll insert an instrument to inflate the abdominal cavity with carbon dioxide (to improve visibility). Then he'll introduce the laparoscope, which holds a tiny camera. Just below the ribs, he'll make two more incisions to insert a pair of grasping forceps. A fourth incision to the right of the midsection allows insertion of laser equipment. Next, he'll excise the gallbladder with a laser beam and use the forceps to deliver the now-detached gallbladder through one of the incisions.

Advise the patient that she may experience minor discomfort at the laparoscopic insertion site and mild shoulder pain for up to 1 week — either from diaphragmatic irritation caused by abdominal stretching or from residual carbon dioxide.

Other care measures

Inform the nonsurgical patient that repeated episodes of biliary colic caused by gallstones may warrant hospitalization, NG tube insertion, and I.V. therapy for hydration and antibiotic administration. Explain that treatment to remove the stones usually begins soon after the episode subsides.

Encourage the patient to keep follow-up appointments and to take medications as directed to help prevent recurrent biliary colic and complications.

Hepatitis

Because hepatitis can lead to permanent liver damage, your teaching must stress the need for strict compliance with treatment. Your first priority, though, may be to demystify the disease for the patient and his family. Because viral hepatitis is contagious and must be reported to the local public health authorities, many people erroneously associate it with unsanitary conditions or with socially unacceptable behavior. Reassure the patient that having hepatitis doesn't mean that he's dirty or immoral.

Before teaching a patient about hepatitis, make sure you are familiar with the following topics:
• how hepatitis affects the liver
• what causes hepatitis
• types of viral hepatitis: A (HAV); B (HBV); C (HCV); and D (HDV)
• signs and symptoms, transmission, and complications of hepatitis, including chronic hepatitis
• diagnostic tests, such as liver function studies, hepatitis profile, and liver biopsy
• importance of rest and diet
• restrictions on alcohol consumption and drug use
• proper hygiene and other measures to prevent the spread of viral hepatitis
• sources of information and support.

ABOUT THE DISORDER

Tell the patient that hepatitis is an inflammation of the liver, which interferes with normal liver function and causes his signs and symptoms. Confirm that initial symptoms of hepatitis include malaise, fever, anorexia, nausea, headache, and abdominal pain. As the disease progresses, jaundice — a yellowish discoloration of the skin and the whites of the eyes — usually develops as well as itching, dark urine, and light-colored stools.

Inform the patient that hepatitis may result from a viral infection or, less commonly, from alcohol, drugs, or an unrelated disease such as leukemia. Explain that the term "viral hepatitis" means hepatitis caused by a virus — most commonly hepatitis virus A, B, C (also called non-A, non-B), or D.

Complications
Emphasize that strict adherence to the treatment plan is essential for liver regeneration. Incomplete regeneration can lead to cirrhosis — progressive destruction of the liver, characterized by scarring, fibrosis, and fatty deposits. Point out that cirrhosis can, in turn, lead to conditions that may bring on hemorrhage, coma, and even death.

Even with satisfactory compliance, viral hepatitis can still lead to complications. About 10% of patients with hepatitis B remain infected with the virus 6 months after the initial infection. These patients are said to have chronic hepatitis. Furthermore, hepatitis C is associated with an increased risk of liver cancer. Explain that development of these complications is influenced by the patient's age when first infected, his immune status, and the severity of the acute infection.

DIAGNOSTIC WORKUP
Inform the patient that a diagnosis of hepatitis hinges on the patient's signs and symptoms and on the results of a number of studies (such as liver function tests and possibly a liver biopsy) that reflect the functional status of the liver. (See *Teaching patients about gastrointestinal tests,* pages 101 to 109.)

If viral hepatitis is suspected, tell the patient that the doctor will order a hepatitis profile. A blood sample will be analyzed to identify the specific virus responsible for his disorder.

TREATMENTS
Explain that no specific treatment exists for hepatitis. Educate the patient about the importance of rest and a proper diet to help the liver heal and to minimize complications. Point out that the liver takes 3 weeks to regenerate and up to 4 months to return to normal functioning. If the patient

has viral hepatitis, emphasize measures to help prevent the disease from spreading.

Activity guidelines
In the early stages, fatigue will motivate the patient to rest. As he begins to feel better, rest is still important, but it may be difficult for the patient to comply with activity restrictions. Nonetheless, urge him to curtail unnecessary activity. For instance, help him find ways to minimize job demands, food shopping, child care, and stair climbing. Explain that he'll need to reduce his schedule for at least 3 weeks, depending on the severity of the illness. Emphasize that exertion and stress during recovery can lead to complications or relapse.

Dietary modifications
Inform the patient that good nutrition promotes liver regeneration. Because the patient may experience anorexia, nausea, or vomiting, help him build an appealing meal plan based on frequent small meals. Inform him that a well-balanced diet can meet his nutritional needs. If appropriate, refer him to a dietitian.

 TIPS AND TIMESAVERS: Encourage the patient to consume at least 1 gal (4 L) of fluid a day. If he is anorectic, drinking sufficient fluids may be especially difficult. Suggest that he try fruit juices or soft drinks containing ice chips. Stress that alcohol consumption is strictly forbidden.

Advise the patient to weigh himself daily. Instruct him to notify the doctor of any weight loss greater than 5 lb (2.3 kg).

Medication
Inform the patient that there's no specific drug therapy for hepatitis. If he has viral hepatitis, explain that anyone exposed to the disease through contact with him should receive immune globulin or the hepatitis B vaccine as soon as possible after exposure. Help him to identify those at risk.

Preventing the spread of hepatitis

To prevent the patient from transmitting hepatitis to others, educate him about how the disease is spread.

Hepatitis A

Inform the patient that hepatitis A is spread when fecal matter from an infected person contaminates food or water. This can happen when an infected person handles food after using the bathroom and doesn't wash his hands or when raw sewage contaminates food supplies or the water used to prepare foods. Common sources of such contamination include infected restaurant workers, sewage leaks into a water supply, or raw shellfish from polluted waters.

How the patient infects others

Explain that when the patient has a bowel movement, some of the hepatitis virus passes out of his body into his stools. This infected fecal matter will contaminate any food or water it comes in contact with. In turn, anyone who eats or drinks the contaminated food or water can develop hepatitis A.

Prevention guidelines

Advise the patient to wash his hands thoroughly after every bowel movement and before handling food or preparing meals. Also warn him not to share food, eating utensils, or toothbrushes.

Hepatitis B, C, or D

Tell the patient with one of these hepatitis types that the disease is spread by contact with the blood of an infected person. Point out that the hepatitis virus is present in the patient's blood and in any of his body fluids that contains visible blood. If any of his blood enters another person's bloodstream (for example, during a blood transfusion), that person can catch hepatitis from the patient.

Also inform him that if his blood or body fluids come in contact with a break in another person's skin (such as a cut or rash) or with the mucous membranes of another person's mouth, vagina, or rectum, that person can develop hepatitis.

Prevention guidelines

Instruct the patient to wash his hands thoroughly and frequently. Warn him not to share food, eating utensils, or toothbrushes. If he injects drugs, tell him not to share the needle with anyone. Also instruct him not to have sex with anyone and not to donate blood until the doctor determines that he is no longer contagious.

 WARNING: Because some drugs can bring on a relapse of hepatitis, advise the patient to check with the doctor before taking any medication, including nonprescription drugs.

Other care measures

If the patient has viral hepatitis, teach him and his family ways to avoid spreading the disease. Emphasize the importance of thorough hand washing in all forms of viral hepatitis. (See *Preventing the spread of hepatitis.*)

Tell the patient that viral hepatitis is a reportable disease. This means the doctor must notify the local public health department so the occurrence can be recorded. An increase in the number of hepatitis cases reported in a particular area may alert public health officials to potential sewage contamination of the water supply or to contamination of a common food source such as a restaurant. As a result, public health authorities may contact the patient to investigate the circumstances of his infection.

Stress the importance of continued medical care. Advise the patient to see the doctor again about 2 weeks after a diagnosis is made. At this time, the doctor will determine if the patient's fluid intake is adequate and will perform additional blood tests to evaluate liver function. After this, the patient will need a follow-up appointment once a month for up to 6 months. Then, if chronic hepatitis develops, the patient must visit the doctor at regular intervals to monitor the course of the disease.

Finally, refer the patient to the American Hepatitis Association or the American Liver Foundation for further information. (See Appendix 2.)

Hiatal hernia

Even in its mildest form, hiatal hernia can disrupt the patient's life as he tries to cope with recurring malaise and persistent difficulty swallowing. To help him control his condition, teaching must emphasize the direct relationship between his symptoms and his meals, activities, and medications.

Before teaching a patient about hiatal hernia, make sure you are familiar with the following topics:
• explanation of hiatal hernia as muscle weakness of the diaphragm opening that encircles the distal esophagus and stomach
• diagnostic tests, such as barium swallow, endoscopy, and esophageal manometry
• meal scheduling, size, and contents
• use of antacids, cholinergics, and other drugs to relieve symptoms and prevent complications
• preoperative instructions for hernia repair, if necessary
• patient positioning, cessation of smoking, and avoidance of activities that increase intra-abdominal pressure
• how to recognize warning signs of complications — esophagitis and ul-

ceration, respiratory distress, aspiration pneumonia, cardiac dysfunction, and mucosal erosion.

ABOUT THE DISORDER

First, clarify any confusion about terms for this disorder by explaining that "esophageal," "hiatus," "hiatal," and "diaphragmatic" hernia are all names for the same condition. Then inform the patient that a hiatal hernia usually results from a weakening or enlargement of the diaphragm opening that encircles the distal esophagus. This defect allows part of the stomach to protrude into the chest cavity when intra-abdominal pressure rises — for example, with coughing or bending from the waist.

Explain that with these pressure changes, the stomach contents and secretions push upward into the esophagus, causing gas or heartburn. Reflux (regurgitation) of secretions can also erode the lining of the esophagus. (See *What happens in hiatal hernia,* page 98.)

Tell the patient that the cause of the muscle weakness that leads to hiatal hernia may be congenital weakness, abdominal or chest injury, or loss of muscle tone from aging, pregnancy, or obesity.

Complications

Emphasize that neglecting the treatment plan will increase the patient's chance of experiencing reflux and heartburn and developing complications (such as irritation of the esophageal lining) leading to esophageal inflammation or ulcer as well as respiratory distress, aspiration pneumonia, or heart dysfunction from pressure on the lungs and heart.

DIAGNOSTIC WORKUP

Tell the patient that the doctor diagnoses hiatal hernia based on typical signs and symptoms and on the results of diagnostic tests that evaluate for mucosal damage — barium swallow, endoscopy, and esophageal manometry. For information on these

What happens in hiatal hernia

Hiatal hernia includes two classic types: sliding (which accounts for over 90% of adult hernias) and rolling, or paraesophageal, hernia.

Sliding hernia
In this hernia, the stomach slips upward into the chest cavity, displacing organs and causing esophageal spasm when the patient lies down or when activities, such as bending or sneezing, increase intra-abdominal pressure. When the patient stands or the pressure subsides, the stomach usually slides back into the abdomen.

Rolling hernia
In this hernia, the stomach sphincter remains below the diaphragm, and the fundus rolls up beside the esophagus when intra-abdominal pressure rises or the patient lies down.

Some patients have a combined hernia, in which both types occur.

Hernia signs and symptoms
About 50% of patients experience signs and symptoms, especially heartburn. Belching and bloating may occur from increased swallowing — an attempt to remove acid from the esophagus. Reflux may cause aspiration pneumonia.

Other possible signs and symptoms include pain, dyspnea, and tachycardia — effects of rising intrathoracic pressure when part of the stomach slides into the thoracic cavity. Accompanying esophageal spasm may cause severe pain radiating to the back, shoulder, or arm.

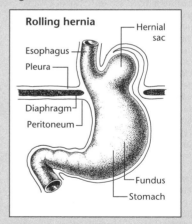

tests, see *Teaching patients about gastrointestinal tests,* pages 101 to 109.)

TREATMENTS
Teach the patient about treatment measures, including modifications in activity and diet, and medication to control stomach bulk and acidity. Let the patient know that if these measures prove ineffective, he may require surgery to reduce the hernia and return the stomach to its normal position.

Activity guidelines

Advise the patient to restrict activities that increase intra-abdominal pressure, such as strenuous exercise, heavy lifting, bending, and coughing.

Dietary modifications

Inform the patient that modifying the timing, size, and content of meals helps to control both the amount of acid secreted during digestion and stomach bulk. Instruct him to avoid beverages and foods that may intensify symptoms. If he's overweight, point out that a weight-loss program built around the twin goals of limiting food intake and exercising can ease symptoms.

Medications

Inform the patient that he will need medications for hiatal hernia indefinitely, even after surgical repair. Teach him about medications used to treat hernia symptoms. If the doctor prescribes antacids, explain that they relieve reflux by neutralizing stomach acid. If he prescribes cholinergics, explain that these drugs ease reflux by increasing esophageal sphincter tone. The doctor may also prescribe a histamine$_2$-receptor blocker to decrease stomach acidity.

Because straining and vomiting increase intra-abdominal pressure, the patient may need to use stool softeners to prevent straining during bowel movements. The doctor may also prescribe antinausea drugs to help prevent vomiting and promote stomach emptying.

Antacids

Tell the patient that liquid antacids are more effective than tablets. Inform him that most liquid antacids taste better cold. Instruct him to shake a liquid antacid well before taking it.

If he must take chewable antacids, tell him to keep them handy. Instruct him to chew the tablet well before swallowing and to follow the dose with a full glass of water. Let him know that he can mix both the liquid and tablet forms with beverages or food if preferred.

Advise the patient to check with the doctor before making any changes in the way he takes medication. If he experiences diarrhea or constipation, the doctor may prescribe a different antacid, combination therapy, or a stool softener.

Surgery

If medication and changes in activity and diet fail to relieve the patient's symptoms, the doctor may recommend surgery to repair the hiatal hernia. Severe stricture and ulcerative esophagitis, hemorrhage, and pulmonary aspiration of gastric contents are also indications for surgery.

Explain that surgery will restore the stomach to its normal position, reducing the hernia, as well as strengthen the lower esophageal sphincter. Tell the patient to expect laxatives and enemas the evening before the surgery to clean the bowel and prevent postoperative complications.

Briefly describe the procedure (such as fundoplication) that the doctor will use to repair the hernia. Also describe what to expect after surgery, such as a sore throat, a nasogastric tube, and possibly chest tubes. Tell the patient that his food intake may be limited to fluids for the first 24 hours.

Explain that postoperative complications are rare but do occur. Complications generally involve the gastric pouch and include erosion, ulcers, bleeding, pressure on the left lung, and production of a volvulus. Tell the patient to notify the doctor immediately if he experiences difficulty swallowing or reflux.

Other care measures

Instruct the patient to avoid wearing constrictive clothing, such as a longline bra or a girdle. Recommend methods to avoid straining with bowel movements, such as modifying the diet to include high-fiber foods and citrus fruits and, if prescribed, taking laxatives or stool softeners.

Discuss stress-reduction techniques, such as walking, yoga, and deep-breathing exercises, emphasizing that these can help reduce the discomfort that accompanies hernia.

 TIPS AND TIMESAVERS: To relieve heartburn, advise the patient to elevate his head with two or three pillows or to place 8 to 10 blocks under the head of the bed. Also suggest that he sleep on his right side.

Discourage smoking because it alters pancreatic secretions that neutralize gastric acid in the duodenum and will increase discomfort.

Make sure the patient can recognize the warning signs and symptoms of complications. Instruct him to contact the doctor immediately if he has signs or symptoms of:
• esophagitis — difficulty swallowing, chest pain, and bloody sputum
• gastritis — abdominal pain, belching, and nausea and vomiting
• aspiration pneumonia — fever, difficulty breathing, rapid respiration, and pain with inspiration.

Peptic ulcer disease

Peptic ulcer disease affects more than 10% of the American population during their lifetime. Although peptic ulcer disease can lead to serious complications, most patients can achieve a good outcome if they comply with prescribed treatment. Compliance — and acceptance of teaching — depends largely on the patient's understanding of his responsibility for managing the disease. That's why thorough teaching is crucial.

Before teaching a patient about peptic ulcer disease, make sure you are familiar with the following topics:
• definition of a peptic ulcer
• explanation of the two types of peptic ulcer disease — duodenal and gastric
• warning signs and symptoms of such complications as hemorrhage,

perforation, peritonitis, and intestinal obstruction
• diagnostic tests, such as the basal gastric secretion test, upper GI endoscopy, gastric acid stimulation test, and upper GI and small-bowel series
• dietary modifications to neutralize acid and reduce gastric motility and secretions
• medications used to relieve symptoms — antacids, anticholinergics, $histamine_2$-receptor antagonists, proton pump inhibitors, antibiotics, and antianxiety agents
• possible surgical procedures, such as gastroenterostomy and vagotomy
• how to manage dumping syndrome
• therapeutic rest, exercise, stress management, and smoking cessation
• sources of information and support.

ABOUT THE DISORDER

Although the patient already knows that a peptic ulcer causes intense pain, he may not know that an ulcer is an erosion of the stomach lining. Inform him that a peptic ulcer may occur in the duodenum (the first part of the small intestine) or the stomach. For many years this erosion was thought to result from contact with acidic gastric secretions (pepsin or hydrochloric acid). But recent studies have identified a bacterium, called *Helicobacter pylori*, as the predominant cause of ulcers.

Point out that peptic ulcers usually have a chronic, recurrent course. Not all patients have signs and symptoms, while others have them only when complications occur. The pain from an ulcer may feel like a burning, gnawing, or aching sensation or soreness, an empty feeling, or hunger.

Complications

Inform the patient that an unchecked, unhealed ulcer can cause life-threatening complications, such as massive hemorrhage, perforation of the stomach wall, peritonitis, hemorrhage, abdominal or intestinal infarction, or shock.

(Text continues on page 109.)

Teaching patients about gastrointestinal tests

TEST AND PURPOSE	TEACHING POINTS
Barium swallow (esophagography) • To help diagnose hiatal hernia, diverticula, and varices • To detect strictures, tumor, ulcers, or polyps in the pharynx and esophagus	• Explain that this test examines the pharynx and esophagus through X-ray films taken after a barium swallow, which clearly outlines these structures. Tell the patient that the study takes 30 minutes. • Describe pretest restrictions: The patient must not eat or drink for 6 to 8 hours before the test and must not smoke on the morning of the test. Also, he should not use an enema the evening before or morning of the test. • Discuss pretest preparations: The patient will remove jewelry, dentures, hair clips, and other objects that may obscure details on the X-ray films. • Explain what happens during the test: The patient will lie on an adjustable table and will be asked to swallow thick and thin mixtures of barium sulfate. Describe barium's chalky taste, adding that it can be flavored to make it more palatable. If the doctor wants to accentuate small strictures or demonstrate dysphagia, the patient will swallow a special barium marshmallow (soft white bread soaked in barium). Tell him that as the barium outlines his pharynx and esophagus, the table will be adjusted so the doctor can take films from several angles. • Tell the patient what happens after the test: He will resume his normal diet and medications as ordered, and will receive a laxative to help expel the barium. Stress the importance of barium elimination, since retained barium may harden, causing obstruction or impaction. Mention that he will have chalky stools for 1 to 3 days as the barium passes through the bowel. Advise him to call the doctor if his stools aren't chalky.
Basal gastric secretion test • To evaluate epigastric pain	• Inform the patient that this test helps evaluate stomach pain by measuring the stomach's acid secretion when he's fasting. Tell him that the test takes about 90 minutes. • Explain pretest restrictions: The patient must withhold antacids, anticholinergics, cholinergics, cimetidine, reserpine, adrenergic blocks, and adrenocorticosteroids, as ordered, for 24 hours before the test. He must restrict food for 12 hours and fluid and smoking for 8 hours before the test. • Explain what happens during the test: A flexible tube will be passed through the patient's nose into his stomach. Assure him that the tube will be lubricated to ease its passage; however, he may feel some discomfort and may cough or gag as *(continued)*

Teaching patients about gastrointestinal tests *(continued)*

TEST AND PURPOSE	TEACHING POINTS
Basal gastric secretion test *(continued)*	the tube is advanced. Then the patient will lie in various positions as his stomach contents are suctioned through the tube for analysis. Assure him that this won't hurt. ● Discuss what happens after the test: The patient may have a sore throat. He may resume his normal diet and, as ordered, his medications.
Cholangiography (percutaneous and postoperative) ● To determine the cause of upper abdominal pain that persists after cholecystectomy ● To evaluate jaundice ● To determine the location, extent, and often the cause of mechanical obstruction	● Tell the patient that this radiographic test examines the biliary ducts after injection of a contrast medium. Tell him that it takes about 30 minutes. ● Describe preparation for the test: The patient must fast for 8 hours before the procedure but should continue any prescribed drug regimen. Inform him that he'll be awake during the test, which may be uncomfortable, and that he'll receive medication to help him relax. ● Explain what happens during the test: The doctor will drape and clean an area on the patient's abdomen, then inject a local anesthetic to minimize discomfort from the test. Warn the patient that the injection will sting briefly. Instruct him to hold his breath as the contrast medium is injected into the liver. (If he undergoes this test postoperatively, the dye is injected through a T tube inserted into the common bile duct after surgery.) Warn him that this injection may cause a sensation of pressure and right upper back discomfort. Tell him to report immediately any adverse effects: dizziness, headache, hives, nausea, and vomiting. Instruct him to lie still, relax, breathe normally, and remain quiet as X-ray films are taken of the biliary ducts. ● Discuss what happens after the test: The patient's vital signs will be checked frequently for several hours, and he must remain in bed on his right side for at least 6 hours. Tell him that he may resume his normal diet.
Computed tomography of the biliary tract, liver, or pancreas ● To detect abnormalities of the biliary tract, liver, or pancreas, such as tumors, abscesses, cysts, and hematomas	● Tell the patient that this test examines the biliary tract, liver, or pancreas through computerized X-rays. Inform him that it is painless and takes about 1½ hours. ● Discuss pretest restriction: The patient must not have food or fluids after midnight before the test but should continue any drug regimen as ordered. ● Explain what happens during the test: The patient will lie on a table while X-rays are taken. Tell him to lie still, relax, breathe normally, and remain quiet because movement will blur the X-ray

Teaching patients about gastrointestinal tests *(continued)*

TEST AND PURPOSE	TEACHING POINTS
Computed tomography of the biliary tract, liver, or pancreas *(continued)* • To detect or evaluate pancreatitis • To determine the cause of jaundice	images and prolong the test. If the doctor is using an I.V. contrast medium, inform the patient that he may experience discomfort from the needle puncture and a localized feeling of warmth on injection. Instruct him to report immediately any adverse effects: nausea, vomiting, dizziness, headache, or hives. Assure him that these reactions are rare. • Tell the patient that he may resume his normal diet after the test.
Endoscopic retrograde cholangiopancreatography (ERCP) • To evaluate tumors and inflammation of the pancreas, gallbladder, or liver • To locate obstructions in the pancreatic duct and hepatobiliary tree • To help determine the cause of jaundice	• Explain that this test examines the liver, gallbladder, and pancreas through X-ray films. Inform the patient that these films are obtained with a flexible tube passed through the mouth into the intestine. Tell him that the test takes 30 to 60 minutes. • Describe preparation for the test: The patient must restrict food and fluids after midnight before the test but should continue prescribed drugs as ordered. He'll be asked to urinate before the test because ERCP can cause urine retention. • Discuss what happens during the test: The patient will lie on an X-ray table, and an I.V. line will be inserted into his hand or arm to administer medication. Inform him that he'll be awake; explain that although the test is uncomfortable, he'll receive a sedative to help him relax. Before tube insertion, the patient's throat will be sprayed with a local anesthetic. Tell him that the spray tastes unpleasant and will make his mouth and throat feel swollen and numb, causing difficulty swallowing. Instruct him to let the saliva drain from the side of his mouth. Tell him that he'll have a mouthguard to protect his teeth from the tube. Assure him he'll have no difficulty breathing. After tube insertion, the patient will receive I.V. medication to relax the small intestine. Instruct him to report immediately any adverse effects: dry mouth, thirst, tachycardia, blurred vision, nausea, vomiting, itching, or flushing. Once the small intestine relaxes, he'll be asked to assume various positions to advance the tube to the pancreas and hepatobiliary tree. Inform him that he may experience warmth or flushing when the contrast medium is injected. The patient's vital signs will be checked frequently. He'll be allowed to eat when his gag reflex returns, usually in about 1 hour. He may have a sore throat for several days.

(continued)

Teaching patients about gastrointestinal tests *(continued)*

TEST AND PURPOSE	TEACHING POINTS
Endoscopy and manometry • To assess damage to the esophageal lining in patients with suspected hiatal hernia	• Inform the patient that endoscopy assesses damage to the esophageal lining and takes several minutes to half an hour. • Describe pretest restrictions: The patient should not eat or drink for 6 to 12 hours before the test. If esophageal manometry will also be performed, he must also restrict alcohol and stop taking cholinergics or anticholinergics, as ordered, for 24 hours before the test. • Discuss what happens before the test: If the patient wears dentures, he should remove them. Tell him that about 1 hour before the test, he will receive a sedative to help him relax. • Explain what happens during the test: The patient will be placed on a table. He will be given a gargle or throat spray containing a local anesthetic to suppress the gag reflex. The doctor will then ask him to swallow the endoscope tube. Advise him to breathe through his mouth with a panting motion while swallowing, to reduce discomfort. The doctor will then examine the esophagus with the tube's fiber-optic device. Stress that the patient must remain still to prevent the endoscope from perforating the esophagus. If the doctor will be examining the stomach and duodenum, the patient will be asked to lie on his side. Explain that a suction machine will keep his mouth and throat free of secretions. During the procedure, a small brush may be inserted through the tube to obtain samples of the mucosal lining for cytology. Manometry (measurement of esophageal sphincter pressure) may also be performed to evaluate the function of the esophagus and of the sphincter between the esophagus and stomach. For manometry, the patient will swallow a catheter attached to a small pressure transducer and then sip water to stimulate esophageal peristalsis. • Discuss what happens after the test: The patient may have a sore throat for several days. Suggest that he use a throat spray or lozenges to ease discomfort. Warn him that he may cough up a small amount of blood during the first day. Instruct him to notify the doctor if he has difficulty swallowing, since this may be a sign of laryngeal or pharyngeal swelling. Also tell him to notify the doctor if he vomits (especially if the vomit contains blood) or if he experiences fever, shoulder or substernal pain, or shortness of breath.

Teaching patients about gastrointestinal tests (continued)

TEST AND PURPOSE	TEACHING POINTS
Gastric acid stimulation test • To aid diagnosis of duodenal ulcer, Zollinger-Ellison syndrome, pernicious anemia, and gastric cancer	• Explain to the patient that this test determines if his stomach is secreting acid properly. Tell him that it takes about 1 hour. • Instruct the patient to stop taking antacids, anticholinergics, cholinergics, cimetidine, reserpine, adrenergic blockers, or adrenocorticosteroids, as ordered, 24 hours before the test. Tell him to restrict food, fluids, and smoking after midnight before the test. • Explain what happens during the test: A flexible tube will be passed through the patient's nose into his stomach. The tube is lubricated to ease its passage; however, he may feel some discomfort and may cough or gag as the tube is advanced. Then he'll receive a subcutaneous injection of a medication (pentagastrin) to stimulate stomach acid secretion. Tell him to report at once any adverse effects: abdominal pain, nausea, vomiting, flushing, dizziness, faintness, or numbness of the extremities. Next, the doctor will obtain several samples of stomach contents for analysis. • Discuss what happens after the test: The patient may have a sore throat. Tell him that he may resume his normal diet and medication as ordered.
Liver-spleen scan • To detect abnormalities of the liver and spleen, such as tumors, cysts, and abscesses • To help diagnose diseases of the liver, such as cirrhosis and hepatitis • To demonstrate enlargement of the liver or spleen • To assess liver and spleen condition after abdominal trauma	• Inform the patient that this noninvasive test examines the liver and spleen through pictures taken with a special scanner or camera. Tell him that it takes about 1 hour. • Explain what happens during the test: The patient will receive an injection of a radioactive substance (usually technetium sulfide 99m) through an I.V. line in his hand or arm to allow better visualization of the liver and spleen. Tell him to report immediately any adverse effects: flushing, fever, light-headedness, or difficulty breathing. Assure him that the injection contains only trace amounts of radioactivity and rarely produces adverse effects. If the test uses a rectilinear scanner, he'll hear a soft, irregular, clicking noise as the scanner moves across his abdomen. If the test uses a gamma camera, he'll feel the camera lightly on his abdomen. Instruct him to remain still, relax, and breathe normally. He may be asked to hold his breath briefly to ensure good-quality pictures.

(continued)

Teaching patients about gastrointestinal tests *(continued)*

TEST AND PURPOSE	TEACHING POINTS
Oral cholecystography • To detect abnormalities of the gallbladder, such as gallstones, tumors, and inflammation	• Tell the patient that this test examines the gallbladder through X-rays taken after ingestion of a contrast medium. Mention that it takes about 30 to 45 minutes (or longer if a fat stimulus is to be given, followed by another series of films). • Describe preparation for the test: If ordered, the patient eats a low-fat breakfast and lunch the day before the test and a fat-free evening meal. After the evening meal, he can have only water, but should continue any ordered drug regimen. He's given a cleansing enema, and 2 to 3 hours before the test, he's asked to swallow six tablets, one at a time, at 5-minute intervals. The enema and tablets help outline the gallbladder on the X-ray film. Tell him to report immediately any adverse effects of the tablets: diarrhea, nausea, vomiting, abdominal cramps, or dysuria. • Explain what happens during the test: The patient will lie supine on an X-ray table while films are taken of his emptying gallbladder and the patency of the common duct. • Discuss what happens after the test: The patient should drink plenty of fluids to help eliminate the dyelike substance in the tablets. If test results are normal, he will resume his usual diet. If another cholecystogram is necessary, he'll stay on a low-fat diet. If test results indicate a problem, he'll receive a special diet.
Percutaneous liver biopsy • To help diagnose cirrhosis, metastatic diseases, and granulomatous infection	• Explain to the patient that this test diagnoses liver disorders through examination of liver tissue. Inform him that the doctor obtains a small liver specimen by inserting a needle. Tell him that the test takes about 15 minutes. • Instruct the patient to restrict food and fluids for at least 4 hours before the test. • Explain what happens during the test: The patient will be awake. Although the test is uncomfortable, assure him that he'll receive medication to help him relax. Inform him that the doctor will drape and clean an area of his abdomen and will inject a local anesthetic, which may sting and cause brief discomfort. Then the patient will be asked to hold his breath and lie still as the doctor inserts the biopsy needle into the liver. Tell the patient that the needle may cause a sensation of pressure and some discomfort in his right upper back. Assure him that the needle will remain in his liver only about 1 second.

Teaching patients about gastrointestinal tests *(continued)*

TEST AND PURPOSE	TEACHING POINTS
Percutaneous liver biopsy *(continued)*	• Describe what happens after the test: The patient's vital signs will be checked frequently for several hours. He must remain in bed on his right side for 2 hours and maintain bed rest for 24 hours. He may experience pain for several hours. Also tell him that he may resume his normal diet.
Ultrasonography of the gallbladder, biliary system, liver, spleen, or pancreas • To help diagnose disorders of the gallbladder and biliary system (such as cholelithiasis and cholecystitis), liver (such as cirrhosis and hepatitis), and pancreas	• Explain that this test examines body structures by means of sound waves and that it takes about 15 to 30 minutes. • Describe preparation for the test: The patient must restrict food and fluids for 8 to 12 hours before the test. If he's having ultrasonography of the gallbladder and biliary system, instruct him to eat a fat-free meal the evening before the test before starting his fast. • Discuss what happens during the test: As the patient lies on a table, a technician will apply conductive gel or oil to his abdomen. Then the technician will move the transducer across the patient's abdomen. Assure him it won't be uncomfortable. Instruct him to lie still, relax, breathe normally, and remain quiet. Explain that any movement will distort the picture and prolong the test. He may also be asked to hold his breath or inhale deeply. If he's having ultrasonography of the gallbladder, he may receive an injection of a drug (sincalide) to stimulate gallbladder contraction. Tell the patient to report immediately any adverse effects: abdominal cramping, nausea, dizziness, sweating, or flushing. • After the test, the patient may resume his normal diet.
Upper GI endoscopy (esophagogastroduodenoscopy) • To identify abnormalities of the esophagus, stomach, and small intestine, such as esophagitis, inflammatory bowel disease, Mallory-Weiss syndrome, lesions, tumors, gastritis, and polyps	• Tell the patient that this test examines the esophagus, stomach, and duodenum using a flexible tube inserted into the intestine through the mouth. Mention that it takes about 30 minutes. • Describe preparation for the test: The patient must not eat or drink for 6 hours before the test but should continue any prescribed medications as ordered. If the test is an emergency procedure, tell the patient that his stomach contents will be suctioned to permit better visualization. • Explain what happens during the test: The patient will lie on an X-ray table and an I.V. line will be inserted into his hand or arm to administer

(continued)

Teaching patients about gastrointestinal tests (continued)

TEST AND PURPOSE	TEACHING POINTS
Upper GI endoscopy (esophagogastro-duodenoscopy) (continued)	medications, if needed, during the test. Inform him that although he will be awake, he'll receive a sedative to help him relax. Before tube insertion, the patient's throat will be sprayed with an anesthetic. Advise him that the spray tastes unpleasant and will make his mouth feel swollen and numb, causing difficulty swallowing. Tell him that he'll be positioned so that saliva drains safely from the side of his mouth, and a mouthguard will be used to protect his teeth from the tube. As the doctor advances the tube, the patient may be asked to assume various positions. Tell him he can expect to feel abdominal pressure and fullness or bloating as the doctor gently introduces air for a better view of internal structures. • Describe what happens after the test: The patient's vital signs will be checked frequently for 8 hours. He can resume eating when his gag reflex returns — usually in about 1 hour. He may have a sore throat for several days.
Upper GI and small bowel series • To help diagnose hiatal hernia, diverticula, varices, regional enteritis, and malabsorption syndrome • To detect strictures, ulcers, or polyps in the esophagus, stomach, and small intestine	• Tell the patient that this test examines the esophagus, stomach, and small intestine through X-ray films taken after swallowing barium, which clearly outlines these structures. Inform him that the test requires several films to be taken up to 1 hour apart, so the entire study may take up to 6 hours. Advise him to bring an activity to help pass the time. • Describe preparation for the test: The patient must eat a low-residue diet for 2 to 3 days and must restrict food, fluids, and smoking after midnight before the test. The doctor also may instruct him to stop taking medications for up to 24 hours before the test. The patient will receive a laxative the afternoon before the test and up to three cleansing enemas the evening before or the morning of the test. Explain that the presence of food or fluid may obscure details of the structures being studied. • Explain what happens during the test: The patient will lie on a movable table and will be asked to swallow small amounts of barium several times during the test. Tell him that the barium has a milkshake consistency and a chalky taste. Inform him that the doctor may compress his abdomen to ensure proper coating of the stomach and intestinal walls with barium. Also explain that the

Teaching patients about gastrointestinal tests *(continued)*

TEST AND PURPOSE	TEACHING POINTS
Upper GI and small bowel series *(continued)*	table will be adjusted to various positions so the doctor can take films from several angles. • Discuss what happens after the test: The patient may resume his normal diet and medication as ordered. He will receive a laxative or enema to help expel barium. Stress the importance of barium elimination, since retained barium may harden, causing intestinal obstruction or impaction. Explain that barium will lightly color his stools for 24 to 72 hours after the test.

DIAGNOSTIC WORKUP

Tell the patient that the doctor diagnoses peptic ulcer disease based on signs and symptoms and the results of diagnostic tests. These tests may include basal gastric secretion test, upper GI endoscopy, gastric acid stimulation test, and upper GI and small-bowel series. (See *Teaching patients about gastrointestinal tests*, pages 101 to 109.)

TREATMENTS

Inform the patient that treatment focuses on resting the stomach so that the ulcer can heal. Specific measures include dietary changes, medications, and stress reduction or lifestyle changes. If these measures fail or if complications develop, the patient may require surgery.

Dietary modifications

Point out that no firm evidence proves that any diet speeds ulcer healing or prevents ulcer recurrence. Therefore, the doctor is likely to recommend that the patient eliminate only those foods that cause distress (such as fruit juices or spicy or fatty foods). However, advise the patient to avoid pepper and coffee; pepper is the only food that objective studies suggest is harmful, and coffee (even decaffeinated coffee) may produce ulcerlike stomach upset in some persons.

The doctor also may instruct the patient to avoid caffeine-containing soft drinks, tea, chocolate, nicotine, and alcohol. Encourage the patient to snack between meals.

Medications

Inform the patient that in light of the recent studies identifying *H. pylori* as the main cause of peptic ulcers, doctors are still debating which drugs to use. However, most believe the best approach is a combination of traditional antiulcer medications and antibiotics.

If the doctor prescribes traditional medications, inform the patient that these suppress gastric acid production or shield the GI tract lining. Agents that suppress gastric acid secretion — proton pump inhibitors and histamine$_2$-antagonists — are the most widely prescribed. The doctor may also prescribe antianxiety drugs to promote rest and relaxation.

Antacids

Inform the patient that antacids relieve pain by neutralizing gastric acid. Warn him not to take systemic antacids such as sodium bicarbonate because they are absorbed into the circulation and can cause acid-base imbalance.

Histamine$_2$-antagonists

Inform the patient that histamine$_2$-

antagonists, such as cimetidine (Tagamet) and famotidine (Pepcid), work by inhibiting the production of histamine, thus decreasing gastric acid secretion. Caution him that over-the-counter formulas of H_2-antagonists have much lower dosage levels than the prescribed version and may not be effective.

Proton pump inhibitors

Inform the patient that proton pump inhibitors such as omeprazole (Prilosec) are more potent than H_2-antagonists. Explain that these drugs block the formation of gastric acid. Before prescribing one of these agents, the doctor, pharmacist, or nurse practitioner will review the patient's current medications closely because proton pump inhibitors can interact with certain medications.

Other drugs

If the patient will take sucralfate (Sulcrate), tell him that this drug combines with proteins to form a protective coating in the base of the ulcer, thus relieving symptoms and promoting ulcer healing. Instruct him to take sucralfate with a full glass of water 1 hour before meals. If he's also taking cimetidine, instruct him to take sucralfate 2 hours before or after cimetidine. Advise him not to take sucralfate with an antacid.

If the patient will take misoprostol (Cytotec), inform him that this medication helps protect the GI lining by decreasing acid secretion. Tell the patient to take this drug with food.

 WARNING: Caution women of childbearing age that misoprostol may induce miscarriage. To prevent miscarriage, advise such a patient to have a serum pregnancy test within 2 weeks before starting this medication, to use an effective contraceptive during therapy, and to tell her doctor if she is pregnant or plans to become pregnant. If pregnancy is suspected, misoprostol should be discontinued immediately.

Recently, the FDA approved a combination agent for treating peptic ulcer: omeprazole (Prilosec) plus the antibiotic clarithromycin (Biaxin). This drug combination is designed to eradicate *H. pylori.*

Anticholinergics reduce gastric acidity. However, they are now rarely used, except as an adjunct when H_2-antagonists fail to control peptic ulcer disease.

WARNING: Advise the patient with an ulcer to avoid taking preparations that contain corticosteroids, aspirin, or another nonsteroidal anti-inflammatory drug such as ibuprofen (Motrin). Explain that these drugs inhibit mucus secretion and leave the GI lining vulnerable to injury from gastric acid. Recommend using an alternative such as acetaminophen (Tylenol) to relieve pain.

Surgery

Surgery may be necessary if conservative treatments fail or if complications develop. Explain the type of surgery the patient will undergo. In vagotomy, the surgeon severs the nerves that stimulate gastric secretion. Vagotomy may be accompanied by removal of part of the stomach or removal of the ulcerated area.

If the patient will be undergoing planned surgery, inform him that he'll have cleansing laxatives and enemas the evening before and a nasogastric tube inserted on the morning of surgery. Explain that both measures prevent complications during surgery. Also inform him that he'll have a drain at the incision site for 1 to 2 days after surgery to remove any accumulated fluid, and he may be fed through a gastrostomy tube. He'll probably resume eating several days after surgery, starting with clear liquids and gradually advancing to solid foods.

Tell the patient that he will probably resume normal activities several weeks after he is discharged. Remind him to continue avoiding poorly tolerated foods, to adhere to his medication schedule, to follow stress man-

Understanding dumping syndrome

If your patient has had a gastric resection with pyloric removal, prepare him for dealing with dumping syndrome, which may begin about 2 weeks after surgery and typically occurs between 15 and 30 minutes after eating. Lasting about 1 hour, the syndrome causes abdominal cramps, diaphoresis, diarrhea, palpitations, fainting, a fast pulse, and weakness.

What causes the problem

Explain that after gastric resection, food and fluid, which the stomach can no longer store, empty rapidly and in large amounts into the small intestine. To accommodate the onrush, the bowel draws fluid from the vascular system. Then the jejunum distends with food and fluid, and intestinal peristalsis and motility increase.

Managing symptoms

To minimize or prevent signs and symptoms, recommend that the patient:
• eat four to six small meals a day
• maintain a normal intake of fats and proteins (they leave the stomach more slowly and attract less fluid into the intestine)
• avoid foods with concentrated carbohydrates (they attract more fluid into the intestine)
• drink fluids between meals, not with meals
• avoid overly hot or cold foods and fluids
• lie down for 30 minutes to 1 hour after eating
• take medication to slow intestinal motility, if prescribed.

Reassure the patient that the syndrome usually resolves within a year after surgery. However, a few patients may have long-term problems and require reconstructive surgery.

agement techniques, and to abstain from smoking. If appropriate, describe the signs and symptoms of dumping syndrome and teach him to minimize or prevent this problem by properly managing his diet. (See *Understanding dumping syndrome*.)

Other care measures
Teach about necessary lifestyle changes, bearing in mind that the patient with ulcer disease may be assertive and independent and thus find these changes difficult to accept. Explain that emotional tension can trigger an ulcer attack and prolong healing, and suggest that the patient identify stressors and develop ways to eliminate them or reduce their effect. Guide him in adjusting his work and home schedules to establish a realistic pattern of work and sleep. Also urge him to give up smoking because

smoking interferes with the effects of all peptic ulcer medications.

Instruct the patient to watch for and immediately report signs and symptoms of life-threatening complications, such as hemorrhage, obstruction, and perforation. Signs and symptoms of hemorrhage include:
• bloody or black, tarry stools
• bloody or coffee-ground vomitus
• chills
• sweating
• weak, rapid pulse
• fast, irregular, shallow breathing
• dizziness on standing
• restlessness.

Indications of intestinal obstruction include:
• a foul taste in the mouth
• a coated tongue
• abdominal fullness or distention worsening after meals and at night

- nausea and vomiting of foul-smelling gastric contents
- colicky pain
- visible bulging in the abdominal wall
- anorexia
- weight loss.
  Perforation may lead to:
- fast pulse
- rapid, shallow breathing
- facial flushing
- fever
- dizziness
- sweating
- black, tarry stools
- a swollen abdomen
- severe pain in the shoulders or stomach.

To help the patient cope with ulcer disease, refer him to the Digestive Disease National Coalition, the National Digestive Disease Information Clearinghouse, or the National Ulcer Foundation. (See Appendix 2.)

5

Neurologic conditions

Alzheimer's disease

Although researchers have made some strides in their efforts to determine the cause and develop treatments or a cure for Alzheimer's disease, this degenerative brain condition now affects approximately 3 million Americans. What's more, that number is expected to quadruple by the year 2040. Necessitating aggressive, long-term teaching and support measures, Alzheimer's disease exacts a staggering economic burden on the health care system and takes a heavy emotional toll on family members.

The primary teaching goal consists of preparing the family to meet the spiraling demands of patient care. You'll direct most of your teaching to the primary caregivers. Offer them emotional support as you explain the inexorable course of this degenerative dementia and the measures they can take to relieve its physical, emotional, and social strains.

Expect family members to wonder why the patient's personality has changed so dramatically. Address their concerns by discussing the pathophysiology of Alzheimer's disease and its possible causes. Point out the difficulty in diagnosing the disease, explaining that diagnosis involves various examinations and tests to rule out other illnesses.

To prepare the family for the patient's progressive deterioration, discuss Alzheimer's signs, symptoms, and stages. Review dietary adjustments and medications to help manage symptoms, and explain how to decrease patient stress and create a safe environment. Not to be overlooked — provide suggestions to help the caregiver avoid burnout.

Before teaching the patient or his family about Alzheimer's disease, make sure you're familiar with the following topics:
• pathophysiology and possible causes of the disease
• signs and symptoms of the disease
• stages of the disease
• diagnostic workup, including patient and family history; physical, neurologic, and psychiatric examinations; laboratory tests; and magnetic resonance imaging (MRI), electroencephalography (EEG), and other tests
• need for activity and exercise to maintain mobility and help prevent complications
• dietary adjustments if patient experiences restlessness, dysphagia, or coordination problems
• medication to relieve depression, behavioral problems, and seizures and experimental drugs to help improve cognitive function
• home care planning — establishing a daily routine, providing a safe home environment, and avoiding overstimulation
• tips for the caregiver, including the importance of adequate rest, good nutrition, and private time
• sources of information and support.

ABOUT THE DISORDER

Inform the patient (if appropriate) and his family that Alzheimer's disease is a degenerative disorder of the brain that causes progressive nerve atrophy in the frontal lobe of the cerebral cortex. Characteristic pathologic changes include neurofibrillary tangles (large, irregular fibrous strands found throughout the nerve cell) and

The many faces of Alzheimer's disease

Although memory loss is commonly associated with Alzheimer's disease, families may not realize that this is only one of its many devastating signs and symptoms. Inform them that the following intellectual, personality, and stress-tolerance deficits are also signs and symptoms of Alzheimer's disease.

Intellectual deficits
- Inattention to time
- Decreased attention span, increased distractibility
- Difficulty making decisions
- Inability to solve problems
- Inability to plan and complete activities
- Inability to perform routine, sequential motor activities, such as dressing, bathing, or eating
- Increased activity (purposeless, repetitive, and compulsive) coupled with decreased performance
- Altered perception of visual and auditory cues

Personality deficits
- Inappropriate affect
- Lack of inhibitions (involving emotional lability, need for immediate gratification, inability to control temper, tactlessness)
- Self-preoccupation and increased refusal to participate
- Confabulation, perseveration, paranoia, delusions, hallucinations, and social withdrawal
- Expression of hostility or helplessness when deficits are mentioned

Stress-tolerance deficits
- Confusion
- Nighttime awakening, pacing, and wandering
- Fatigue and loss of energy
- Avoidance behavior
- Anxiety
- Violence

senile or neuritic plaques (extracellular clusters of degenerated nerve terminals), which hinder cerebral cortex function. Other abnormalities include reduced oxygen metabolism, decreased blood flow in the brain, thickened capillary walls in the cerebral cortex, absence of the perivascular neural plexus, and loss of brain cells. Explain that the cause of Alzheimer's disease isn't known, but several factors are suspected: a deficiency in the brain's neurotransmitter substances, viruses, genetic predisposition (first-degree relatives have four times the risk of developing the disease), and environmental toxins (such as aluminum).

Review the signs and symptoms of Alzheimer's disease. Describe the subtle, early signs such as forgetfulness. Emphasize that the disease is more than just memory loss — it produces progressive changes in the patient's

intellect, personality, sensation, motor skills, and overall functioning. (See *The many faces of Alzheimer's disease*.)

Explain that the disease progresses in stages, but at an unpredictable rate. Eventually, though, the patient will suffer complete memory loss and total physical deterioration. (See *How Alzheimer's disease progresses*.)

Complications
Reinforce the need to take precautions as the disease progresses, to prevent the patient from injuring himself (by his own violent behavior, wandering, or unsupervised activity). Point out that insufficient exercise and activity may lead to immobility and its complications, such as pneumonia and other infections. Stress that malnutrition and dehydration may occur if the patient forgets or refuses to eat. In the final disease stage,

INSIGHT INTO ILLNESSES

How Alzheimer's disease progresses

Counsel family members to expect progressive deterioration in the patient with Alzheimer's disease. To help them plan future patient care, discuss the stages of this relentless and inevitably progressive disease.

Bear in mind that family members may refuse to believe that the disease is advancing, so be sensitive to their concerns. If necessary, review the information again when they're more receptive.

Forgetfulness
Explain that in early stages of Alzheimer's disease, the patient becomes forgetful, especially of recent events. He frequently loses everyday objects such as keys. Aware of this loss of function, he may compensate by relinquishing tasks that might reveal his forgetfulness. Because his behavior isn't disruptive and may be attributed to stress, fatigue, or normal aging, he usually doesn't consult a doctor at this stage.

Confusion
Describe what happens as the disease progresses: The patient has increasing difficulty with activities that require planning, decision making, and judgment (such as managing personal finances, driving a car, or performing his job). However, he does retain everyday skills such as personal grooming.

Point out that social withdrawal occurs when the patient feels overwhelmed by a changing environment and his inability to cope with multiple stimuli. Travel is difficult and tiring. Forewarn the family that as the patient becomes aware of his progressive loss of function, he may become severely depressed.

Emphasize that safety becomes a concern when the patient forgets to turn off appliances or can't recognize unsafe situations, such as boiling water. At this point, the family may need to consider day care or a supervised residential facility.

Decline in activities of daily living
Tell the family that at this stage, the patient loses the ability to perform activities of daily living, such as eating or washing, without direct supervision. Weight loss may occur. The patient withdraws from the family and increasingly depends on the primary caregiver. Communication becomes difficult as the patient's understanding of written and spoken language declines.

Explain that agitation, wandering, pacing, and nighttime awakening are linked to an inability to cope with a multistimuli environment. The patient may mistake his mirror image for a real person (pseudohallucination). Inform caregivers that because they must be constantly vigilant, they may suffer physical and emotional exhaustion as well as a sense of loss and anger.

Total deterioration
Point out that in the final stage of Alzheimer's disease, the patient no longer recognizes himself, his body parts, or other family members. He becomes bedridden, and his activity consists of small, purposeless movements. Verbal communication stops, although he may scream spontaneously. Complications of immobility may include pressure sores, urinary tract infections, pneumonia, and contractures.

patients typically are confined to bed and generally die from complications related to immobility.

DIAGNOSTIC WORKUP

Inform the patient (if appropriate) and family that no tests directly diagnose Alzheimer's disease; it can be confirmed with certainty only on autopsy through microscopic evaluation of brain tissue.

Instead, the doctor will take a thorough patient and family history and the patient will undergo several examinations and tests to rule out other diseases that cause dementia. Assessments typically include physical and neurologic examinations and a neuropsychological interview. Thorough and accurate assessment promotes an accurate and early diagnosis. Because several doctors may be involved in the diagnosis, be sure to clarify to the patient (if appropriate) and family who will perform each examination and where it will be done.

The patient will also undergo laboratory and other diagnostic tests, including MRI, EEG, cerebral blood flow studies, and cerebrospinal fluid (CSF) analysis. (See *Teaching patients about neurologic tests.*)

 WARNING: Forewarn the family that the diagnostic workup may be lengthy, requiring several trips to the hospital. Tell them that the process may overwhelm the patient, leading to deterioration in his behavior and intellectual performance. Reassure them that health care professionals will make every effort to minimize the patient's stress before and between the tests.

Patient and family history

Explain that the doctor will ask the family questions about the patient's short-term memory, judgment, and decision making and whether the patient shows increased fatigue or personality changes. In Alzheimer's disease, the patient history typically reveals a progressive decline in cognitive function, not a stepwise decline as in

other types of dementia. Mention that a medication history can rule out the possibility of drug toxicity — the most common, and most easily corrected, cause of confusion and dementia in elderly patients.

Physical examination

Inform the family that the patient will undergo a complete physical examination to rule out confusion caused by an underlying illness, such as heart failure or pneumonia.

Neurologic examination

Advise the family that a neurologic examination (lasting about 2 hours) will assess specific deficits characteristic of Alzheimer's disease. Examples of such deficits include an impaired sense of smell (usually an early symptom), impaired stereognosis (inability to recognize and understand the form and nature of objects by touching them), gait disorders, tremor, and loss of recent memory. Peculiar or inappropriate speech is also common. (In one study, 90% of Alzheimer's patients answered questions with intrusions or inappropriate repetition of their responses to earlier questions.) Explain that the patient may be asked to make calculations, solve problems, and answer questions about current events.

Tell the family that the doctor may perform a "snout reflex" test to rule out a focal problem such as a tumor. This test involves tapping or stroking the patient's lips or the area just under his nose. Point out that the snout reflex is normal in early infancy but suggests diffuse organic brain disease in adults. Therefore, grimacing or puckering the lips is a positive sign for Alzheimer's disease.

Is the patient aware of his deficits? If so, warn the family that during the tests he may become frustrated and angry and refuse to answer questions. The patient with more advanced disease may become agitated or belligerent. Tell the family that the patient with memory loss may be even more confused and restless after the tests.

(Text continues on page 125.)

Teaching patients about neurologic tests

TEST AND PURPOSE	TEACHING POINTS
Cerebral angiography (cerebral arteriography) • To detect disruption or displacement of the cerebral circulation by occlusion or hemorrhage	• Inform the patient that this test, which takes about 2 hours, highlights the brain's blood vessels on an X-ray as a dyelike substance circulates through them. It detects disruption or displacement of the cerebral circulation by occlusion or hemorrhage. • Explain what happens during the test: A technician will shave and clean the injection site — the carotid or femoral artery — and may immobilize the patient's head with tape or straps. If the carotid artery will be used, inform the patient that he may have his face covered with a drape and his arms immobilized to maintain a sterile field. • Describe what happens during the test: The patient must lie still on an examining table and may feel discomfort from this prolonged motionlessness. The doctor will inject a local anesthetic and insert a catheter at the appropriate site for dye injection. During the injection, the patient may sense pressure, warmth, a transient headache, nausea, or a salty taste. Tell him to report any of these sensations. Immediately after the injection, he'll hear clacking sounds as the X-ray equipment takes pictures. Explain that multiple dye injections may be required to completely visualize the blood vessels. Instruct him to lie still to avoid blurring the films but to comply if the doctor tells him to move an arm or a leg. • Discuss what happens after the test: The catheter is removed, and pressure is applied to the puncture site for about 15 minutes, followed by a pressure dressing and an ice pack. The patient's pulses are checked frequently to monitor his circulation. He must hold his head and neck (for the carotid approach) or leg (for the femoral approach) straight for 4 to 12 hours. He can resume his usual diet but should increase fluid intake for the rest of the day to help expel the contrast medium.
Cerebral blood flow (CBF) studies • To measure CBF • To detect abnormalities in cerebral perfusion • To evaluate the effectiveness of certain cerebral operations	• Explain that these CBF studies measure blood flow to the brain and help detect abnormalities. Inform the patient that the test takes about 30 minutes, is painless, and exposes him to less radiation than a chest X-ray. • Describe what happens during the test: The patient will lie still on a table and will have a frame placed around his head. He may inhale a radioactive gas, such as xenon, technetium, or krypton. Or he may receive an I.V. injection of the radioactive substance and breathe through a mask or

(continued)

Teaching patients about neurologic tests *(continued)*

TEST AND PURPOSE	TEACHING POINTS
Cerebral blood flow (CBF) studies *(continued)*	dome while the isotope-sensitive detector probes measure the blood flow rate. Explain that he can resume his usual activities immediately after the test.

Cerebrospinal fluid (CSF) analysis
• To help detect infection, multiple sclerosis, or cancer
• To help detect obstruction of the subarachnoid space around the spinal cord
• To inject medication or contrast medium into the central nervous system
	• Explain that this test involves removal and laboratory analysis of CSF. Tell the patient that it takes about 15 minutes. Inform him that he'll feel some pressure during the procedure as the needle is inserted, and he may become uncomfortable from the position assumed during the test.
	• Describe preparation for the test: For a *cisternal puncture,* instruct the patient to restrict food and fluids for 4 hours before the test, if ordered. Explain that he'll assume a sitting position with his chin resting on his chest, or he'll be positioned on his side at the edge of a bed with a small pillow placed beneath his forward-bending head. After cleaning and possibly shaving the upper neck area, the doctor will inject a local anesthetic.
	    For a *lumbar puncture,* tell the patient that he will be seated with his head bent toward his knees or will lie on the edge of a bed or table, with his knees drawn up to his abdomen and his chin resting on his chest. After cleaning the lumbar area, the doctor will inject a local anesthetic. Tell the patient to report any tingling or sharp pain.
	• Explain what happens during the test: In a *cisternal puncture,* the patient will be instructed to remain still as the doctor inserts a hollow needle into the midline of the vertebral column below the occipital bone. In a *lumbar puncture,* the doctor inserts a hollow needle into the subarachnoid space surrounding the spinal cord. Tell the patient to hold still to avoid dislodging the needle. Also tell him that he may be asked to breathe deeply or to straighten his legs, and that the doctor may apply pressure to the jugular veins.
	• Describe what happens after the test: After a *cisternal puncture,* the doctor removes the needle and applies an adhesive bandage. The patient briefly lies flat on his abdomen while the puncture site seals. Then he can resume his usual activities.
	    After a *lumbar puncture,* the doctor removes the needle and applies an adhesive bandage. The patient lies flat for 4 to 24 hours to prevent head-

Teaching patients about neurologic tests (continued)

TEST AND PURPOSE	TEACHING POINTS
Cerebrospinal fluid (CSF) analysis (continued)	ache. His head should be even with or below the level of his hips. Point out that although he must not raise his head, he can turn from side to side. Also tell him to increase his fluid intake for the rest of the day to help replenish CSF and to prevent a headache.
Computed tomography (CT) scan ●To identify structural abnormalities, edema, and lesions, such as nonhemorrhagic infarction, hematomas, aneurysms, and tumors, in the brain and spinal cord	●Explain that a CT scan produces X-ray images of the brain or spinal tissue. Tell the patient that it takes about 30 to 60 minutes and causes no discomfort, although he may feel chilled because the equipment requires a cool environment. If the doctor will be using a contrast medium, tell the patient to restrict food and fluids for 4 hours before the test. ●Explain what happens during the test: A technician will position the patient on an X-ray table and place a strap across the part of the body to be scanned to restrict movement. The table will then slide into the circular opening of the scanner. If a contrast medium is ordered, the patient will receive it through an I.V. site; the infusion takes about 5 minutes. Instruct the patient to tell the technician immediately if the infusion causes discomfort, a feeling of warmth, or itching. (The technician can see and hear him from an adjacent room.) Also tell the patient that he will hear noises from the scanner and may notice the machine revolving around him. ●Describe what happens after the test: The patient can immediately resume his usual activities and diet. Advise him to increase his fluid intake for the rest of the day to help expel the contrast medium.
Digital subtraction angiography (DSA) ●To evaluate the patency of cerebral vessels and to determine their position ●To detect and evaluate lesions and vascular abnormalities	●Explain to the patient that DSA visualizes the blood vessels in his head and neck. Tell him that the test will take about 30 to 45 minutes. Inform him that he may experience a feeling of warmth or a metallic taste on injection of the contrast medium. Instruct him to restrict solid food for 4 hours before the test. ●Explain what happens during the test: The patient is positioned on an X-ray table and an I.V. needle or catheter is inserted. Caution him to lie still during the test. After the doctor injects a contrast medium, the patient will be instructed to lie still while a series of X-ray images is taken. Instruct him to tell the doctor immediately if he feels any discomfort or shortness of breath.

(continued)

Teaching patients about neurologic tests *(continued)*

TEST AND PURPOSE	TEACHING POINTS
Digital subtraction angiography (DSA) *(continued)*	• Describe what happens after the test: The doctor removes the needle or catheter. If the I.V. route was used, the patient can resume his normal activities. For the intra-arterial route, he'll need to restrict movement in his arm or leg for 4 to 12 hours. Encourage him to increase his fluid intake for the rest of the day to help expel the contrast medium.
Electroencephalography (EEG) • To evaluate the brain's electrical activity in such disorders as seizures • To help identify the brain area in which the patient's seizures originate and determine the frequency with which they occur • To aid diagnosis of intracranial lesions, such as abscesses and tumors	• Explain to the patient that the EEG records the electrical activity of his brain. Assure him that the test is painless and that the electrodes won't give him an electric shock. Tell him that it takes about 45 minutes. • Depending on the type of EEG ordered (such as sleep, sleep deprivation, or photic stimulation), explain the necessary restrictions. Instruct the patient to wash his hair 1 to 2 days before the test to remove hair spray, cream, or oil. • Describe what happens during the test: The patient will be positioned comfortably in a reclining chair or on a bed. After lightly abrading the patient's skin to ensure good contact, a technician will apply paste and attach electrodes to the patient's head and neck. Tell the patient to remain still throughout the test. Review the activities he may be asked to perform, such as breathing deeply and rapidly for 3 minutes (hyperventilating) or sleeping, depending on the type of EEG. • Explain what happens after the test: The technician will remove the electrodes. He'll also remove the paste, using acetone. (This may sting where the skin was scraped.) Tell the patient to wash his hair to remove residual paste; then he can resume his usual activities.
Closed-circuit television EEG • To obtain further information about electrical brain activity	• If the routine EEG produces insufficient information, tell the patient that the doctor may request more extensive monitoring over an extended period using closed-circuit television EEG. • Tell him that a log may be kept to help determine what triggers his seizures. Mention that the monitoring is painless and won't give him an electric shock. Tell him how long monitoring will last. If the test will use special scalp electrodes, instruct the patient to wash his hair beforehand. • If special electrodes are to be used, describe how they will be inserted. Fluoroscopy will help guide transsphenoidal electrode insertion. A trocar will be used to pass a very thin wire through the pterygoid

Teaching patients about neurologic tests *(continued)*

TEST AND PURPOSE	TEACHING POINTS
Closed-circuit television EEG *(continued)*	fossa. Tell the patient to expect some discomfort, and mention that he'll have a wire extending from his upper cheek area. Subdural or depth electrodes require surgical insertion, involving an open flap craniotomy or burr holes; the electrodes will extend from the patient's skull. Explain that heavy, cast-like dressings will protect them from dislodgment. Tell the patient that he may have bathroom privileges, but otherwise he'll be confined to an area within the video camera's range (usually in bed). Reassure him that after the electrodes are removed, he can resume his normal activities.
Electromyography (EMG) • To evaluate neuromuscular disorders such as myasthenia gravis	• Explain that EMG measures the electrical activity of specific muscles. Tell the patient that it takes about 1 hour. • Describe what happens during the test: The patient will either lie down or sit up, depending on the muscle to be tested. A technician will clean the skin over the muscle. Tell the patient he may experience some discomfort as a needle attached to an electrode is inserted into the muscle. Then another electrode is placed on the patient's limb to deliver a mild electrical charge. This may cause discomfort as each muscle is stimulated to test its response at rest and during voluntary contraction. Tell the patient to remain still during the test, except when asked to contract or relax a muscle. Also explain that an amplifier may cause crackling noises whenever his muscle moves.
Evoked potential studies (evoked responses) • To aid diagnosis of nervous system lesions and abnormalities • To assess neurologic function	• Tell the patient that the electrodes are removed after the test and that he can resume his usual activities. • Explain to the patient that evoked potential studies measure his nervous system's electrical response to a visual, auditory, or sensory stimulus. Tell him that the test lasts about 1 hour and is painless. Instruct him to wash his hair 1 to 2 days before the test. • Describe what happens during the test: The patient will be positioned on a bed or table or in a reclining chair. Emphasize that he must lie still during the test. Mention that a technician will clean his scalp and apply paste and electrodes to his head and neck. Also tell him he may hear noises from the test equipment. Tell him that he'll be asked to perform various activities, such as gazing at a

(continued)

Teaching patients about neurologic tests *(continued)*

TEST AND PURPOSE	TEACHING POINTS
Evoked potential studies (evoked responses) *(continued)*	checkerboard pattern or a strobe light or listening with headphones to a series of clicks. Or he may have electrodes placed on an arm and leg, and may be asked to respond to a tapping sensation. • Discuss what happens after the test: The technician will remove the electrodes. The patient can resume his normal activities. Tell him to wash his hair to remove residual paste.
Magnetic resonance imaging (MRI; nuclear magnetic resonance scan) • To aid diagnosis of intracranial and spinal lesions • To rule out intracranial lesions as the cause of dementia • To evaluate for neurologic abnormalities • To detect diffuse axonal and brainstem injuries • To help determine the cause of seizures	• Explain that this test evaluates the condition of the brain or spinal cord. Tell the patient that it takes about 1 hour and causes no discomfort. Reassure him that it will not expose him to radiation. However, because it will expose him to a strong magnetic field, he should report any metal objects in his body (such as a pacemaker, aneurysm clips, hip prosthesis, bullet fragments, or an implanted infusion pump), which could make him ineligible for the test. Tell the patient he may receive a sedative. • Explain what happens during the test: The patient will be positioned on a table that slides into a large cylinder housing the MRI magnets. His head, chest, and arms will be restrained to help him remain still. Stress that lying still prevents blurring of the images. Mention that a technician can see and hear him from an adjacent room. Tell the patient he'll hear a loud knocking noise while the machine is running. If the noise bothers him, he may be given earplugs or pads for his ears. A radio encased in the machine, or earphones may help block the sound (but he will still hear some noise). Mention that he may feel some discomfort from being enclosed within the large cylinder. Ask him if he is claustrophobic. • Tell the patient he can resume his normal activities after the test.
Nerve conduction studies • To determine the velocity of impulses traveling along a nerve • To aid diagnosis of diseases that affect	• Explain to the patient that nerve conduction studies measure the speed at which electrical impulses travel along a nerve. Tell him that the test takes about 1 hour. Inform him that he may experience discomfort during needle insertion and delivery of each stimulus. • Describe what happens during the test: The patient will lie on a bed or sit on a chair, depending on the nerve to be tested. The technician will clean the patient's limb and tape surface electrodes to

Teaching patients about neurologic tests *(continued)*

TEST AND PURPOSE	TEACHING POINTS
Nerve conduction studies *(continued)* the peripheral nervous system, such as Guillain-Barré syndrome	the skin at the distal end of the nerve. The doctor will then insert the needle at various sites along the nerve route, and with each insertion will deliver a slight electrical charge. Tell the patient to keep still during the test because movement may distort results, prolonging the test. •Explain what happens after the test: The technician will remove the electrodes and needle. The patient can then resume his usual activities.
Neuropsychological tests •To evaluate cognitive function •To help distinguish organic from psychiatric disorders	•Explain that a battery of neuropsychological tests evaluates simple to complex mental and verbal abilities. It also includes a personality inventory. Tell the patient (or his family) that the tests take about 1 to 2 hours. Explain that a battery of written and oral tests will be administered and that the patient may be asked to perform such activities as making calculations, solving problems, and answering questions about current events. Forewarn the patient or his family that these tests may produce fatigue and frustration. (A short rest period is usually all that's needed before testing can continue.) •Tell the family that after the test, the patient with memory loss may show increased confusion and restlessness.
Oculoplethysmography •To aid detection and evaluation of carotid occlusive disease	•Explain that this test indirectly evaluates carotid blood flow. Tell the patient that it will take only a few minutes. •Describe preparation for the test: The patient will be asked to remove any contact lenses. He will have anesthetic drops instilled in his eyes, which may cause burning. •Discuss what happens during the test: The patient's head will be placed in a frame. He'll have eyecups placed on his eyes (held in place with light suction) and photoelectric cells clipped to his earlobes. Tell him to remain still and avoid blinking during the test. If he's also having ophthalmic artery pressure studies, mention that he'll briefly lose his vision when suction is applied to his eyes. •Discuss what happens after the test: The doctor will remove the eyecups and head frame. Tell the patient not to rub his eyes or replace his contact lenses for at least 2 hours. Also tell him to blink and to protect his eyes until the effects of the anesthetic drops wear off.

(continued)

Teaching patients about neurologic tests (continued)

TEST AND PURPOSE	TEACHING POINTS
Positron emission tomography (PET) scan (positron emission transaxial tomography) • To evaluate cerebral perfusion • To evaluate cerebral glucose metabolism and thus aid diagnosis of tumors and disorders that alter cerebral metabolism, such as Alzheimer's disease, Parkinson's disease, multiple sclerosis, and cerebrovascular accident	• Inform the patient that a PET scan evaluates brain cell function by measuring how rapidly brain tissue consumes radioactive isotopes. Tell him that the test takes about 1 hour, is painless, and involves minimal radiation exposure. • Explain what happens during the test: The patient will lie on a moving table with his head immobilized and placed inside a ring-shaped opening in the machine. He'll be given a radioactive tracer either by inhalation or by I.V. injection. If the doctor chooses the inhalation method, the patient will inhale a radioactive tracer through a mask. Tell him to breathe normally; he won't smell or taste anything odd. If the doctor uses the I.V. method, tell the patient that he may feel a warm sensation during the tracer's injection. Advise him to report any discomfort to the technician. With either method, tell the patient he'll have a dome-shaped hood placed over his head and face to prevent the exhaled tracer from circulating in the room. Stress the importance of lying still to avoid blurring the images. • If the I.V. method is used, explain that the doctor will remove the needle after the test and collect a blood sample. Then the patient can resume his normal activities.
Single-photon emission tomography (SPECT) scan • To study cerebral blood flow	• Tell the patient that a SPECT scan will help determine the cause of his seizures. Mention that it takes about 1 hour. • Explain that before the test, the patient may receive a dose of salty-tasting Lugol's solution (depending on the tracer agent) and an I.V. amine tracer. • Describe what happens during the test: The patient will lie on a narrow metal table and will feel the table move. A large disklike machine will move around his head as it makes images of the tracer agent flowing through the brain. Stress the importance of lying still to ensure accurate results. • Tell the patient that he can resume his usual activities after the test.

Teaching patients about neurologic tests *(continued)*

TEST AND PURPOSE	TEACHING POINTS
Transcranial Doppler studies • To measure the velocity of blood flow through certain cerebral vessels • To detect and monitor the progression of cerebral vasospasm • To determine whether collateral blood flow exists before surgical ligation or radiologic occlusion of diseased vessels • To help determine brain death	• Inform the patient (or his family) that these studies provide information about the presence, quality, and changing nature of circulation to an area of the brain. Inform him that the test takes about 30 minutes and is painless. Mention that he'll lie on a table or in his bed and that he'll rest his head on a foam cushion. • Explain what happens during the test: The technician will apply gel in front of the patient's ear, over his eye, or on the back of his head. Tell him to expect light pressure in that area as the technician places a microphone-like probe against his head; he'll hear a swishing sound as the probe senses the blood flowing through the vessels. Stress the importance of lying still to ensure accurate results. • Tell the patient that he can resume his normal activities after the test.
Wada's (amobarbital) test • To determine hemispheric dominance for speech, memory, and other specific activities	• Explain that this test can help determine the cause of a seizure. Tell the patient that the test takes 1 to 2 hours, depending on whether both sides of the brain are tested. • Describe what happens during the test: The patient will be positioned on an X-ray table. The doctor will insert a catheter into the femoral artery and, aided by fluoroscopy, guide it to the carotid artery. He will then inject the amobarbital and ask the patient to perform tests related to memory, speech, and cognitive functions. Tell the patient that drug effects disappear in about 20 minutes. If the other cerebral hemisphere is to be tested, the doctor will reposition the catheter to the other carotid artery and repeat the drug infusion and performance tests. • Discuss what happens after the test: The patient will be instructed to lie in bed for 2 to 12 hours with his leg kept straight. He may have an ice pack over the catheter insertion site.

Neuropsychological interview
Explain that a neuropsychological interview helps rule out severe depression, which is often mistaken for dementia or Alzheimer's disease in elderly patients. All of these conditions cause apathy, unresponsiveness, and memory loss. Point out that this is a lengthy test (4 to 6 hours) and may greatly upset the patient.

TREATMENTS
Tell the family that Alzheimer's disease has no cure, but various treat-

ments may temporarily improve the patient's quality of life and make caring for him easier. Such treatments focus on stress reduction, safety measures, drug therapy, diet modification, and physical activity.

Activity guidelines

Explain that adequate exercise and activity will help maintain the patient's mobility and prevent complications, such as pneumonia or other infections. Exercise also promotes a normal day and night routine.

 TIPS AND TIMESAVERS: Encourage family members to find physical activities that satisfy and occupy the patient. Such activities include repetitive chores, such as folding towels, scrubbing the floor, sweeping, or indoor stationary bicycle riding. Repetitive motions decrease the patient's stress level by eliminating the need for him to make decisions about what to do next.

Dietary modifications

Stress the importance of a well-balanced diet with adequate fiber. If the patient is hyperactive, advise the family to increase his caloric intake with between-meal supplements. But tell them to avoid giving him stimulants, such as caffeinated coffee, tea, cola, and chocolate.

Recommend limiting the number of foods on the patient's plate so he won't have to make decisions. If he has coordination problems, advise the family to cut his food and to provide finger foods, such as fruit and sandwiches. To prevent injury, suggest using plates with rim guards, built-up utensils, and cups with lids and spouts.

If the patient has difficulty swallowing, advise the family to serve semisoft foods. Suggest freezing liquids to a slush or mixing them with other foods. If the patient can't swallow or has no interest in food, nasogastric or gastrostomy tube feedings may be necessary; instruct the family accordingly.

If the patient puts almost anything in his mouth, whether it's food or not, encourage the family to keep preferred foods handy.

Medication

The doctor may order medications to manage the patient's signs and symptoms. For example, antipsychotics and antidepressants control behavioral changes, and neuroleptics control seizures. Caution the family to check with the doctor before giving the patient any unprescribed drugs (especially sedatives) because drug action may be enhanced in Alzheimer's disease.

If the patient has trouble swallowing, advise crushing tablets or opening capsules and mixing them with a semisoft food. However, caution the family always to check with the pharmacist before crushing tablets or opening capsules because specially formulated drugs shouldn't be altered. Mention that, in many cases, flavorful oral suspensions may be available that will ease administration problems.

Investigational drugs

Inform the family that researchers are investigating combinations of several drugs, including choline chloride, lecithin, tacrine hydrochloride, and physostigmine salicylate (Antilirium), to try to slow the disease process. (These substances appear to have little or no benefit when used alone.) For example, choline chloride and lecithin — both precursors for acetylcholine synthesis — are being given together to improve cognitive function by increasing acetylcholine availability. The cholinesterase inhibitors tacrine hydrochloride and physostigmine salicylate are being used to prolong acetylcholine action in the brain and thus enhance cognitive function.

Other care measures

Encourage the family to grant the patient as much independence as possible while ensuring his — and others' — safety. To combat the patient's confusion, emphasize maintaining a routine in *all* his activities. If the patient panics or becomes belligerent, advise the family to remain calm and to try distracting him.

Recommend dividing the patient's daily tasks into short, simple steps and then guiding him through them. Tell the family to use activities that stimulate or calm him appropriately. Suggest repetitive tasks, such as sanding wood and listening to music.

Also advise the family to avoid overstimulating the patient before bedtime and to limit fluids about 3 to 4 hours before bedtime, so the patient won't need to get up to urinate. Warn them that if he develops irregular sleep patterns and wanders at night, he may harm himself and others. If necessary, tell the family to lock doors and windows, barricade stairways, and use night-lights. If the patient is confused about his surroundings, tell the family to use pictures to guide him.

Teach the family about home safety measures, such as storing medication out of the patient's reach and removing throw rugs. If necessary, remind them to remove handles and buttons from appliances.

 TIPS AND TIMESAVERS: If the patient has coordination problems, suggest using Velcro straps instead of buttons and loafers or shoes with elastic shoelaces.

Stress that the patient can't control his behavior, although sometimes he may respond appropriately. And even if the patient no longer recognizes his family, urge them to keep including him in their activities.

Last, emphasize to the family the importance of taking some time for themselves. Refer them to a local Alzheimer's support group and to the Alzheimer's Association for further information and support. (See Appendix 2.)

Cerebrovascular accident

Cerebrovascular accidents (CVAs, or strokes) occur 550,000 times a year in the United States. CVA is the third leading cause of death in the United States and the leading cause of disability and neurologic deficits.

As defined by the National Survey of Stroke, a CVA is a syndrome of sudden or rapid-onset neurologic findings lasting more than 24 hours and arising from thrombotic or embolic occlusion of a cerebral artery resulting in infarction, or from spontaneous vessel rupture leading to intracerebral or subarachnoid hemorrhage.

The teaching demands of the CVA patient may range from simple to complex, depending on the extent of residual disabilities. Typically, CVA poses difficult but not insurmountable teaching challenges. First, you'll teach the patient about his disorder and, as necessary, help him understand diagnostic procedures and such treatments as drug therapy or surgery. To support his sense of independence, you'll discuss how he can compensate for any temporary or permanent neurologic deficits. You'll also describe preventive measures that will decrease risk of recurrence.

The CVA patient may feel depressed about his condition and the prospects of a lengthy rehabilitation. As you teach ways to avoid serious setbacks in rehabilitation, anticipate such periods of discouragement for him and his family.

Before teaching a patient about CVA, make sure you are familiar with the following topics:
• type of CVA the patient has suffered
• risk factors for CVA
• diagnostic tests, such as computed tomography (CT) scan and cerebral angiography
• explanation of the type of surgery, if necessary — craniotomy, carotid endarterectomy, extracranial-intracranial bypass, or ventricular shunt

• the importance of rehabilitation in minimizing neurologic deficits
• balanced program of activity and rest
• communication tips for the patient and his family
• dietary adjustments, such as semi-soft foods for dysphagia
• use of assistive feeding devices
• use of a cane or a walker, if needed
• home safety tips
• sources of additional information and support.

ABOUT THE DISORDER

Explain to the patient that a CVA is commonly, but not necessarily, associated with atherosclerosis — a condition that causes an interruption in blood supply to the brain. A blood clot or plaque can block an artery, producing tissue *ischemia* (decreased blood supply) and *infarction* (death of tissue to the affected area from lack of blood supply). If an internal carotid artery — one of the blood vessels in the neck — becomes blocked because of atherosclerosis, a clot may form, halting oxygen flow to the brain. Or a vessel may rupture, causing increased intracranial pressure from *hemorrhage* and, possibly, brain herniation.

Explain the patient's type of CVA. In *ischemic cerebral infarction,* partial or complete arterial occlusion impairs cerebral perfusion, halting delivery of oxygen, glucose, and other nutrients to affected brain cells, which then stop functioning. Transient ischemia may last from a few minutes to 24 hours. This focal neurologic deficit, called a *transient ischemic attack* (TIA, or "little stroke"), resolves completely without permanent damage. The most underreported form of CVA, TIAs can be visualized on MRI or with improved CT scan images. Signs and symptoms of TIA may range from brief vision loss to serious neurologic deficits associated with a CVA.

A *reversible ischemic neurologic deficit* (sometimes called stroke with full recovery) resembles TIA except that recovery takes longer than 24 hours.

Stroke-in-evolution indicates that neurologic deficits are worsening, whereas *completed stroke* indicates that the deficits are stable, neither increasing nor dramatically resolving.

In an *intracerebral hemorrhage* (ICH), a ruptured intracerebral artery (usually resulting from hypertension) produces a focal area of bleeding into brain tissue. ICH usually causes sudden loss of consciousness that progresses to a coma. The patient advances to respiratory arrest unless appropriate measures are taken to arrest the bleeding. This type of CVA has the highest mortality and morbidity. Patients with altered clotting mechanisms, those receiving anticoagulants, patients with a history of thrombocytopenia, drug abusers, hemophiliacs, and patients with acquired immunodeficiency syndrome are at increased risk for ICH. Crack cocaine users have suffered CVAs from an extreme rise in blood pressure (up to 400 mm Hg in some cases).

Explain that neurologic deficits can be specific or widespread, depending on the brain area affected. Inform the patient that some of his signs and symptoms may be temporary, depending on the cause of his CVA.

Complications

When possible, let the patient know that participation in a rehabilitation program is important for maximum recovery. Inform him that a program that includes range-of-motion exercises, cognitive retraining and socialization, speech therapy, and maintenance of normal eating, elimination, and grooming habits will begin as soon as possible.

Point out that an altered level of consciousness and immobility heighten the risk of complications. Also explain that the patient may have another CVA if he fails to address risk factors.

DIAGNOSTIC WORKUP

The patient will undergo a complete neurologic workup, beginning with a detailed history and physical examination. Blood tests may be performed to evaluate clotting. As appropriate, teach the patient about such scanning tests as CT scans, positron emission tomography, single-photon emission computed tomography, and magnetic resonance imaging. (See *Teaching patients about neurologic tests,* pages 117 to 125.)

Assist in preparing the patient for such studies as angiography and other tests to identify abnormalities and evaluate cerebral blood flow. Teach him about other tests the doctor may order to evaluate a CVA, including cerebral blood flow studies, oculoplethysmography, neuropsychological tests, and transcranial Doppler studies.

TREATMENTS
Provide instruction about CVA treatments, which aim to limit the extent of brain injury and prevent or treat complications. For optimal effectiveness, treatment of brain ischemia must occur as soon as possible — within 90 minutes to 6 hours of onset of CVA symptoms.

Interventions for CVA commonly include physical rehabilitation, dietary and drug regimens to help decrease risk factors, possible surgery, and care measures to help the patient adapt to specific deficits, such as speech impairment or paralysis.

Rehabilitation
Inform the patient and family that the rehabilitation program will include physical medicine (using such physical agents as heat, cold, light, water, and exercise), occupational therapy, and assistive devices or braces to help improve the patient's mobility and independence. The patient may also be a candidate for muscle strengthening and conditioning exercises, swallowing exercises, speech therapy, and gait training.

Teach the patient how to perform special mobilization techniques. If the *Bobath method* is prescribed, inform him that it aims to restore function on both sides of the body and to incorporate the affected side into weight bearing. In this method, the patient progresses from simple movements to more complex ones. If he will undergo *proprioceptive neuromuscular facilitation,* inform him that this system of therapeutic exercise reduces spasticity by training him in specific body movements against resistance. The goal is to help him develop greater control over voluntary motor movements.

Activity guidelines
Instruct the patient and family to follow the prescribed exercise program. Teach them how to perform passive range-of-motion exercises. Reinforce the need to take well-timed rest periods and to use protective devices to prevent injury and promote safety.

To help the patient manage daily activities, provide the following suggestions:
• To help distinguish left from right, urge the patient to wear a watch or bracelet on the left wrist as a "landmark." Or, he can mark the left shoe sole with an *L* or tag the inside left trouser leg or sweater sleeve with colored tape to differentiate left from right.
• If the patient has problems with spatial relations, suggest using maps or colored dots to mark a daily route. Advise the family to keep the environment as uncluttered as possible — for example, keeping only a few items on the nightstand. Also suggest *pointing* to objects to give verbal clues, such as "*in* the wastebasket" or "*under* the desk."
• If the patient's apraxia makes dressing himself difficult, recommend buttoning shirts (or blouses) from the bottom up. Some patients find it easier to match buttonholes that way.
• Whatever the task, urge the family to praise the patient's efforts. Discouragement can be disabling in itself. A patient with a right-sided lesion will understand encouraging words; a patient with a left-sided lesion may respond to nonverbal encouragement such as a pat on the back.

Making eating easier

If your patient has had a CVA that affects his ability to eat, he may find eating easier and more enjoyable if he uses special glasses, cups, plates, and utensils. Here are some tips to help him use these devices.

Glasses and cups

If the patient has trouble holding a glass, advise him to use an unbreakable plastic tumbler instead. Plastic is lighter and less slippery than glass. Or he can use terry cloth sleeves over glasses to make them easier to grasp.

The patient can also choose from many specially designed cups. For instance, he can use a cup with two handles, which is easier to keep steady than a cup with one handle. Or he can try a pedestal cup or a T-handle cup, which is easy to grasp. He can also try a cup with a weighted base, which helps prevent spills.

Cup with V-opening

If the patient has a stiff neck, recommend using a cup with a V-shaped opening on its rim. He can easily tip this cup to empty it without bending his neck backward.

decrease spills. If he has decreased sensation or feeling in his hands, advise him to use an insulated cup or mug to avoid burning himself.

Drinking straws

Flexible or rigid straws, either disposable or reusable, come in several sizes. Some straws are wide enough for the patient to drink soups (cooled to room temperature) and thick liquids through them. To hold the straw in place, instruct the patient to use a snap-on plastic lid with a slot for the straw.

Dishes

If possible, advise the patient to use only unbreakable dishes. To keep a plate from sliding, suggest that he place a damp sponge, washcloth, paper towel, or rubber disk under it. Also tell him to consider using a plate with a nonskid base or place mats made of dimpled rubber or foam. Suction cups attached to the bottom of a plate or bowl also help prevent slipping.

Be sure to tell your patient about plate guards. These helpful devices block food from falling off the plate,

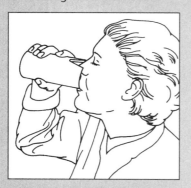

If the patient's hands are unsteady, he may find it easier to hold a cup with a large handle. Or he can drink from a lidded cup with a lip to help

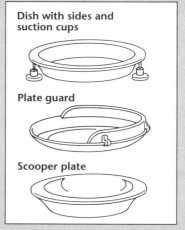

Dish with sides and suction cups

Plate guard

Scooper plate

Making eating easier *(continued)*

so it can be picked up easily with a fork or spoon. Instruct him to attach the guard to the side of the plate opposite the hand he uses to feed himself.

A scooper plate has high sides that provide a built-in surface for pushing food onto the utensil. Eating from a sectioned plate or tray may also be convenient.

Flatware

If the patient's hand is weak or his grip is shaky, recommend that he try ordinary flatware with ridged wood, plastic, or cork handles — all easier to grasp than smooth metal handles. Or suggest that he try building up the handles with a bicycle handlebar, a foam curler pad, or tape (this also works for holding

pens and pencils, toothbrushes, or razors). He can also try strapping the utensil to his hand.

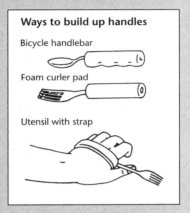

Ways to build up handles

Bicycle handlebar

Foam curler pad

Utensil with strap

Dietary modifications

If the patient is obese or has elevated serum levels of cholesterol, lipoproteins, or triglycerides, you may need to reinforce a weight-loss diet or one low in saturated fats. If he has difficulty swallowing or has one-sided facial weakness, advise him to eat semisoft foods and to chew on the unaffected side of his mouth.

Instruct the patient to sit upright when eating and to tilt his head slightly forward. Recommend that his family or other caregiver prepare solid foods in a blender and freeze liquids to a slush or mix them with other foods. If the patient has partial arm paralysis, suggest that he use feeding aids, such as specially adapted plates with rims and built-up utensils. (See *Making eating easier.*)

 TIPS AND TIMESAVERS:
Remind the patient and family that even if he has learned to feed himself at home, he may have difficulty eating in a restaurant. One solution: Take his utensils to the restaurant rather than risk his social withdrawal.

Medication

Teach the patient about the goals of drug therapy — preventing further thrombus formation, enhancing blood flow to the brain, and protecting brain cells. Medications may include antiplatelet drugs, such as aspirin, dipyridamole, and ticlopidine. Be sure the patient, family, or other caregivers know the names of all prescribed drugs, along with their dosages and possible adverse effects.

If the doctor prescribes aspirin, inform the patient that aspirin has been shown to help prevent CVA recurrence. If the patient will be taking large doses of aspirin for a prolonged period to prevent blood clotting, tell him to watch for such adverse effects as unusual bleeding, bruising, rashes, tinnitus, hearing loss, nausea, vomiting, stomach upset, bleeding gums, and bloody or black, tarry stools.

If the doctor prescribes dipyridamole (Persantine, Pyridamole), tell the patient that this drug prevents blood clotting. Instruct him to stay alert for such adverse effects as bleeding, bruising, rash, tinnitus, hearing loss, nausea, vomiting, diarrhea, headache, dizziness, weakness, flushing, and fainting.

Ticlopidine hydrochloride (Ticlid), a newer antiplatelet agent, has been shown to reduce CVA recurrence by up to 50% in the first year. Teach the patient taking this drug to stay alert for the adverse effects listed previously for aspirin. Stress that he must undergo blood studies for the first 3 months of therapy to check for serious adverse reactions.

Thrombolytic agents

The doctor may prescribe a thrombolytic agent such as alteplase (Activase) to promote neurologic recovery and reduce the chance of lasting disability. For maximal effectiveness, such therapy must begin within 3 hours of symptom onset. Also, the patient's history must be carefully evaluated for contraindications, such as intracerebral hemorrhage, other evidence of bleeding, recent head injury or surgery, and uncontrolled hypertension.

Other agents

The doctor may prescribe a calcium channel blocker such as nifedipine (Procardia) within 18 hours of onset of symptoms. Tell the patient that this drug can reduce neurologic deficits by aiding circulation and easing brain ischemia.

Surgery

Depending on the cause and extent of the CVA, the patient may undergo carotid endarterectomy to remove atherosclerotic plaques or another procedure, such as hematoma evacuation, embolectomy, or angioplasty.

Carotid endarterectomy

Tell the patient scheduled for this procedure that the skin on his neck will be thoroughly cleaned and shaved. If he will receive a cervical block anesthetic, tell him that he'll be awake during surgery; if he will receive a general anesthetic, tell him that he'll sleep during surgery.

Mention that after surgery, dressings will cover the incision and that he may experience a transient numbness and tightness in the incision area and soreness or a lump in his throat. Reassure him that these effects of swelling should disappear in a few days. Inform him that he'll be able to resume his usual daily activities the day after surgery, barring complications.

Other care measures

Involve both the patient and his family in devising new communication methods if necessary, supporting his recovery, and boosting his efforts to be self-sufficient. Also teach the patient how to prevent another CVA.

Alternative communication methods

For a patient with a speech deficit, recommend other communication methods, such as writing or using a picture board. Review prescribed speech and language therapy, and reinforce the importance of continuing it.

Instruct the family to speak slowly to the patient in normal tones. If the patient has receptive aphasia (difficulty understanding speech), recommend that the family use gestures to clarify their message. If he has expressive aphasia (difficulty forming words and putting sentences together), encourage them to take their time and not rush his response or jump in and finish his sentences. Also advise them not to react to the patient's frustration. Tell them to give him short, simple directions, cues, and lists.

 WARNING: Inform the family that the patient may overestimate his abilities, claiming he can perform tasks (for example, driving a car) that in fact he cannot. Explain the importance of carefully monitoring his abilities without frustrating his efforts for independence. Tell them to let him try most activities — short of those that could injure him or others or could cause excessive frustration or fatigue.

(Text continues on page 137.)

Walking with a cane

Dear Patient:

You can use the following guidelines for walking with a cane if your *left* leg is weaker. If your *right* leg is weaker, start with the cane on your left side, and adapt the instructions. You may want to draw the step patterns for yourself.

1. First, be sure you're wearing non-skid, flat-soled, supportive shoes, and check that they fit securely. Avoid wearing sandals or clogs because they do not support your weight properly. Next, check your cane's rubber tip to be sure it has no cracks or tears and is wearing evenly. Also, make sure the tip fits securely and evenly on the cane's end.

If possible, remove throw rugs and avoid walking on slippery, wet, or waxed floors or on gravel driveways. Also, try to walk close to a wall so you have something to lean against if you drop your cane.

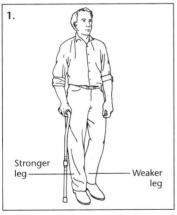

2. Now, position the cane about 4 inches (10 centimeters) to the side of your stronger leg, as shown. Distribute your weight evenly between your feet and your cane.

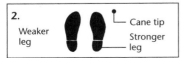

3. Shift your weight to your stronger leg and move the cane about 4 inches in front of you.
4. Move your weaker foot forward so it's even with the cane.
5. Shift your weight to your weaker leg and the cane. Now, move your stronger leg forward, ahead of the cane. If you've done this step correctly, your heel will be slightly beyond the tip of the cane.
6. Next, move your weaker foot forward, so it's even with your stronger foot. Then move your cane in front of you about 4 inches.

Repeat these steps. As you proceed, remember to keep your head erect, shoulders back, and back straight. Your abdomen should be in, and your knees slightly flexed.

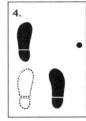

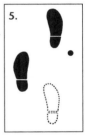

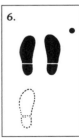

Teaching your patient how to use a walker

If the patient needs a walker, the doctor will order either a stationary or a reciprocal walker, depending on the patient's needs.

Types of walkers

A *stationary walker* is inexpensive, very stable, and usually lightweight. It consists of an adjustable metal frame with handgrips and four legs. Most stationary walkers have no movable parts, although some models are available with small front wheels. Some models also fold up for travel and easy storage.

Reciprocal walker

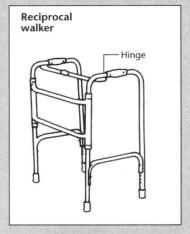

Hinge

Stationary walker

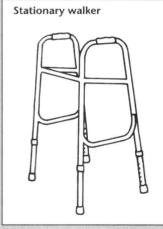

A *reciprocal walker* consists of a metal frame with handgrips, four legs, and a hinge mechanism that allows one side to be advanced ahead of the other. Its height is usually adjustable from 27" to 37" (69 to 94 cm), and some models fold up for storage and travel. The reciprocal walker is flexible and "walks" with the patient.

Familiarizing the patient with his walker

Advise the patient to put on the shoes he'll be wearing when he uses the walker. Then instruct him to stand up straight with his feet close together, relax his shoulders, and put the walker in front of and partially around him.

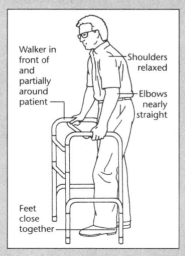

Walker in front of and partially around patient

Shoulders relaxed

Elbows nearly straight

Feet close together

Teaching your patient how to use a walker *(continued)*

Next, tell the patient to grasp the sides of the walker and look at the position of his elbows — they should be nearly straight. If they're not, instruct him to adjust the walker's height by pushing in the button on each of the walker's legs and sliding the tubing up or down as appropriate. Make sure that the button locks back into place and that the patient has adjusted the legs to the same height.

Now, instruct the patient to try the walker. He should be able to move it without bending over. If he still doesn't feel comfortable, help him to adjust the height again.

Coping with a fall

If the patient falls while using a walker, instruct him to first call for help before trying to get up. If no help is available, tell him to use the following method to help himself up.
1. Look around the room for a low, sturdy piece of furniture such as a coffee table. Inch backward toward the table by pushing your hands down on the floor and lifting your buttocks up. As you do this, pull the walker with one hand.
2. When you get to the table, place your walker near it. Then reach back and place both hands on the table top. Next, press down on the table

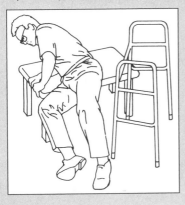

top and lift your buttocks onto the table.
3. Place the walker in front of you and raise yourself to a standing position by pushing your hands down on the handgrips.

Remind the patient that it's nor-

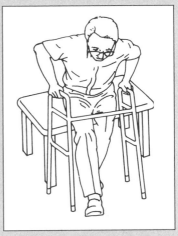

mal to feel a little dizzy when he first stands up. Advise him to take a moment to gain his balance before walking. If dizziness doesn't go away or seems excessive, he should lower himself back onto the table and call for help. Or, he may wish to sit for awhile before attempting to stand up.

Using a three-point gait

If the doctor recommends a three-point gait, instruct the patient to follow these steps for using this gait with his walker.

Moving the weaker leg

Place the walker slightly in front of you. Distribute most of your weight between your stronger leg (footstep shown in solid black) and the walker, but try to support some weight on your weaker leg as well. Now, shift

(continued)

Teaching your patient how to use a walker *(continued)*

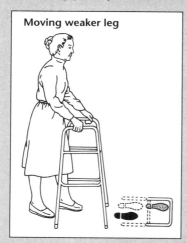

Moving weaker leg

all of your weight to your stronger leg while you lift and advance your weaker leg (patterned footstep) and the walker as far as 8" (20 cm).

Moving the stronger leg

Next, shift your weight to your weaker leg and the walker while you move your stronger leg as far as 8" (20 cm) forward.

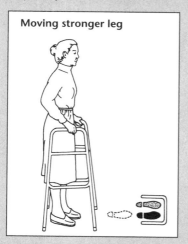

Moving stronger leg

Repeat these steps, moving first the walker and your weaker leg and then your stronger leg. Never attempt to put all of your weight on your weaker leg.

Sitting down and getting up with a walker

Provide the following directions to help your patient sit down in a chair and then stand up while using a walker.

Sitting down

1. Begin by choosing a sturdy armchair. Stand with your back to the chair and with the walker directly in front of you.

2. Place the back of your stronger leg against the seat of the chair. Carefully lift your weaker leg slightly off the floor. Now grasp the chair's armrest with the hand on your weak side. Shift your weight to your stronger leg and the hand grasping the armrest. Then grasp the other armrest with your free hand.

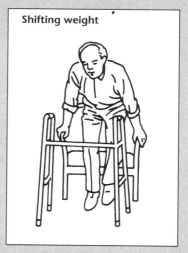

Shifting weight

Teaching your patient how to use a walker *(continued)*

3. Balancing yourself between both arms, gently lower yourself into the chair and slide backward. After you're seated, place the walker beside your chair.

Getting up
1. Pull the walker in front of you. Slide forward in the chair.
2. Place the back of your stronger leg against the seat. Then move your weaker leg forward. Now, placing both hands on the armrests,

push yourself to a standing position. Support your weight with your stronger leg and the opposite hand. Then grasp the walker's handgrip with your free hand.
3. Grasp the free handgrip with your other hand. Now, distribute your weight evenly between your hands and your stronger leg. Take a moment to get your balance. Steady yourself, take a deep breath, and you're off.

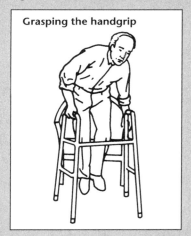

Grasping the handgrip

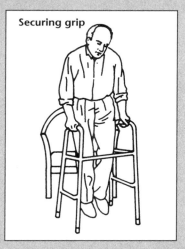

Securing grip

Also inform the family that the patient may be emotionally labile — crying or laughing at seemingly inappropriate times. Explain that he can't control these reactions.

Safety measures
Recommend installing grab bars near the toilet and bathtub, removing throw rugs, and securing carpets — or removing them entirely if the patient uses a walker or wheelchair. If the patient needs to use a cane, give him a copy of the patient teaching aid *Walking with a cane,* page 133. If he must use a walker, provide the in-

structions in *Teaching your patient how to use a walker,* which begins on page 134. If he has sensory losses, suggest lowering the water heater's temperature to prevent burns.

Establishing routines
To prevent confusing the patient who has difficulty generalizing, advise the family to follow a routine and minimize changes.

Other compensatory strategies
If the patient has a *one-sided deficit,* encourage him to bathe and dress the affected side first. Suggest calling at-

tention to that side with a watch or a ring. If the patient has *homonymous hemianopia,* tell him to scan his environment by carefully looking from side to side.

CVA prevention

Teach the patient and family about correcting risk factors for CVA. For example, if the patient smokes, refer him to a stop-smoking program. As appropriate, teach him to maintain his ideal weight; to follow his prescribed diet, exercises, and stress-reduction program; and to check with the doctor before taking any nonprescription drugs. If the patient is a woman of childbearing age, tell her to avoid using oral contraceptives.

Keep up the patient's and family's morale, which may flag if the patient's rehabilitative progress fluctuates. Remind them that response to CVA treatment varies among patients. Encourage them to contact a local support group and to obtain additional information from the local branch of one of the organizations listed in Appendix 2.

Finally, urge the patient to obtain a medical identification bracelet or necklace if he's taking anticoagulants or antiplatelet drugs.

Parkinson's disease

An estimated 1 million Americans — most of them over age 55 — suffer from Parkinson's disease. About 35,000 new cases are diagnosed each year. An effective teaching plan can help the patient retain control over his life for as long as possible. For instance, it can help him learn to perform daily activities despite motor deficits that disrupt coordination and movement.

To keep the patient active and independent, you'll need to emphasize the importance of complying with long-term drug therapy and supportive treatments, such as a diet and exercise program. As the patient's symptoms change, you'll need to modify your teaching to fit his needs.

Before teaching the patient about Parkinson's disease, make sure you are familiar with the following topics:
• explanation of the disease's progressive course
• diagnostic tests such as cerebrospinal fluid (CSF) analysis
• exercise program and precautions
• dietary modifications
• drug therapy
• surgery, if appropriate
• home safety modifications
• self-help aids for dressing and walking
• sources of information and support.

ABOUT THE DISORDER

Describe Parkinson's disease as a progressive, degenerative disorder of the central nervous system affecting the brain centers that regulate movement. Tell the patient that destruction of neurons in the substantia nigra leads to deficient production of dopamine and excessive production of acetylcholine — chemicals that relay messages across the nerve pathways. The dopamine deficiency involves the area of the brain responsible for control of voluntary muscle movements and posture. As a result, most symptoms relate to problems with posture and movement.

Discuss bradykinesia

Inform the patient that the characteristic signs — tremors, bradykinesia (slowness of movement), and rigidity (increased muscle tone) — usually have a gradual onset and may vary in severity from one patient to another. Point out that Parkinson's disease initially affects one side of the body but eventually involves both sides. Tremors begin in the fingers, increase during stress or anxiety, and subside with purposeful movement and sleep. Describe how bradykinesia changes the gait so that the body tilts forward while the arms remain at the sides (instead of swinging with walking). The patient may also notice muscle rigidity or widespread stiffness when performing any activity.

If the patient complains of other symptoms, such as oily skin, increased perspiration, insomnia, or mood changes, tell him that these are part of the disorder. As Parkinson's disease progresses, facial expressions become stiff and masklike and the patient stops blinking the eyes. He may drool because of difficulty in swallowing and in moving saliva to the back of the mouth. Typically, patients develop a stooped, forward-leaning, shuffling, propulsive gait with short, rapid, accelerating steps.

Provide a preview

Tell the patient that his speech may become slow and monotonous, with poor articulation. Forewarn him and his family that the disorder may lead to dementia, which may be indistinguishable from the mental deterioration seen in Alzheimer's disease. (See *Recognizing signs and symptoms of Parkinson's disease,* pages 140 and 141.)

Complications

Emphasize that noncompliance with drug therapy and other treatments can lead to poorly controlled signs and symptoms and, possibly, injury caused by postural and coordination difficulties. For instance, the patient with poorly controlled symptoms may be unable to stop and start walking; also, he may experience orthostatic hypotension, which may lead to falls.

Point out that failure to follow an exercise program may result in decreased mobility and such complications as pneumonia, pulmonary emboli, and urinary tract infections. Tell the patient that if he doesn't faithfully perform his facial exercises, difficulty swallowing may develop (or worsen), leading to weight loss and aspiration pneumonia. Also, lack of facial mobility may hamper communication, contributing to social isolation and depression.

Also discuss *parkinsonian crisis,* pointing out that this medical emergency causes a sudden and severe increase in bradykinesia, muscle rigidi-ty, and tremors. The patient may experience increases in his heart rate and respirations, fever, and muscle paralysis that impedes swallowing or compromises his airway. If Parkinson's disease results from encephalitis, the patient may experience *oculogyric crisis* — fixation of the eyes in one position, generally upward, for minutes or even hours.

DIAGNOSTIC WORKUP

Parkinson's disease has no specific test diagnoses and is diagnosed from clinical findings. However, the doctor may order a computed tomography scan or magnetic resonance imaging to rule out such abnormalities as tumors. The patient may also undergo positron emission tomography or single-photon-emission computed tomography. Tell the patient that these tests help detect tumors and disorders that alter cerebral metabolism. (See *Teaching patients about neurologic tests,* pages 117 to 125.)

More likely, though, the patient will undergo CSF analysis. The doctor also may order urinalysis to measure dopamine levels, which are reduced in Parkinson's disease. Cineradiographic swallowing studies may show an abnormal pattern and delayed relaxation of the cricopharyngeal muscles.

To help rule out disorders that mimic Parkinson's disease, the doctor may observe the patient's response to dopaminergic drugs. He also checks the patient's medication history for drugs that can cause parkinsonlike symptoms, such as haloperidol and phenothiazines; in Parkinson's disease, these symptoms won't subside when the drugs are discontinued.

TREATMENTS

Because Parkinson's disease has no cure, treatment aims to relieve signs and symptoms and keep the patient functional as long as possible. To achieve this goal, the patient must exercise daily, modify his diet, and take prescribed medications. Some patients may require surgery.

Recognizing signs and symptoms of Parkinson's disease

When a loved one develops Parkinson's disease, family members need to know what to expect. By describing what will happen at each stage of the disease, you may lessen their anxiety.

Early unilateral features
Explain that at first, the family may notice changes in the patient's posture, gait, facial expression, or speech. Early signs usually affect only one side of the body. A tremor in the arm — the most common sign — usually occurs at rest. Also, the patient may lean slightly toward the unaffected side.

Describe other early signs, including a blank facial expression and slight muscle rigidity that increases in resistance to passive muscle stretching. Muscle rigidity and tremors may also occur in the leg on the affected side, along with mild edema of the foot and ankle.

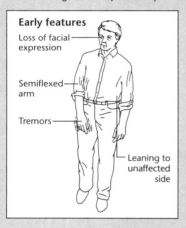

Early features
Loss of facial expression
Semiflexed arm
Tremors
Leaning to unaffected side

Later bilateral involvement
Explain that as signs of Parkinson's disease gradually spread from one side of the body to the other, the patient assumes a stooped posture. He may complain of fatigue and weakness as bradykinesia progressively affects all body movements. Gradually, his movements lose their spontaneity, becoming carefully executed. Eye blinking, arm swinging while walking, and expressive facial and hand gestures disappear. This

Activity guidelines
Inform the patient that moderate daily exercise can improve his mobility, help reduce the risk of contractures, promote respiration and circulation, aid bowel function, lessen muscle rigidity, and increase strength. If possible, encourage him to perform active range-of-motion (ROM) exercises. Otherwise, teach a caregiver how to perform passive ROM exercises. Instruct the patient to exercise when he feels rested and movement seems easiest, such as in the late morning or soon after taking medication.

Review specific exercises, using pictures when helpful. Provide a checklist to help structure an exercise routine. (See *Teaching patients how to do*

stretching exercises, pages 142 and 143.) Instruct the patient to start his program slowly and build up gradually. Enlist the family's help in encouraging him to exercise.

 WARNING: Caution the patient not to exercise excessively because fatigue will interfere with daily activities.

Dietary modifications
Teach the patient about the importance of maintaining a stable protein level. Explain that excessive dietary protein can affect the action of levodopa, an amino acid used to treat Parkinson's disease; insufficient protein, on the other hand, may cause nutritional imbalance.

loss of motor function may force the patient to stop working. Although still able to care for himself, he may become depressed and withdrawn.

During this period, encourage family members to include the patient in their activities to maintain his sense of value and belonging. To preserve independence, encourage them to allow the patient to do as much for himself as possible.

Gait problems and disability

Inform the patient and family that the hallmarks of the later stage include progressively pronounced gait disturbances. The patient walks more slowly in small, mincing steps and may unexpectedly find himself locked in a position, unable to move.

As his disability increases, he will need assistance for all activities of daily living. Although tremors may not worsen, muscle rigidity and bradykinesia will affect every aspect of his life, from getting out of bed in the morning to eating.

Eventually motionless and unable to stand, the patient will be left with

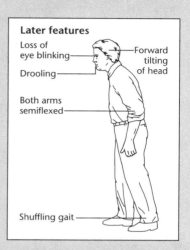

Later features

Loss of eye blinking

Drooling

Forward tilting of head

Both arms semiflexed

Shuffling gait

little remaining voluntary motor function. Bradykinesia will cause soft, monotonous speech, a masklike facial expression, and constant drooling. Neurogenic bladder and diminished thoracic excursion will leave the patient susceptible to infection.

Tell the patient to avoid caffeine, which may worsen his symptoms. Because his intestinal motility may decrease, advise him to drink adequate amounts of fluid and to eat more high-fiber foods, especially if he's troubled by constipation.

 TIPS AND TIMESAVERS: If the patient has difficulty chewing or swallowing, recommend semisoft foods (applesauce, mashed potatoes, solid foods prepared in a blender) to help ensure adequate nutrition and minimize the risk of aspiration.

To prevent choking, suggest freezing liquids to a slush or mixing them with other foods such as cereals. Instruct the patient to sit up straight,

move food to the back of his mouth, tilt his head slightly forward, and then swallow.

If the patient eats slowly, advise eating small, frequent meals. Instruct an obese patient in a weight-reduction diet. Explain that his weight affects his mobility and absorption of his medications.

Medication

Inform the patient that drug therapy aims to control his symptoms. The doctor may prescribe:
• levodopa or levodopa-carbidopa to replace the neurotransmitter dopamine
• anticholinergics, such as trihexyphenidyl or benztropine, and antihis-

Teaching patients how to do stretching exercises

The doctor may prescribe exercises to help your patient maintain flexibility and muscle strength. Tell him to do each exercise 1 to 5 times daily at first, and then to gradually increase to 10 to 20 times daily. If he's unable to do these exercises standing up, he can do most of them sitting down.

Facial muscle exercises
Instruct the patient to raise his eyebrows and then lower and squeeze them together. Next, tell him to open his eyes wide and then close them tight.

Now tell him to wrinkle his nose, and follow this by opening his mouth wide in a big "O" and then closing it tight. Instruct him to shift his jaw from side to side. Finally, tell him to give a big smile and then purse his lips as though trying to whistle. Instruct him to repeat the exercises.

Neck exercises
Have the patient begin by turning his head from side to side. Next, tell him to bend his head down and back. Instruct him to repeat the exercises.

Shoulder exercises
Tell the patient to raise his shoulders toward his ears as high as he can. Then tell him to lower them. Have him repeat this a few more times.

Arm and shoulder exercises
Tell the patient to raise his arms over his head. Then have him swing his arms down, extending them behind his back. Repeat.

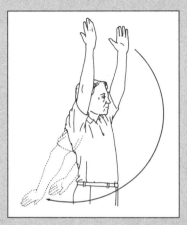

Trunk exercises
Instruct the patient to place his hands on his hips, and then twist his body at the waist from side to side, keeping his hips and legs in place. Repeat.

Hip and knee exercises
As the patient holds onto a counter or a sturdy piece of furniture, instruct him to raise his right knee toward his right shoulder. Then have him lower it and then raise his left knee toward his left shoulder.

tamines such as diphenhydramine to increase inhibition of central motor neurons
• bromocriptine, an ergot derivative, which acts as a dopamine agonist
• the antiviral agent amantadine, which promotes dopamine synthesis and release.

 WARNING: Caution the patient never to abruptly discontinue his medication.

Doing so may bring on a parkinsonian crisis, intensifying his symptoms.

Tell the patient that the doctor may increase the dosage as the disease progresses. However, emphasize that the patient must not increase medication dosages on his own because this may lead to drug toxicity.

Initially, drug therapy may cause nausea and vomiting. Reassure the patient that such reactions will disap-

Instruct him to lower the knee and repeat these movements.

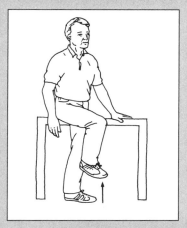

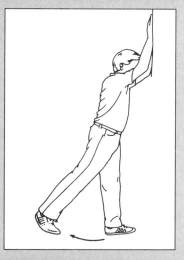

Next, have the patient stand facing a wall, about 8" (20 cm) away. Tell him to place his hands on the wall until they're above his head and then raise his right leg up behind him, keeping his knee straight. Instruct him to do the same with the left leg. Repeat.

Knee exercises

Have the patient sit and straighten his right knee, extending his right leg out in front of him. Then have him bend his right leg back under the chair as far as he can. (Tell him to keep his ankle flexed to avoid a muscle spasm.) Have him repeat

with the left leg. Tell him to perform this exercise several times.

Ankle and foot exercises

With the patient sitting, tell him to make circles with his right foot — first in one direction and then in the other. Have him repeat with the left foot. Tell him to do this a few more times.

Ankle and toe exercises

With the patient sitting, tell him to extend his leg and point his toes toward the floor. Then have him point them up toward his nose. Tell him to try this several more times.

pear in a few months. Suggest that he take medications after meals to decrease nausea.

If the patient has an intellectual impairment or memory difficulties, instruct him and his family to premeasure his medication doses for the day in separate containers, each marked with the scheduled administration time. If the patient has difficulty swallowing, suggest that he

crush pills or open capsules (unless he's taking an experimental sustained-release form of medication) and then mix the medication with a food that's easy to swallow, such as applesauce.

Surgery

If medication fails to relieve unilateral tremors, stereotaxic thalamotomy may be performed. Tell the patient who will undergo this surgery that first his head will be shaved and cleansed. Then a metal frame will be attached to his head to hold it still and to guide the surgeon.

Inform the patient that after he's given a local anesthetic, the surgeon will make a burr hole in his skull and create a surgical lesion in the thalamus on the side *opposite* the tremors. This lesion will block the transmission of nerve impulses that cause the tremors. To clarify the procedure, discuss how the right side of the brain controls the left side of the body, and vice versa.

Tell the patient that he'll experience some pressure and discomfort when the doctor applies the head frame. During surgery, he'll be asked to follow commands, such as raising an arm, and to answer questions as a test of memory and speech. Explain that he may have a headache after surgery, in part because of the prolonged immobility of his neck and shoulder muscles.

If your patient is scheduled for adrenal medullary autologous transplant (currently under research), follow your hospital's protocol for teaching him. The surgery involves removal of one of the adrenal glands (usually the left) and implantation of a section of the adrenal medulla into the brain tissue (usually the caudate nucleus). The patient must undergo both laparotomy and craniotomy.

Other care measures

Help the patient preserve his independence by teaching him how to adjust his daily activities to his current ability.

Enhancing mobility

Tell the patient that sitting in a chair that has arms will make it easier to obtain sufficient support. Elevating the back of a favorite chair by shortening the front legs 1" to 2" (2.5 to 5 cm) will make it easier to get up. Suggest tying a sheet to the foot of his bed to help the patient pull himself into a sitting position. Remind him to rise slowly to avoid orthostatic hypotension.

To help the patient maintain balance and forward momentum, instruct him to walk with a wide-based gait and to swing his arms. (See *Walking with a wide-based gait.*) If appropriate, show him how to use a weighted cane or a walker.

Also teach him how to unlock a position if he becomes temporarily fixed in it. Common unlocking techniques include turning the head, opening the mouth, placing an arm behind the back or across the chest, tapping a leg with the hand, bending the knees slightly, or raising the toes. Advise the patient to use these techniques cautiously to avoid losing his balance and falling.

To prevent falls, recommend removing throw rugs and unstable furniture and moving furniture against the walls to widen traffic paths. Also tell the patient to wear sturdy shoes with good support and traction.

Combating oily skin and increased perspiration

Explain to the patient the importance of daily bathing. Instruct him to avoid oil-based soaps or lotions, and tell him to use an antiperspirant deodorant on his hands if he has sweaty palms.

Dealing with urinary urgency

Tell the patient to remain near a bathroom or to keep a urinal nearby. If he has difficulty sitting and standing, suggest that he install a raised toilet seat and grab bars.

Making dressing easier

Advise the patient to wear clothing with zippers rather than buttons or to use Velcro strips. Loafer-style shoes or elastic shoelaces solve the problem of tying and untying shoes.

Coping with dysarthria

Instruct the patient to take his time pronouncing each word. If his voice is too soft, tell him to breathe deeply before beginning each sentence. Tell him that reading aloud (especially poetry) and singing can help his articulation, inflection, and voice projection.

Reducing stress
Teach the patient to explore a relaxation technique compatible with his lifestyle. Avoid recommending progressive muscle relaxation, which may increase rigidity and tremors. Simple techniques, such as deep breathing and visualization, can be used spontaneously throughout the day.

Teach a family member simple massage techniques to help reduce the patient's stress at the end of the day. Point out that stress may result from excessive intake of sugar and caffeine and from prolonged exposure to loud noise, bright lights, or extreme temperatures.

Teaching family members
Instruct the family to be alert for signs of depression in the patient, such as anorexia, insomnia, and disinterest in his surroundings. Tell them to encourage the patient's participation in family discussions, even though facial rigidity may cause him to look disinterested.

The emotional or financial crises brought on by the illness may severely strain family relationships. Encourage family members not to neglect themselves. Don't hesitate to suggest counseling, and encourage them to draw on community resources as well as family and friends. Refer both the patient and family to a local group or national organization for information and support. (See Appendix 2.)

Finally, urge the patient to wear a medical identification bracelet or necklace at all times.

Seizures
Seizures can take a significant toll on the patient and his family. Advances in electroencephalographic (EEG) monitoring and neuroimaging techniques have increased the number of patients undergoing new treatments for seizures, such as surgery and investigational drugs (gabapentin and lamotrigine).

Walking with a wide-based gait

Walking with a wide-based gait and swinging the arms will help your patient to maintain balance and keep moving forward. Instruct him to follow these step-by-step guidelines to practice this technique. Remind him to look ahead when walking and not at his feet.
1. Have the patient start by positioning his feet 8" to 10" (20 to 25 cm) apart. Tell him to stand as straight as he can.
2. Now instruct him to lift his foot high with his toes up, taking as large a step as possible.
3. As he brings his foot down, tell him to place his heel on the ground first and roll onto the ball of his foot and then his toes. Instruct him to perform the same steps with the other foot. Then have him repeat these movements.
4. Instruct the patient to swing his right arm forward when moving his left leg. Have him swing his left arm forward when moving his right leg.

Despite these advances, a cure for seizures remains elusive, and myths and misconceptions about seizures and epilepsy still abound. The patient's prospects of leading a productive life may hinge on successful teaching about seizure-triggering factors and the importance of strict compliance with long-term drug therapy. You'll need to point out that the patient's drug therapy may change, depending on his symptoms and other factors. What's more, you'll need to teach about possible activity restrictions, precautions for an imminent seizure, preparation for diagnostic tests, and, if appropriate, surgery.

Remember to include family members in your teaching. They'll need to know how to help the patient during a seizure and how to promote his pursuit of a normal life.

Before teaching a patient about seizures, make sure you are familiar with the following topics:
• how the brain's abnormal electrical activity leads to seizures
• the patient's specific type of seizure — generalized convulsive; generalized nonconvulsive; simple partial; complex partial; or partial, secondarily generalized
• diagnostic tests, such as EEG and computed tomography scans, to help determine the seizure's cause
• importance of diet in providing energy for normal neuron function
• drugs and their administration, including the risks of overmedication and undermedication
• preparation for craniotomy, if necessary
• trigger factors, including fatigue and hypoglycemia
• precautions to take for an imminent seizure
• how the family or other caregivers should manage a seizure
• importance of wearing a medical identification bracelet
• sources of information and support.

ABOUT THE DISORDER
Explain to the patient that a seizure is a sudden change in normal brain activity caused by an abnormal, uncontrolled electrical discharge from brain cells. The seizure results in distinctive changes in behavior and body function, which may take the form of alterations in sensation, behavior, movement, perception, or consciousness.

Tell the patient that some people experience a one-time seizure following an acute disorder of the central nervous system (for instance, a head injury) or as a result of fever, drug or alcohol withdrawal, or metabolic disturbances (such as a low blood glucose level). In contrast, the term *epilepsy* indicates a chronic condition characterized by recurrent seizures.

Inform the patient that the cause of seizures can't always be determined.

The site of the increased brain activity determines the patient's signs and symptoms.

Explain the patient's type of seizure: generalized convulsive; generalized nonconvulsive; simple partial; complex partial; or partial, secondarily generalized.

A *generalized convulsive* seizure such as a tonic-clonic (or grand mal) seizure involves the entire brain and, therefore, the entire body in convulsive activity. *Generalized nonconvulsive* seizures include atonic and absence (petit mal) seizures.

In a partial seizure, the abnormal activity occurs in one part of the brain. A *simple partial* seizure usually has one associated manifestation, such as a jerking motion of a leg. A *complex partial* seizure has more than one manifestation, such as a jerking motion of an arm and loss of consciousness. Some types of partial seizures may spread and become *secondarily generalized.*

Inform the patient that he may experience more than one type of seizure. Also tell him that during the initial seizure phase, he may notice an *aura* — a sensory phenomenon, such as seeing stars or smelling roses — but not every person who has a seizure experiences one.

Complications
Emphasize the need for strict adherence to the drug regimen to prevent overmedication or undermedication. Point out that overmedication may intensify adverse reactions, whereas undermedication can increase the duration, frequency, and number of seizures, making the risk of injury greater.

Inform the patient that complying with therapy may help him avoid *status epilepticus* — a state of continuous or rapidly recurring seizures in which the patient doesn't completely recover neurologic function between seizures. Point out that patients who don't comply with the medication regimen are most susceptible to this medical emergency. Status epilepticus can result in cerebral anoxia, aspiration, hyperthermia, exhaustion, serious injury (such as fractures), and even death.

DIAGNOSTIC WORKUP

Teach the patient about tests to help determine the underlying cause of his seizures, such as skull X-rays, EEG, closed-circuit television EEG, computed tomography scan, positron emission tomography scan, single-photon emission tomography scan, magnetic resonance imaging, cerebral blood flow studies, and Wada's (amobarbital) test. (See *Teaching patients about neurologic tests,* pages 117 to 125.)

If the patient has been taking anticonvulsant medications, tell him he will undergo periodic blood testing to monitor blood levels of the prescribed drug and detect any blood dyscrasias resulting from drug therapy.

If serum electrolyte tests are ordered, inform the patient that these tests can rule out metabolic disorders associated with seizures, such as hypoglycemia and hypocalcemia.

TREATMENTS

Emphasize strict compliance with the anticonvulsant drug regimen to control seizures. Also explain the significance of a balanced diet and regular meals in preventing seizures. If necessary, prepare the patient for a craniotomy. Explain its purpose, what happens during surgery, and preoperative and postoperative care. Be sure to educate the patient and his family about seizure triggers and what to do if a seizure occurs.

Dietary modifications

Instruct the patient to eat regular meals and to check with the doctor before dieting. Point out that maintaining adequate blood glucose levels provides the necessary energy for neurons to work normally. Dieting or skipping meals may lead to decreased glucose levels (hypoglycemia). This can cause unstable neurons to malfunction, triggering a seizure. Teach the patient to recognize the signs and

symptoms of hypoglycemia, so he can eat a snack when needed.

Medication

Many doctors prefer *monotherapy* — use of a single medication — in the medical management of epilepsy. Such therapy minimizes potential drug interactions and limits adverse reactions. It also promotes compliance through its simplicity, and is cheaper than multidrug therapy.

Make sure the patient understands that anticonvulsant drugs can't cure seizures, but they will control them. Advise him to take the medication exactly as ordered — both undermedication and overmedication can cause seizures. Explain that the doctor will regulate drug dosage according to blood drug levels, so the dosage may periodically change (for example, with age or illness).

 WARNING: If illness prevents the patient from taking his oral medication, tell a family member or other caregiver to contact the doctor immediately. The doctor may decide to administer medication by another route.

Tell the patient what to do if he misses a dose. However, caution him not to apply missed dose instructions for an anticonvulsant drug to any other drug he is taking (because instructions vary with each drug's half-life). Forewarn him that he may have withdrawal seizures if he abruptly stops taking his anticonvulsant medication.

Explain to the patient that he'll be taking medication as long as the doctor determines he's at risk for seizures. Even if the patient has a prolonged seizure-free period, he must never stop taking an anticonvulsant without the doctor's supervision. The length of time the patient will need such medication (a few years or for life) depends on many factors, such as the cause of seizures and the patient's response to treatment.

Surgery

A patient with disabling, medically intractable epilepsy may be a candidate for surgical intervention. Inform

Guidelines for preventing seizures

If your patient has epilepsy, teach him how to control the factors that can trigger a seizure. Here are some suggestions:

● Instruct the patient to take the *exact* dose of medication at the times prescribed. Missing doses, doubling doses, or taking extra doses can cause a seizure.

● Supply information on balanced, regular meals, and stress the importance of good nutrition. Explain that low blood glucose levels (hypoglycemia) and inadequate vitamin intake can lead to seizures.

● Caution the patient to limit alcohol intake. Alcohol can reduce the seizure threshold and should not be consumed without the doctor's approval.

● Urge the patient to get enough sleep. Excessive fatigue can bring on a seizure.

● Tell the patient to treat a fever early during an illness and to avoid hyperthermia because it may lead to seizures.

● Teach the patient to stay alert for odors that may trigger an attack. Advise him and his family to note any strong odors occurring at the time of a seizure and to report these to the doctor.

● Help the patient learn how to control stress. If appropriate, suggest relaxation techniques, such as deep-breathing exercises.

● Tell the patient to avoid factors known to trigger seizures in some patients — for example, flashing lights, hyperventilation, loud noises, heavy musical beats, video games, and television.

the patient that the most common curative surgery is a temporal lobectomy, which removes the part of the brain where seizures originate without causing neurologic or cognitive deficits.

If the patient will undergo extratemporal resection in the frontal, parietal, or occipital lobes, inform him that this procedure will remove the seizure-producing focus of the brain without causing neurologic deficits. If he will undergo a corpus callosotomy, tell him this surgery will prevent the spread of the epileptic discharge from one brain hemisphere to the other.

Other care measures
Encourage the patient to try to identify factors that trigger his seizures. (See *Guidelines for preventing seizures.*) Also, tell the patient that he may experience seizures even if he takes anticonvulsants as prescribed.

Safety measures
Encourage the patient to pursue normal activities if possible — but remind him of safety considerations. Tell him

what to do if he suspects a seizure is coming on. Also make sure the family knows what to do if a seizure occurs. (See *Helping a seizure victim.*) If the patient is a child, instruct the parents to notify day care or school authorities of their child's condition. Also stress the importance of the patient wearing a medical identification bracelet or necklace at all times.

Point out that, in many states, patients with uncontrolled seizures are not permitted to drive a motor vehicle. Even though this may cause the patient to feel stigmatized and dependent, stress the serious consequences of violating laws designed to protect the patient and others in the community. Provide information on community services that offer alternative methods of transportation.

Psychosocial support
Patients with epilepsy commonly confront psychosocial challenges that can be as debilitating as the medical condition. The unpredictability of seizures can create problems at home,

Helping a seizure victim

A person with epilepsy may have a seizure at any time, in any place. During a seizure, he may lose consciousness and fall down. To prepare the family to help, provide them with the following instructions.

During the seizure

Tell the family to turn the patient on his side and remove hard or sharp objects from the area. They should loosen restrictive clothing, such as a collar or a belt, and place something soft and flat under the patient's head.

Remind them *never* to force anything into the patient's mouth, especially fingers. Advise them to ask onlookers to leave the area. If family members suspect that the patient

has swallowed his own vomit, they should call a doctor immediately.

After the seizure

Advise the family to allow the patient to lie quietly. As he awakens, they should gently call him by name, and reorient him to his surroundings and to recent events.

If the patient has an injury, such as a badly bleeding tongue, he should be taken to the doctor's office or to a hospital emergency department.

Urge a family member to write an accurate description of the seizure as soon as possible. The doctor may request certain information, including the seizure's duration and the patient's activity immediately before, during, and after the seizure.

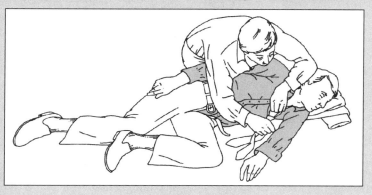

at work, or in interpersonal relationships.

Encourage the patient's family to provide emotional support to help the patient adjust to epilepsy without making him feel dependent. Refer the patient and family to appropriate associations for support and information. (See Appendix 2.)

Traumatic brain injury

Approximately 1 million Americans a year suffer traumatic brain injury. About 50,000 of them die, and another 100,000 sustain irreversible brain damage. Victims — a large percentage of whom are males ages 15 to 30 who were drinking alcohol around the time of injury — may require multiple high-tech interventions. Although these advanced diagnostic and treatment measures have improved survival rates and reduced disabilities, the patient may still face a long and difficult recovery.

Your teaching about traumatic brain injury may range from simple to involved. For example, the patient with a mild concussion may need only a few home care instructions. In contrast, after a severe head injury, all aspects of the patient's life may change. You'll be challenged to provide teaching that encompasses the care of many body systems. What's more, a patient's response to treatment is unpredictable — and sometimes unfavorable.

Begin your teaching by explaining the patient's injury and the diagnostic workup. If the patient is severely compromised and unable to communicate, you'll focus your teaching on his family. When the patient's condition stabilizes, you'll address such treatment measures as activity and dietary guidelines, medications, and procedures to monitor and reduce increased intracranial pressure (ICP). If the patient has a moderate to severe head injury, you'll also need to teach him and his family about rehabilitation and long-term care.

Before teaching a patient about traumatic brain injury, make sure you are familiar with the following topics:
• explanation of traumatic brain injuries and their classification
• diagnostic tests, such as computed tomography (CT) scan, magnetic resonance imaging (MRI), evoked potential studies, and neuropsychological testing
• complications, such as hypoxia and increased ICP
• activity restrictions
• dietary modifications, including fluid restrictions and semisoft foods for dysphagia
• prescribed medications to reduce ICP or prevent seizures
• preparation for such procedures as ICP monitoring or barbiturate coma
• explanation of craniotomy, if necessary

• importance of rehabilitation in minimizing neurologic deficits; need for family involvement in rehabilitation
• other care measures, such as adapting to neurologic deficits, home safety tips, and postconcussion instructions
• sources of information and support.

ABOUT THE DISORDER
Explain to the patient or his family that a traumatic brain injury is a traumatic insult to the skull and brain — not a distinct disease process. Point out that such an injury can cause varying degrees of damage to the skull and the brain. Primary injuries — those occurring at the time of impact — include skull fractures, concussion, contusion, scalp laceration, brain tissue laceration, and tear or rupture of cerebral vessels.

Inform the patient or his family that most traumatic brain injuries result from trauma that causes the head's momentum to stop suddenly, flinging the brain against the inside of the skull (*coup injury*), or that causes the brain to rebound, striking the opposite wall of the skull (*contrecoup injury*).

Point out that signs and symptoms depend on which brain areas were injured. Using simple terms, discuss brain structure and function, correlating the patient's dysfunctions with injury to specific brain areas.

Next, discuss the patient's injury type and classification. (See *Classifying traumatic brain injuries.*) If necessary, clarify the doctor's explanation of the patient's injury and discuss its implications. Be sure to point out that a patient with a severe head injury but no other apparent visible trauma may present a misleading picture to others. For instance, family members may remark, "He just looks like he's sleeping." If the patient is elderly, emphasize that the effects of a brain injury may be confused with those of normal aging.

Complications
Inform the patient or family that a brain injury raises the body's metabolic rate, increasing the oxygen needs of all body organs. Without

INSIGHT INTO ILLNESSES

Classifying traumatic brain injuries

Tell the patient and his family that health care professionals can classify traumatic brain injuries in several different ways. Explain that classification may be based on:

• severity of injury (mild, moderate, severe)
• skull integrity (open or closed)
• type of injury (concussion, contusion, laceration)
• mechanism of injury (direct impact, acceleration, deceleration).

An *acceleration injury* results from impact with a moving force, such as a baseball bat. In a *deceleration injury,* the head hits an immovable object such as a dashboard.

As shown in the illustrations below, head injury may also be classified by cerebral involvement — focal or diffuse.

Focal brain injury

If the patient has a focal brain injury, inform him that cerebral damage, which usually results from direct impact, is well delineated.

Examples of focal head injuries include hematomas, contusions, and skull fractures.

Focal injuries can cause permanent deficits. However, the risk for complications may be decreased if the patient's injury (for example, from a skull fracture) also falls in the open-skull category because an open skull accommodates cerebral swelling.

Diffuse brain injury

In a diffuse brain injury, many brain areas are damaged. Typical causes of this type of injury include an indirect blow to the head or a combination of direct and indirect impact. Examples include concussions and diffuse axonal injuries, in which axons tear as the brain jostles against the skull.

Diffuse injuries are associated with closed head injuries and rarely cause outward signs of trauma. However, generalized swelling and increased intracranial pressure may occur inside the skull.

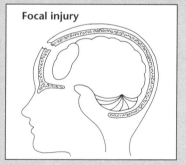

Focal injury

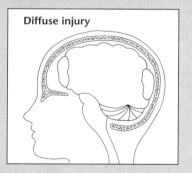

Diffuse injury

supportive treatment, hypoxia may develop, causing further brain damage, permanent disability, and even death. Other possible complications include systemic hypotension, hyper-

capnia, sustained increased ICP, cerebral edema, respiratory problems, and infection.

Add that head trauma can cause diabetes insipidus and syndrome of inappropriate antidiuretic hormone. Explain that these complications affect the entire body by disrupting fluid and electrolyte balance.

For patients who need prolonged convalescence, review common complications of immobility: contractures, pressure sores, pneumonia, and atelectasis.

DIAGNOSTIC WORKUP

Help prepare the patient for several phases of tests — first to evaluate his injury and later to measure his recovery. Baseline studies may include X-rays of the skull and cervical spine, CT scans and, possibly, MRI and evoked potential studies. (See *Teaching patients about neurologic tests,* pages 117 to 125.)

Explain that diagnostic tests help determine the extent of the patient's injury. Mention that neuropsychological testing may be ordered once the patient's condition stabilizes.

TREATMENTS

Discuss the treatment plan with the patient and his family. Instruct them about physical rehabilitation, dietary measures, and drug regimens. If necessary, teach them about cranial surgery or such procedures as ICP monitoring. Review other care measures to help compensate for neurologic deficits.

Briefly describe methods, such as mechanical ventilation, steroid therapy, careful maintenance of fluid balance, and barbiturate administration, that may be used to treat brain swelling, increased metabolic demands, and increased ICP.

Activity guidelines

Inform the patient or family that his activity level depends on his condition. If he's unstable and seriously impaired, his activities may be limited to turning and range-of-motion (ROM) exercises. Teach his family turning and repositioning techniques and passive ROM exercises. Explain that these exercises help to prevent muscle atrophy and provide the

brain with important information about the patient's position. Also teach the caregiver about providing appropriate stimuli and maintaining a safe environment.

If the patient is paralyzed, teach the family how to position him to maintain proper body alignment and prevent musculoskeletal problems.

If the patient is allowed out of bed, prepare him for some initial discomfort. Reassure him that physical activity will help him sleep better and prevent pulmonary complications. Mention that brain injury can interfere with the brain's sleep-control center, and that physical activity will enhance normal sleep.

When the patient is able to sit in a chair or ambulate, show the family the proper transfer and ambulation techniques. Stress the importance of proper body mechanics to prevent patient falls and injury to the caregiver.

If the doctor orders physical therapy, reinforce the program's principles and instructions. Motivate the patient to work hard in physical therapy, reminding him that all efforts will pay off in increasing strength and motor control.

Dietary modifications

Point out that a brain injury induces a hypermetabolic state that depletes the body's glycogen and protein stores. This condition can induce muscle wasting because the muscles are used as an energy source. To help counteract this state, emphasize the importance of a high-calorie, protein-rich diet. Reinforce the dietitian's instructions.

Advise the patient to sit upright and tilt his head slightly forward when eating. If he has dysphagia or facial weakness on one side, recommend that he eat semisoft foods and chew on the unaffected side of his mouth. Suggest preparing solid foods in a blender and freezing liquids to a slush or mixing them with other foods.

Tips and timesavers: If appropriate, teach the patient how to use feeding aids such as utensils with built-up handles.

A patient with a severe brain injury may be unable to eat. Explain to the family that nutrition will be provided intravenously by total parenteral nutrition or by tube feeding through a nasogastric or gastrostomy tube. If one of these feeding methods will continue at home, instruct caregivers on its use.

The patient with high ICP may have to restrict fluid intake. Teach the patient or family how to measure and record how much fluid he takes in and how much he eliminates.

Medication
If the patient's condition is critical, teach the family about drugs used to control symptoms and prevent complications. Explain that the patient may receive high doses of a glucocorticoid, such as dexamethasone or methylprednisolone, to reduce brain swelling, stabilize cerebral blood flow, and restore autoregulation.

If the patient has increasing ICP, the doctor may order an osmotic diuretic such as mannitol. Explain that this I.V. medication helps to reduce ICP by moving fluid out of the cells and into the vascular system, where it can be eliminated as urine. Mannitol begins to reduce ICP in 10 to 15 minutes; its effects last 2 to 6 hours.

For the patient with a moderate to severe brain injury, explain that brain injury can reduce the brain's seizure threshold, causing potentially serious complications. Discuss anticonvulsants, if ordered. Explain that a common anticonvulsant such as phenytoin may prevent seizures.

Procedures
If appropriate, teach the patient and family about ICP monitoring to detect early signs of increased ICP, a potentially dangerous complication. If the patient requires barbiturate coma to treat increased ICP, help prepare him for this procedure.

ICP monitoring
Tell the patient and family that this procedure measures the pressure exerted by brain tissue, blood, and cerebrospinal fluid (CSF) against the skull. Explain that monitoring can detect small increases in ICP before clinical danger signs develop.

Describe which of the three types of monitoring the patient will undergo. In *ventricular catheter monitoring,* a small polyethylene catheter is inserted into the lateral ventricle. In *subarachnoid screw monitoring,* an ICP screw and transducer wick is introduced into the subarachnoid space. In *epidural sensor monitoring* — the least invasive method — a fiberoptic sensor is placed in the epidural space. In all three procedures, pressure readings appear on a display monitor or chart recorder.

Clarify measures the doctor may order to reduce ICP — typically medication adjustments or decreased fluid intake. Or he may attach a catheter to the monitoring device to drain excess CSF, thereby decreasing pressure.

Barbiturate coma
If the patient has a sustained increase in ICP that can't be corrected by conventional treatments, the doctor may order a barbiturate coma. If the patient's deteriorating condition limits communication, inform the family that the procedure reduces the patient's metabolic rate and cerebral blood flow, which helps to reduce increased ICP.

Tell the family that the patient will receive a loading dose of a barbiturate, then a continuous I.V. infusion of the drug. Warn them that the patient will be unresponsive once the coma is induced. He must be placed on a respirator (if this has not already been implemented) and will be carefully watched for resultant changes in blood pressure, loss of muscle tone, and effectiveness of therapy.

Reassure the family that a barbiturate coma includes careful monitoring and necessary supportive care. Inform them that the doctor will discontinue this therapy as soon as appropriate.

Surgery

If necessary, help prepare the patient for cranial surgery. Explain that a craniotomy involves creating a surgical incision in the skull, exposing the brain for many possible treatments. Alternatively, the neurosurgeon may drill a burr hole into the patient's skull, and then aspirate an epidural hematoma with a fluid clot.

Review preoperative procedures. Tell the patient that his hair will be washed with an antimicrobial shampoo the night before surgery. In the operating room, his head will be shaved and he'll receive a general anesthetic.

Also prepare the patient for postoperative recovery. Tell him that he'll awaken from surgery with his head bandaged to protect the incision or burr hole.

 WARNING: Caution the patient to avoid coughing after surgery because it may cause increased ICP.

Other care measures

Involve both the patient and family in supporting recovery. Before a patient with a concussion is discharged, make sure he has a responsible adult accompanying him. List signs and symptoms that call for medical attention, and review whom to call if his condition worsens. Provide other instructions on postconcussion care. (See *Caring for a patient after a concussion.*)

After a serious brain injury resulting in permanent neurologic deficits, prepare the patient and his family for a lengthy recovery. Help them to cope by explaining proposed rehabilitation programs.

Coping with speech and visual deficits

If the patient has a speech deficit, help him to communicate in other ways, such as writing or using a picture board. Instruct the family to speak slowly to him in normal tones. Recommend that they use gestures to clarify their message if the patient has receptive aphasia. Advise them to give the patient short, simple directions, cues, and lists.

If the patient has a vision deficit, show him how to scan the environment. Teach family members how to approach the patient to avoid startling him. For example, if he has lost peripheral vision, advise family members to approach him from the front, not the side. Demonstrate how to set up meal trays and a living environment for optimal visualization. To prevent injuries, recommend maintaining adequate lighting.

TIPS AND TIMESAVERS: Tell the family that use of contrasting colors in the home, such as dark carpeting and light walls, can enhance the patient's visual functioning.

Managing cognitive deficits

Explain that cognitive deficits may become more evident as the patient spends more time at home. However, reassure the patient and family that cognitive deficits don't constitute an emergency — although they may hinder his ability to work and alter his socialization skills. Help the family appreciate that the patient isn't being lazy or manipulative; rather, he isn't capable yet of performing in any other way.

Warn the family that the patient may overestimate his abilities, claiming that he can perform tasks (for example, drive a car) that in fact he cannot. Discuss ways to monitor the patient's abilities without frustrating efforts toward independence. Suggest that they allow him to try most activities — short of those that could injure him or others or could cause excessive frustration or fatigue.

Forewarn the patient and his family or other caregivers that he may be emotionally labile, crying or laughing at seemingly inappropriate times. Explain that the patient can't control these reactions.

Caring for a patient after a concussion

Although a concussion is a relatively mild brain injury, it can temporarily disrupt normal activities. The patient can continue recovering at home — as long as a family member or other caregiver watches him for the next 24 hours and calls for medical help if necessary. Here are some guidelines the caregiver must follow.

Observing the patient

Instruct the caregiver to set an alarm clock to wake the patient every 2 hours during the first night at home. Tell him to ask the patient his name, where he is, and whether he can identify the caregiver. If the patient doesn't wake up or can't answer the caregiver's questions, he should be taken to the hospital right away.

Reviewing medical instructions

Emphasize that the patient must take it easy and return gradually to his usual activities during the first 48 hours after discharge. He should avoid medicine stronger than acetaminophen (Tylenol) for a headache. He should also avoid aspirin, because it can intensify any bleeding caused by the injury. Suggest that the patient try relieving a headache by lying down but raising the head slightly with pillows.

Also, the patient should eat lightly, especially if nausea or vomiting occurs. (Occasional vomiting isn't unusual, but it should subside in a few days.)

Getting medical help

Instruct the caregiver to call the doctor or return to the hospital at once if the patient experiences:
- increasing irritability or personality changes
- increasing sluggishness
- confusion
- seizures
- persistent or severe headache, unrelieved by acetaminophen
- forceful or constant vomiting
- blurred vision
- abnormal eye movements
- staggering gait.

Recognizing delayed symptoms

Although the patient may feel fine in a few days, new symptoms may emerge later. Called *postconcussion syndrome,* these symptoms may occur up to a year after the injury.

Tell the caregiver and the patient to watch for:
- headache that gets worse with emotional stress or physical activity
- lack of usual energy
- occasional double vision
- dizziness, giddiness, or light-headedness
- memory loss
- emotional changes (feeling irritable or easily upset, especially in crowds)
- feelings of tension and nervousness
- difficulty concentrating
- reduced sex drive
- easy intoxication by alcohol
- loss of inhibitions
- difficulty relating to others
- noise intolerance.

These symptoms should subside. If they get worse or last longer than 3 months, the patient should seek medical advice.

Using mechanical assistance

If the patient needs a walker or a cane, reinforce his efforts to use these devices safely. For safety's sake, recommend installing grab bars near the toilet and bathtub, removing throw rugs, and securing carpets. If the patient has sensory losses, suggest lowering the water heater's temperature to prevent burns.

If the patient's injury impairs his cough reflex, show caregivers how to perform oral suction. Inform them that this will make the patient more comfortable and will help keep him from gagging on his own secretions.

If the patient experiences hypertonic movements after head trauma, discuss any splints and serial casts that may help him maintain a functional position.

Providing psychosocial support

Help the family to recognize that, like the patient himself, they may have feelings of fear, hopelessness, and loss of control. Encourage them to express their feelings. To ensure a therapeutic environment, clarify any confusing care measures. Refer them to appropriate sources of information and support. (See Appendix 2.)

6

Musculoskeletal conditions

Carpal tunnel syndrome

A serious occupational health problem, carpal tunnel syndrome affects people who use their hands repetitively and strenuously. Occupations of those affected range from homemakers and computer operators to assembly line workers, meat cutters, machinists, mechanics, and carpenters.

Your teaching must emphasize that recovery depends on compliance with treatment. You'll need to pinpoint activities that trigger or worsen the disorder and then suggest ways to avoid or modify them. You'll also review medications that reduce pain and inflammation, immobilization devices, surgery, and strengthening exercises.

Before teaching a patient with carpal tunnel syndrome, make sure you are familiar with the following topics:
• anatomy and function of the median nerve and carpal tunnel
• relationship between repetitive wrist activity and carpal tunnel syndrome
• diagnosis, including physical examination and electrophysiologic studies
• how to alter work habits and modify the workplace to reduce symptoms
• how to use protective gloves and splints
• strengthening and stretching exercises for the wrist, hand, and fingers
• medications such as nonsteroidal anti-inflammatory drugs (NSAIDs)
• surgery to relieve carpal tunnel syndrome, if appropriate
• care tips for patients with contributing systemic disorders
• sources of information and support.

ABOUT THE DISORDER

Explain to the patient that carpal tunnel syndrome occurs when the median nerve is compressed where it passes through the carpal tunnel. (See *Locating the carpal tunnel*, page 158.) Inform him that the median nerve controls many movements in the forearm, wrist, and hand, such as turning the wrist toward the body and flexing the index, middle, and ring fingers. Compression of this nerve causes loss of movement and sensation in the wrist and fingers.

Point out that the exact cause of carpal tunnel syndrome is unknown. However, occupations that require rapid, repetitive wrist motions involving excessive wrist flexion or extension predispose a person to this condition. Other suspected risk factors include vitamin B_6 deficiency and edema-causing conditions, such as diabetes, rheumatoid arthritis, pregnancy, renal failure, heart failure, and premenstrual fluid retention.

Review possible symptoms, which include weakness, burning, pain, numbness, or tingling in one or both hands. In severe cases, the patient also experiences:
• paresthesia of the thumb, index, and middle fingers and half of the ring finger
• inability to make a fist
• atrophy of the fingernails
• dry, shiny skin on the hands and fingers.

Vasodilation and venous stasis may cause some signs and symptoms to intensify at night and in the morning. The patient may be able to relieve discomfort by vigorously shaking or dangling his arms at his sides.

INSIGHT INTO ILLNESSES

Locating the carpal tunnel

Give your patient a brief anatomy lesson by showing him the tunnel made by the transverse ligament in this cross section of a right hand.

Also show him where the median nerve and the flexor tendons pass through the tunnel at the wrist to innervate the fingers and the hand. Demonstrate how he can press the nerve to produce the symptoms known as carpal tunnel syndrome.

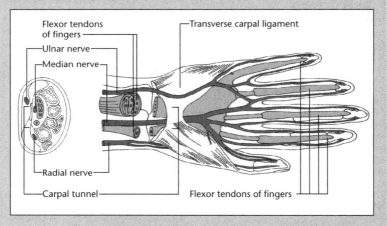

Flexor tendons of fingers — Transverse carpal ligament
Ulnar nerve
Median nerve
Radial nerve
Carpal tunnel — Flexor tendons of fingers

Complications

Emphasize that continued overuse of the affected wrist will increase tendon inflammation, compression, and neural ischemia. Wrist function will then continue to decline and, if left untreated, the patient may experience permanent nerve damage with movement and sensation losses.

DIAGNOSTIC WORKUP

Inform the patient that a physical examination and health history are necessary to diagnose carpal tunnel syndrome. During the physical examination, the doctor may perform Phalen's test and check for Tinel's sign to help gauge the severity of signs and symptoms. To confirm the condition, the doctor may order electrophysiologic tests.

Electrophysiologic tests

Tell the patient that these nerve stimulation procedures use electrical current in amounts too small to be harmful. Reassure him that these tests aren't painful, although they may feel uncomfortable or strange. Explain that before testing begins, a technician may ask about the patient's signs and symptoms.

If the patient is having a *digital electrical stimulation test*, tell him that this test confirms carpal tunnel syndrome. The technician will place electrodes around the index and middle fingers to stimulate the fingers electrically, and will attach an electrode over the median nerve in the wrist to record nerve stimulation. If the median nerve is compressed, the stimulating current will take longer than usual to travel from the fingers to the wrist, or the stimulation may be weak, depending on the degree of compression.

Explain that in the *motor function test* of the median nerve, the technician places stimulating electrodes over the median nerve at the wrist and recording electrodes over the thumb and directly below the thumb on the inside of the hand. The technician then watches for thumb movements. Delayed movement usually signals median nerve compression and carpal tunnel syndrome.

Tell the patient that in *electromyography*, the technician will insert very fine needles into the wrist and thumb to check for irritability (spontaneous electrical activity) of the hand muscles innervated by the median nerve.

TREATMENTS
If the patient's symptoms have been present only for a short time, if they suggest mild carpal tunnel syndrome, or if they're expected to subside on their own (for example, after pregnancy), treatment may begin with conservative measures, such as activity restrictions, rest, massage, immobilization, and medication. These measures help prevent further discomfort and compression of the median nerve.

If symptoms persist, affect both wrists, or cause severe discomfort and disability, the doctor may recommend surgery.

Activity guidelines
Teach the patient that resting the affected wrist or wrists can relieve symptoms of carpal tunnel syndrome. Help him identify the activities that aggravate or trigger his symptoms. Then advise him to eliminate or modify these activities. If he can't eliminate a precipitating activity, suggest that he try slowing his pace and decreasing the activity. Emphasize that rest can relieve only the immediate symptoms; it can't cure the underlying problem. Point out that resuming the activity will cause continued symptoms and damage.

Immobilization
Encourage the patient to use an immobilization device, such as a glove or a splint, if recommended by the doctor. Explain that the device will decrease inflammation, compression, and discomfort. Remind the patient to wear the device continuously (even during sleep, if necessary) as long as he has symptoms.

If the patient will use a splint, review the exercise program that complements splinting therapy. Review the exercises that will help him maintain joint motion, prevent wrist stiffness, and preserve the function and strength of muscles not affected by the wrist movement. (See *Exercises for patients with carpal tunnel syndrome,* page 160.)

Medication
Tell the patient that the drugs most commonly prescribed to treat carpal tunnel syndrome are NSAIDs taken orally and corticosteroids given by injection into the carpal tunnel tendons. If the doctor suspects a vitamin B_6 deficiency, he may also prescribe pyridoxine.

NSAIDs
If the drug regimen includes an NSAID, explain that this drug helps to control pain and reduce inflammation. Instruct the patient to take the medication exactly as prescribed. Caution him that it may take 2 to 4 weeks to reach maximal effectiveness. If the drug regimen includes indomethacin (Indocin), mefenamic acid (Ponstel), phenylbutazone (Butazolidin), or piroxicam (Feldene), advise him to take these medications with food or antacids to avoid stomach upset.

 WARNING: Advise a pregnant patient to avoid all NSAIDs because they may cause dystocia and bleeding complications during delivery.

Corticosteroids
After administering a local anesthetic, the doctor may inject a steroid

Exercises for patients with carpal tunnel syndrome

If the patient must limit his hand motions to relieve carpal tunnel syndrome, he'll need to exercise his wrist, hand, fingers, and thumb daily to maintain muscle tone. The doctor, nurse, or physical therapist will show him how to support, control, and move his hand correctly. Urge him to do his exercises with the affected hand and, if needed, with the other hand. Provide the instructions below.

Wrist and hand exercises

1. Tell the patient to extend his arm (palm down, fingers straight) keeping his palm flat. Then have him slowly raise his fingers as far as they'll comfortably go without flexing his wrist. Now instruct him to slowly lower his fingers as far downward as they'll comfortably go.

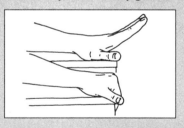

2. With his arm still in the extended position, tell him to wave or rock his hand from side to side and then gently twist his hand from side to side. Next, have him move his hand

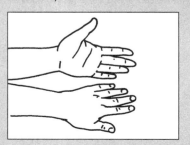

in small circles, first in one direction and then in the opposite direction.

Finger and thumb exercises

1. With a rubber band around the patient's fingers for mild resistance, tell him to spread his fingers as far apart as possible. Then instruct him to bring them back together and make a fist.

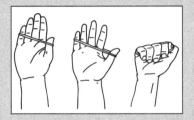

2. Tell the patient to hold up his hand and touch his little finger and thumb together. Have him repeat this movement, touching his other three fingers to his thumb.

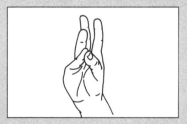

3. Finally, instruct the patient to bend all his fingers up and down, as though waving goodbye.

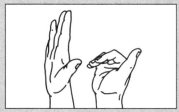

preparation to reduce inflammation. Tell the patient that this will bring almost immediate pain relief, but point out that the relief is temporary.

Pyridoxine
Explain to the patient with vitamin B_6 deficiency that he'll take pyridoxine daily for at least 3 weeks; then the doctor will reevaluate his status. Instruct him to store the drug in a dark bottle protected from light. During pyridoxine therapy, urge him to follow a nutritious diet that includes yeast, wheat germ, liver, whole grain breads and cereals, bananas, and legumes — all good sources of B_6.

Surgery
If the patient's condition doesn't improve after about 6 months of unsuccessful conservative treatment, or if he experiences objective neurologic changes in the hand, surgical decompression of the median nerve at the carpal tunnel is necessary.

Tell the patient scheduled for this surgery that his hand will be immobilized and, with his palm up, a tourniquet will be applied to prevent blood circulation in the surgical field. Once the surgeon has isolated the transverse carpal ligament, the ligament will be transected, the incision closed, and a dressing applied.

Review the postoperative care outlined by the surgeon, which will include appropriate pain management, dressing care, and elevating the hand. Alert him to the signs and symptoms of infection — redness, warmth, swelling, or pus at the incision site — and instruct him to call the doctor immediately if these occur.

Other care measures
Because an underlying systemic condition (such as obesity, pregnancy, diabetes, leukemia, renal disease, or Raynaud's syndrome) can worsen carpal tunnel syndrome, review the patient's history carefully to assess his learning needs. For example, encourage an overweight patient to begin a nutritionally balanced, medically supervised weight-loss program. Urge a diabetic patient to monitor his blood glucose level regularly, to exercise, and to follow his dietary regimen. Inform a pregnant patient that, in many instances, carpal tunnel syndrome resolves on its own after delivery.

Chronic low back pain

Low back pain is nearly as common as the common cold. Experts estimate that 70% to 80% of the world's population will suffer from disabling back pain at some time in their lives. Besides requiring intensive medical and surgical care, chronic back pain often necessitates difficult career and lifestyle changes.

Because chronic back pain can have a far-reaching impact on a patient's lifestyle and productivity, you'll need to provide comprehensive teaching. First, you'll help the patient identify what triggers his back pain. Then, together you'll develop strategies to help him avoid or live productively with recurrent pain. A comprehensive teaching plan can help ensure successful care and help the patient avoid further injury and hospitalization. Remember, too, to provide emotional support; severe, debilitating pain often leads to frustration and depression.

Before teaching a patient about chronic back pain, make sure you're familiar with the following topics:
• explanation of back anatomy
• risk factors and causes of low back pain
• preparation for diagnostic tests, including laboratory tests, computed tomography (CT) scans, magnetic resonance imaging (MRI), and myelography
• proper body mechanics for activities of daily living, such as standing, lifting, sitting, and driving
• exercises to strengthen the back
• drug therapy, including nonsteroidal anti-inflammatory drugs (NSAIDs), muscle relaxants, and other medications

• relaxation, physical therapy, and other pain management techniques
• when to call the doctor
• sources of information and support.

ABOUT THE DISORDER
Explain to the patient that chronic low back pain is defined as back pain that lasts for more than 6 months or recurs every 3 months to 3 years. Inform him that such pain can result from disease or from injury caused by occupational hazards, stress, poor body mechanics, poor posture, obesity, or other factors. These factors, along with normal aging, may be precursors to disorders that cause back pain.

To help the patient understand how back pain arises, inform him that the spinal column consists of 33 vertebrae that extend from the neck to the coccyx. All but the first two vertebrae have a disk between them. Intervertebral disks absorb the shock generated by walking and allow for movement of the spinal column — forward, backward, and sideways. (See *Viewing the vertebrae.*)

Finding the pain source
As the patient begins to understand back structure, he may recognize the difficulties involved in identifying the primary cause of back pain.

Injuries and inflammation
Inform the patient that injury to or inflammation in any one of the spinal structures can cause back pain — for example, pain may result from a herniated disk, a sprained or strained ligament, a torn muscle, or a pinched nerve. Other common causes include arthritis and degenerative disorders.

Explain that an intervertebral disk can withstand only a limited amount of stress. Eventually, stress may force the elastic material from the center of the disk (nucleus pulposus) to *herniate*, or break through the fibrous ring of the vertebrae. The vertebrae then move closer together as the disk compresses, resulting in pain and possible sensory and motor loss as pressure is placed on the nerve roots where they exit between the vertebrae. This condition is called *herniated disk* (also referred to as ruptured disk or herniated nucleus pulposus).

Inform the patient that a ruptured or bulging disk causes irritation and pressure on the spinal nerve roots and may lead to swelling and a shift in the vertebra's alignment. The result is a pinched nerve. (See *What's a pinched nerve?* page 164.)

Psychological stress
Point out that stress results from the body's response to external events. A person who feels pressure from his personal life or job may internalize it. If he does this consistently, his body may respond by displaying physical symptoms, which may include back pain. The back muscles, for instance, may tighten, causing pain. Then a cycle begins: Stress causes tension, which causes pain, which causes more stress, and so on. Unbroken, this cycle can immobilize the patient.

Physical stress
Tell the patient that certain physical factors put him at risk for back pain. These include poor posture and poor body mechanics, a low level of physical fitness, and jobs that require intense physical labor or awkward positioning for prolonged periods (such as driving a truck and nursing).

Understanding back pain
Pain from a back condition may be sudden and intense, dull and diffuse, or deep and aching. It may affect one or both sides of the body (unilateral or bilateral). The location of the pain corresponds to the site of the injury and the nerve roots involved.

Pain may be exacerbated by any activity that increases pressure on the spine, such as sneezing, coughing, and straining. Lying down may relieve the pain.

Lumbar disk disease produces pain and numbness in the lower back (lumbosacral area) with possible radiculopathy (sciatica) to the but-

Viewing the vertebrae

Using an illustration or a skeletal model, show the patient the *lumbar* (or low back) vertebrae. Explain that this area and the *cervical* (neck) vertebrae are the most often injured because these areas have few supportive structures.

Because the lumbar vertebrae are most often used and misused during lifting, pushing, and other labors, they are at increased risk for injury. In contrast, the *thoracic* vertebrae attach to the ribs, which provide support. Thus braced, the thoracic area sustains injury less often.

Show the patient the position of the disks between the vertebrae. Explain that a disk is composed of a fluid-filled center surrounded by a tough, fibrous ring.

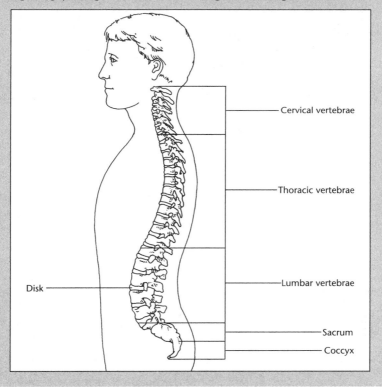

Cervical vertebrae

Thoracic vertebrae

Disk

Lumbar vertebrae

Sacrum

Coccyx

tock, down the back of the thigh and the calf, and to the sides of the foot. Mobility is severely compromised; the patient may have a lopsided gait, difficulty standing upright, or difficulty flexing the foot forward and sideways. The patient commonly finds sitting and climbing stairs excruciatingly painful.

Cervical disk disease may cause pain and numbness in the upper extremities, shoulders, upper chest, back of the head, or back of the neck. Pain may radiate down the neck into

INSIGHT INTO ILLNESSES

What's a pinched nerve?

Normally, spinal nerves pass through a small notch between the vertebrae. Explain to the patient that this notch can be a treacherous point on the nerve's pathway to the spinal cord. Why? Because many conditions can close off part of the notch, thereby trapping, or pinching, the nerve.

Tell the patient that poor posture (for example, swayback) can pinch a spinal nerve by pushing the vertebrae closer together. Add that a tumor, a broken vertebra, or a disk problem can also cause swelling in the area or shift the vertebrae's alignment and pinch the nerve. Make sure the patient understands that a pinched nerve in the lumbar spine typically causes low back pain.

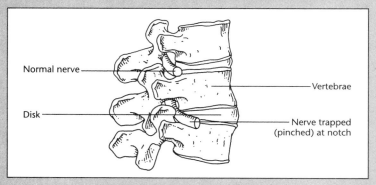

the forearm and the fingers. The patient may report decreased mobility and strength of the arms and neck and may display an abnormal curvature of the spine.

 WARNING: Tell the patient to seek emergency medical help if he experiences warning signs of paralysis — decreased sensation, extreme sensory loss, or altered bowel and bladder function.

DIAGNOSTIC WORKUP
Advise the patient that the doctor will take a thorough history and perform a physical assessment, which may reveal decreased reflexes, muscle wasting, paresthesias, or numbness in the affected area. He also may order laboratory tests and imaging tests, such as CT scans and MRI or, possibly, electromyelography or diskography, to help determine the cause of back pain. (See *Teaching patients about musculoskeletal tests*.)

Laboratory tests may include a complete blood cell count, erythrocyte sedimentation rate, and rheumatoid factor test. Explain that these tests will help determine if a rheumatoid disease such as arthritis is the cause of the patient's pain.

To help evaluate for lumbar disk disease and sciatic nerve involvement, the doctor may perform the straight leg test, sciatic nerve test, and sitting root tests.

(Text continues on page 170.)

Teaching patients about musculoskeletal tests

TEST AND PURPOSE	TEACHING POINTS
Arthrography • To detect abnormalities of the menisci, cartilage, and ligaments of the knee • To detect shoulder abnormalities, such as a torn rotator cuff and anterior capsule derangement • To evaluate the need for surgery	• Explain to the patient that this radiographic test involves injecting air or a radiopaque contrast medium into the joint space. Tell him that it's performed by a doctor in the X-ray department and that it takes about 1 hour. • Describe what will happen during the test: After the patient's joint is anesthetized, the contrast medium will be injected. Forewarn the patient that he may experience a tingling sensation or pressure in the joint. X-rays will then be taken as the contrast medium fills the joint space. The patient will be asked to quickly assume various positions for these X-rays, then to remain as still as possible. If the knee is being studied, tell the patient that he may have to take a few steps. • Explain what will happen after the test: The patient may experience some swelling or discomfort or may hear crepitant noises in the joint. Advise him to apply ice to the joint to reduce swelling and to take a mild analgesic for pain. If symptoms persist more than 2 days, tell the patient to contact the doctor. Advise the patient to rest the joint for at least 12 hours after the test. If the doctor applies an elastic bandage after a knee arthrogram, tell the patient to keep the bandage in place for several days. Teach him how to rewrap it.
Arthroscopy • To detect and diagnose meniscal, patellar, condylar, extrasynovial, and synovial diseases • To monitor disease progression • To perform joint surgery or biopsy • To monitor the effectiveness of therapy	• Explain to the patient that this test allows direct examination of the inside of a joint. Reassure him that it's a safe, convenient approach for surgery, if necessary. Tell him that arthroscopy is usually done in the operating room under general or local anesthesia by an orthopedic surgeon, and that it takes 30 to 60 minutes. • Describe physical preparation for the test: The patient must not eat or drink after midnight before the test. Immediately before the test, he'll receive a sedative and the area around the joint will be shaved. • Explain what will happen during the test: The patient may feel transient discomfort as the local anesthetic is injected (if applicable). The doctor will make a small incision and insert the arthroscope into the joint cavity. • Explain what will happen after the test: The patient will be allowed to walk as soon as he's fully

(continued)

Teaching patients about musculoskeletal tests *(continued)*

TEST AND PURPOSE	TEACHING POINTS
Arthroscopy *(continued)*	awake. Tell him that he'll experience mild soreness and a slight grinding sensation in his knee for a day or two. Instruct him to notify the doctor if he feels severe or persistent pain or develops a fever with signs of local inflammation. Advise against excessive use of the joint for a few days after the test. Tell the patient that he may resume his normal diet, which was discontinued before the test.
Bone biopsy •To distinguish between benign and malignant bone tumors •To detect metastatic bone diseases and infection	•Explain to the patient that this test allows direct examination of a small sample of bone and that it takes 15 to 30 minutes (for needle biopsy) or 30 to 60 minutes (for open biopsy). Mention whether he will receive a local or general anesthetic. •Describe pretest restrictions: If the patient will be receiving a general anesthetic, he mustn't eat or drink for 12 hours before the test. •Explain what will happen during the test: If the patient will undergo needle biopsy with a local anesthetic, the patient will feel a sharp, sticking sensation as the local anesthetic is injected into the skin. The doctor will make a small incision, then insert the needle into the bone. Warn the patient that he'll feel pressure as the needle is advanced into the bone. •Discuss what will happen after the test: The patient will experience some pain and tenderness for 1 to 3 days after a needle biopsy or for 2 to 6 days after an open biopsy. Advise him to call the doctor if pain or tenderness worsens, if drainage from the biopsy site increases, or if fever develops. Tell him that he can resume his normal activities after the test as soon as he's comfortable doing so. If he has undergone open biopsy, tell him the doctor will remove the stitches or sutures in 5 to 10 days.
Bone scan (bone scintigraphy) •To detect or rule out malignant bone lesions when radiographic findings are normal but cancer is confirmed or suspected •To detect occult bone trauma due to pathologic fractures	•Explain to the patient that this painless test can often detect bone abnormalities before conventional X-rays can. •Describe preparation for the test: Tell the patient that fasting before the test isn't necessary. However, he should avoid eating a meal or drinking large amounts of fluids right before the test. •Explain what will happen during the test: After applying a tourniquet on the patient's arm, the doctor will inject a small dose of a radioactive iso-

Teaching patients about musculoskeletal tests (continued)

TEST AND PURPOSE	TEACHING POINTS
Bone scan (bone scintigraphy) (continued) • To monitor degenerative bone disorders • To detect infection	tope. Assure the patient that the isotope emits less radiation than a standard X-ray machine. Mention that a 2- to 3-hour waiting period will follow injection of the isotope. During this time, the patient will need to drink 4 to 6 glasses of fluid. Then he'll be asked to lie supine on a table within the scanner. The scanner will move slowly back and forth, recording images for about 1 hour. Instruct him to lie as still as possible during the test. Tell him that he may be asked to assume various positions on the table.
Computed tomography scan • To aid diagnosis of bone tumors and other abnormalities	• Explain to the patient that this test helps detect bone abnormalities and that it takes 30 to 90 minutes. • Describe pretest restrictions: If the patient is scheduled to receive a contrast medium, he mustn't eat for 4 hours before the test. • Discuss physical preparation for the test: The patient will be asked to put on a hospital gown and to remove all jewelry before the test. Instruct him to empty his bladder just before the test. • Explain what will happen during the test: The patient will be asked to lie on a table within the large tunnel-like scanner. Then he may be given a contrast medium by mouth or by injection. During the test, the table he's lying on will move a small distance every few seconds. Tell him that the scanner will rotate around him and may make a clicking or buzzing noise. Instruct him to remain still during the test. Although he'll be alone in the room, assure him that he can communicate with the technician through an intercom system. • If the patient received a contrast medium, encourage him to drink plenty of fluids after the test.
Diskography • To identify a degenerated or extruding intervertebral disk	• Inform the patient that diskography is an X-ray study of the spine. Tell him that during this study, which uses fluoroscopy, a contrast medium is injected into the disk space. Tell him that it takes about 15 to 30 minutes. • Explain what will happen during the test: The patient will receive a local anesthetic and, possibly, a sedative because the procedure can be uncomfortable. Initially the patient is positioned in a supine position on the radiograph table, then may be repositioned for additional radiographic views.

(continued)

Teaching patients about musculoskeletal tests *(continued)*

TEST AND PURPOSE	TEACHING POINTS
Diskography *(continued)*	Instruct him to remain still and hold his breath. Emphasize that his cooperation will help ensure accurate results. • Discuss what will happen after the procedure: The patient may receive analgesics or local heat application to relieve any pain.
Joint aspiration (arthrocentesis) • To aid in differential diagnosis of arthritis • To identify the cause of joint effusion • To relieve pain and distention resulting from accumulation of fluid within the joint • To administer local drug therapy (usually corticosteroids)	• Explain to the patient that this test removes a fluid sample from within the joint space for analysis. Tell him that it takes about 10 minutes. • Explain what will happen during the test: The patient will be asked to assume a position and then remain still. After cleaning the skin over the joint, the doctor will insert the needle. After withdrawing the fluid, he'll apply a small bandage to the puncture site. • Explain what will happen after the test: Ice or cold packs may be applied to the joint to reduce pain and swelling. If the doctor removed a large amount of fluid, tell the patient that he may need to wear an elastic bandage. Advise him not to use the joint excessively after the test, to help avoid joint pain, swelling, and stiffness. Instruct him to report any increased pain, tenderness, swelling, warmth, or redness as well as fever; these may signal infection.
Myelography • To detect spinal abnormalities, such as tumors, herniated intervertebral disks, fractures, and inflammation	• Explain to the patient that this test reveals obstructions in the spinal canal. Tell him that it's done in the X-ray department and that it takes about 1 hour. • Describe what will happen during the test: The patient will be positioned prone on a tilting X-ray table. After cleaning the skin on the patient's lower back with an antiseptic, the doctor will inject an anesthetic. Warn the patient that he may experience a stinging sensation. Next, the doctor will insert a needle between two vertebrae of the spinal cord and will inject an oil- or water-based contrast medium. Inform the patient that he may feel a transient burning sensation during injection. He may also feel flushed and warm and may experience a headache, a salty taste, or nausea and vomiting. X-rays will be taken as the table is tilted vertically and then horizontally to allow the contrast medium to flow through the spinal canal. After completing the test, the doctor will with-

Teaching patients about musculoskeletal tests *(continued)*

TEST AND PURPOSE	TEACHING POINTS
Myelography *(continued)*	draw the oil-based contrast medium or allow the water-based medium to be absorbed. He'll then apply a small dressing to the puncture site. • Describe what will happen after the test: If an oil-based medium was used, the patient must remain flat in bed for 6 to 8 hours and avoid abrupt movement. He must drink plenty of fluids and can resume his normal diet. If nausea prevents this, explain that he may receive I.V. fluids and an antiemetic. If a water-based medium was used, the patient must sit in a chair or lie with the head of the bed elevated for 6 to 8 hours, and then remain on bed rest for an additional 6 to 8 hours. He must drink plenty of fluids and can resume his normal diet, as tolerated. If the patient is on phenothiazine therapy, tell him that he must temporarily discontinue the drug, as ordered by the doctor. Tell the patient to notify the doctor if he has a headache for more than 24 hours after the test or if he develops weakness, numbness, or tingling in his legs.
Photodensitometry • To measure cortical bone density as an aid in early diagnosis of osteoporosis	• Explain to the patient that this test can detect osteoporosis before it's apparent on conventional X-rays. Tell him that the test takes about 20 minutes. • Mention that during the test his hand will be positioned next to a small piece of aluminum alloy. As X-rays are taken, a computer will compare the density of the bone to that of the aluminum.
Photon absorptiometry (single) • To measure cortical bone density as an aid in early diagnosis of osteoporosis	• Explain to the patient that this painless test can accurately detect osteoporosis, even with bone loss as slight as 1% to 3%. Tell him that the test takes about 20 minutes and causes no discomfort. • Tell him that his arm will be positioned in a cradle and that X-rays will be taken of the radius — a bone in his forearm.
Photon absorptiometry (dual) • To measure trabecular bone density as an aid in early diagnosis of osteoporosis	• Explain to the patient that this painless test can detect osteoporosis before most other tests. Tell him that it takes about 20 minutes and causes no discomfort. • Tell him that he'll be positioned on his back in a tunnel-like machine that will take X-rays of his lumbar spine.

(continued)

Teaching patients about musculoskeletal tests *(continued)*

TEST AND PURPOSE	TEACHING POINTS
Sinography • To determine whether a sinus tract communicates with bone as an aid in evaluating osteomyelitis • To differentiate osteomyelitis from a local abscess	• Explain to the patient that this test explores the course of his sinus tract. • Describe what will happen during the test: The doctor will insert a catheter into the sinus tract, then instill a contrast medium through the catheter. He'll take serial X-rays as the medium flows through the sinus tract. • After the test, tell the patient that the contrast medium will be absorbed into the bloodstream or by the dressing over the sinus tract.
Transiliac bone biopsy • To allow direct examination of osteoporotic changes in bone cells	• Explain that this procedure can reveal osteoporotic changes. • Inform the patient that before the procedure, the skin over the iliac crest will be cleaned and a topical anesthetic applied. • Describe what happens during the procedure: The doctor will make a small incision, introduce a hollow needle, and aspirate a tiny core of bone marrow. Tell the patient to expect brief discomfort. • Tell the patient that after the needle is removed, pressure will be applied to the puncture site for 10 to 15 minutes. Advise him to expect slight soreness over the incision, and instruct him to report additional bleeding or severe pain.

Straight leg test
In this test, the examiner raises the patient's leg while the patient lies on his back. With lumbar disk disease, raising the leg to an angle less than 90 degrees causes pain in the back of the leg.

Sciatic nerve test
In this test, the examiner extends and raises the patient's leg until pain occurs, then lowers it to a comfortable position. He also dorsiflexes the foot to stretch the sciatic nerve. Pain in the posterior aspect of the leg suggests sciatic nerve involvement.

Sitting root test
The patient sits on the examination table with his legs dangling and his chin touching his chest. Then the examiner holds the patient's thigh against the table and asks him to try to straighten the leg. With sciatic nerve involvement, the patient experiences pain before the leg is fully extended.

X-rays
Spinal X-rays are ordered as an adjunct to other diagnostic techniques if the level and extent of the suspected injury warrant this.

TREATMENTS
Inform the patient that the primary treatments for chronic back pain are conservative: bed rest, medication, back strengthening exercises, heat application, traction, physical therapy, and weight reduction, if necessary. If these measures fail, the doctor may recommend more aggressive therapies, such as epidural steroid injection, chemonucleolysis, or surgery.

Activity guidelines

Reinforce activity restrictions prescribed by the doctor. Explain that bed rest limits the motion of the vertebral column, relieves nerve root compression, and reduces disk swelling. Teach the patient to lie in a position that reduces tension on the spine, such as semi-Fowler's or a side-lying position. For added support, recommend that he have a bed board placed under his mattress.

Emphasize that modifying daily activities is crucial to helping him regain his previous level of functioning and to avoiding further injury. Demonstrate the proper position for performing routine activities, such as standing, walking, sitting, driving, lying down, lifting, pulling, and pushing. Have him repeat the demonstration so you can evaluate his understanding. (See *Using good posture to protect the back,* page 172.)

Also urge him to follow his prescribed exercise program. Explain that regular back exercises will increase blood flow to the tissues, strengthen his back and abdominal muscles, and stretch the ligaments that attach muscles to the bone. They will also help him maintain a normal spinal curvature.

Underscore that an exercise program must be conducted under the direction of a doctor or physical therapist. Advise him to consult the doctor before participating in sports. *WARNING:* Caution the patient not to alter his exercise program without appropriate medical supervision.

Dietary modifications

Explain to the overweight patient that excess weight aggravates the strain on his spine. If the doctor prescribes a weight-loss diet, make sure the patient has a written copy of it. When teaching about meal planning, include other family members — especially the one who does most of the cooking.

Medications

The doctor may prescribe drug therapy for acute pain. Therapy may involve a combination of muscle relaxants, analgesics (narcotics or NSAIDs), and steroids to reduce pain and inflammation. Because narcotic analgesics can cause constipation, the doctor may suggest concomitant use of a laxative. Teach the patient that a high-fiber diet and adequate fluid intake also help to prevent constipation.

Epidural steroid injection

If the patient's pain involves the nerve root and isn't relieved by conservative measures, the doctor may recommend injection of an epidural steroid or anesthetic (or both) directly into the spine to reduce pain and muscle spasms. Tell the patient that this treatment may relieve his pain and improve his level of functioning. If it doesn't provide adequate pain relief, he may require another injection in 2 weeks. However, the injection can be repeated only a limited number of times.

Procedures

Discuss adjunctive measures for pain relief: applying local heat or cold to reduce muscle spasms, and using pillows, a bed board, or a firm mattress to ensure comfortable positioning. If the patient has decreased sensation, advise frequent skin checks for safety during heat or cold therapy.

Traction

The doctor may order traction to enhance the effects of bed rest. Explain that traction holds the spine in position and enhances the effects of bed rest. Inform the patient that pelvic-cervical traction reduces muscle spasms and widens the intervertebral space, thus reducing bulging or rupture of the disk. If the patient will be in traction at home, teach him and his family what devices will be used, how traction works, and how long he'll be in traction. Tell him that traction will be discontinued if it doesn't bring satisfactory results.

Chemonucleolysis

If these measures fail to relieve pain from a herniated disk, the doctor may

Using good posture to protect the back

If your patient has chronic back pain, emphasize that good posture is a must — whether he's standing, sitting, or lying down. Point out that it strengthens the abdominal and buttock muscles that support the hardworking back.

Standing and walking

When the patient stands correctly, he should be able to draw an imaginary line from his ear through the tip of his shoulder, middle of his hip, back of his knee, and front of his ankle. He won't be able to do this if he stands with his lower back arched, his upper back stooped, or his abdomen sagging forward.

To correct his posture, instruct the patient to stand 1' away from a wall. Then have him lean back against the wall with his knees slightly bent. Tell him to tighten his stomach and buttock muscles to tilt his pelvis back and flatten his lower back.

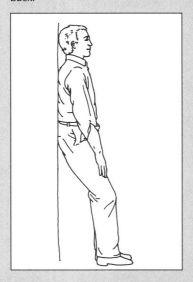

As he holds this position, have him inch up the wall until he's standing. His lower back should still be pressed against the wall. Inform him that this is the posture he should assume when walking.

Sitting

If possible, the patient should choose a hard, straight-backed chair to sit on. Tell him to place a rolled towel or a small pillow behind his lower back. To keep his back from tiring when sitting for a long time, instruct him to raise one leg higher than the other by propping it on a footrest.

Lying down

Advise the patient to sleep on a firm mattress. If he must sleep on a soft mattress, recommend supporting it with a bedboard or a piece of plywood placed underneath it.

The best position for sleeping is lying on the side with the knees bent and a pillow between them. Explain that this position prevents the spine from twisting when he drops his upper leg. Tell the patient not to curl up excessively, though, because this can put too much pressure on his back bones.

Caution the patient not to sleep on his stomach or on high pillows. These positions can strain his back, neck, and shoulders. Sleeping on the back is okay if he keeps a pillow under the knees or places a small pillow or rolled towel under the small of his back.

Lifting and carrying

Instruct the patient to maintain the natural low back curve with his pelvis tucked in while lifting and carrying. Tell him to turn and face the object he wants to lift. As he keeps his feet flat and shoulder-

Using good posture to protect the back *(continued)*

width apart, have him bend his knees, lower himself to the object, and place his hands around it. Then with his knees bent and back straight, tell him to use his arm and leg muscles (instead of his back muscles) to lift the object. Warn him to avoid lifting heavy objects above his waist.

Advise him to carry the object by holding it close to his body. Tell him to avoid carrying unbalanced loads or anything heavier than he can easily manage. Advise him to get help for large or bulky items.

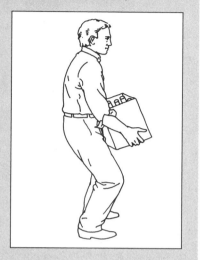

recommend chemonucleolysis as an alternative to surgery. Explain that this procedure involves injection of the enzymes chymopapain or collagenase into the disk to reduce the nucleus pulposus and thereby relieve pain. Usually performed with radiographic visualization, the procedure takes about 45 minutes. Tell the patient that this procedure is 50% to 80% effective, but that total pain relief may not occur for up to 3 months.

Surgery

When conservative measures fail to relieve back pain, the doctor may recommend surgery. Surgery may involve laminectomy, spinal fusion, or diskectomy. (If the patient has signs or symptoms of spinal cord compression, such as incontinence due to a sensory or motor loss of sphincter control, surgery is performed without delay.)

If the patient will undergo *laminectomy,* inform him that the surgeon will remove one or more of the bony laminae (the flattened portion on either side of the vertebra's arch) that

cover the vertebrae. This procedure is most commonly performed to relieve pressure on the spinal cord or spinal nerve roots resulting from a herniated disk.

Inform the patient that after laminae removal, *spinal fusion* — grafting of bone chips between vertebral spaces — may be performed. Spinal fusion also may be done apart from laminectomy in some patients with vertebrae weakened by trauma or disease. Point out that in this procedure, bone chips are taken from the hip or lower leg and placed in the unstable area of the spine, where they fuse with and stabilize the spine.

For a herniated disk, alternative treatments include microsurgical diskectomy and percutaneous automated diskectomy. Tell the patient that in *microsurgical diskectomy,* the surgeon visualizes the herniated disk material and uses microsurgical techniques to remove it through a small incision. He may also remove extruded fragments. If the patient will undergo *percutaneous automated diskectomy,* inform him that the doctor removes the herniated disk using an instrument that cuts and aspirates, and then gently aspirates the disk portion that's causing the pain. The procedure can be done on an outpatient basis using local anesthesia.

After surgery, provide instructions for wound care. Make sure the patient knows how to recognize signs and symptoms of infection: swelling, warmth, discharge, fever, and excessive pain that's not relieved by analgesics. If the patient needs an immobilizer or brace, provide appropriate instructions to both the patient and caregiver.

Reinforce the doctor's postoperative activity restrictions. Make sure the patient understands that he must resume activities *gradually*; for example, he may resume exercising by taking short walks inside his home. Tell him to wear supportive shoes when walking, even in the house.

Finally, refer the patient to appropriate organizations for further information and support, as necessary. (See Appendix 2.)

Fractures

Fractures are the most common orthopedic injury — so common that some patients may not even regard the injury as serious. To correct this misconception, you'll need to emphasize the reasons for complying with therapy to avoid permanent deformity or disability. After all, inadequate or improper care of a fracture can lead to life-threatening complications such as fat embolism (with pelvic and long bone fractures) or compartment syndrome (with elbow, wrist, knee, and ankle fractures).

Before teaching a patient about a fracture, make sure you are familiar with the following topics:
• explanation of the types of fractures and how bones heal
• possible complications, such as fat embolism and compartment syndrome
• diagnostic tests, such as X-rays and computed tomography (CT) scans, if necessary

• limitations on activity and weight bearing
• instructions for cast care, exercises for casted limbs, and crutch walking, if necessary
• analgesics and their possible adverse effects
• procedures and surgery to align displaced bone fragments and immobilize the injury
• tips for preventing accidental fractures
• sources of information and support.

ABOUT THE DISORDER
Explain to the patient that a fracture is a partial or complete break in a bone that occurs when excessive stress is applied to a bone. Typically, the stress results from major trauma. However, an injury called a *stress fracture* can occur when a normal bone is subjected to repeated stress (such as from prolonged standing, walking, or running). If the patient has a bone-weakening disease, such as osteoporosis or a bone tumor, minor trauma or even normal activities may lead to a *pathologic fracture*.

Tell the patient that fractures are classified in several ways, including location, direction of the fracture line, and position of the bony fragments. (See *Classifying fractures*.)

Inform the patient that signs and symptoms of a fracture include pain and tenderness of the injured part, loss of normal limb contours, limb shortening, swelling, bruising, decreased range of motion, abnormal movement, and a crackling noise.

Tell the patient that healing begins almost immediately after the injury occurs. However, the rate of healing depends on the type of fracture. A displaced fracture in which the fragments must be realigned may take months or even years to fully heal. (See *Average healing times for fractures*, page 177.)

Complications
Inform the patient that complications can arise shortly after the injury or may develop later. Help him understand how he will be monitored

INSIGHT INTO ILLNESSES

Classifying fractures

To help your patient understand his injury and its treatment, first teach him about his type of fracture. A fracture may be classified as:
● open — a fracture in which bone fragments penetrate the skin
● closed — a fracture that doesn't penetrate the skin
● complete — an interruption in bone continuity
● incomplete — an incomplete interruption in bone continuity.

Next, describe the fracture's location. For example, in long bones, fractures are described as distal, proximal, or midshaft. Near a joint, fractures are called intracapsular or extracapsular. Within the joint, they're called intra-articular.

As described below, fractures are further classified by the direction of the fracture line and the position of bony fragments. Your patient's fracture may combine several types.

FRACTURE LINE DIRECTION

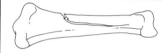

Longitudinal
Fracture line runs parallel to the bone's axis

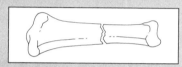

Transverse
Fracture line crosses the bone at a right angle to the axis

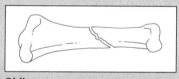

Oblique
Fracture line breaks the bone at a slanted angle to the bone's axis

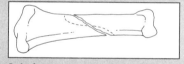

Spiral
Fracture line runs through the bone in a coil-like manner or twists around the bone; usually caused by torsion or a twisting force

BONY FRAGMENT POSITION

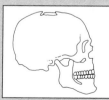

Depressed
Broken bone is driven inward

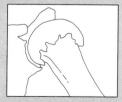

Impacted
One fragment is forced into or onto another fragment

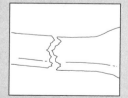

Nondisplaced
Fragments maintain essentially normal alignment

(continued)

Classifying fractures *(continued)*

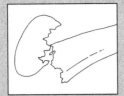

Displaced
Disrupted anatomic bone relationships occur with deformity

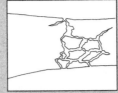

Comminuted
Three or more fragments

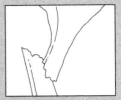

Overriding
Fragments overlap and shorten total bone length

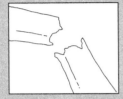

Angulated
Fragments deviate from their normal linear alignment so that they're at angles to each other

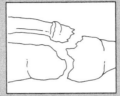

Avulsed
Fragments are pulled from their normal position by forceful muscle contractions or ligamentous resistance

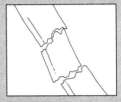

Segmental
Fractures occur in two adjacent areas with an isolated central segment

for possible problems. Explain that some bleeding is normal — but tell him to report excessive bleeding immediately.

Discuss *compartment syndrome* — a serious complication that, if untreated, may obstruct blood supply and cause permanent dysfunction and deformity. Explain that the condition may arise suddenly, right after injury, or gradually, over several days. It's caused by tissue swelling within muscle groups, which compresses nerves and arteries, resulting in muscle ischemia. Without treatment, irreversible muscle damage may occur within 6 hours.

 WARNING: Instruct your patient to immediately report early symptoms of compartment syndrome: worsening pain that's unrelieved by analgesics, increased swelling, or numbness and tingling in the affected limb. Tell him not to elevate the limb or apply ice if these symptoms occur because doing so would further reduce blood supply to the affected area.

If the patient has a long bone fracture, inform him that he'll be monitored for another complication — *fat embolism*. Explain that this potentially life-threatening complication may occur as the bone marrow releases fat into a vein. The fat may then lodge in the lungs, obstructing breathing, or may pass into the arteries, eventually affecting the central nervous system.

DIAGNOSTIC WORKUP
Inform the patient that X-rays can diagnose most fractures. Typically, X-rays of the suspected fracture are taken from two angles; X-rays are also taken of the joints above and below the fracture. The doctor may also

order a CT scan. (See *Teaching patients about musculoskeletal tests,* pages 165 to 170.)

TREATMENTS
Explain that treatment of a fracture aims to restore function and motion to the injured part. Stress the importance of complying with doctor's orders, such as activity and weight-bearing restrictions. Encourage the patient to eat a well-balanced diet to obtain essential nutrients for bone healing. As appropriate, teach him about therapeutic exercise, medications, traction, surgery, and how to care for the cast and use crutches.

Activity guidelines
Inform the patient that the doctor will provide specific guidelines on activity restrictions so that the fracture will heal properly. Tell him that the doctor or physical therapist will decide when he should begin a program of passive and active range-of-motion exercises as well as when he can start to use his injured body part.

Reinforce the doctor's recommendations on restricting weight bearing on the injured limb, and review instructions on using crutches or other assistive devices for ambulation.

Dietary modifications
Stress the importance of a nutritious diet that includes foods rich in vitamin C (citrus fruits and tomatoes), calcium (dairy products, salmon, and broccoli), vitamin D (found in fortified milk and produced by sun-exposed skin), and vitamin A (carrots, sweet potatoes, and other yellow or orange fruit or vegetables). Explain that these foods promote healing, calcium absorption, and bone remodeling.

Medication
Inform the patient that the doctor may prescribe a narcotic or nonnarcotic analgesic to reduce pain. The most frequently prescribed nonnarcotic analgesics are acetaminophen

Average healing times for fractures

"How long will it be until my broken bone heals?" Expect to hear that question often from patients with fractures. Using the chart below, give your patient an estimate of the healing time for his fracture. Remind him, though, that his own fracture may require more or less time to mend than average. Emphasize that he can speed his recovery by complying with his prescribed treatment and rehabilitation.

BONE	HEALING TIME (WEEKS)
Collar bone	6
Upper arm	
Neck	6
Shaft	12
Forearm	
Both bones	12
One bone	6
Hand	6 to 10
Finger	3
Hip	12
Upper leg	16 to 24
Lower leg (tibia)	
Plateau	8
Shaft	16 to 24
Ankle	8 to 12
Lower leg (fibula)	
Shaft	8
Ankle	8
Heel	8 to 12
Foot	8
Toe	3

and nonsteroidal anti-inflammatory drugs (NSAIDs) such as ibuprofen.

Tell the patient taking an NSAID that the drug may cause stomach upset and GI bleeding. Instruct him to call the doctor immediately if he has any signs of bleeding, such as black, tarry stools or bloody vomitus.

If the patient is taking a narcotic such as codeine, tell him that this medication may cause constipation. Advise him to consult his doctor about using a stool softener.

 WARNING: If the patient is taking a narcotic, caution him to avoid driving and other activities that require alertness until the effects of the drug are known.

If the patient has an open fracture, the doctor will prescribe antibiotics. Tell the patient to take the drug exactly as directed and to complete the entire course of prescribed therapy.

Procedures

Explain that the first step in healing the fracture is to correct the alignment of bone fragments — a procedure called *reduction.* The next step is to immobilize the injury with a cast, splint, or other support to prevent dislocation of the bone fragments and to aid healing.

Closed reduction

For most fractures, closed reduction is the preferred treatment. Inform the patient that the doctor will manipulate the injured body part to lock the ends of the bone fragments together and restore normal alignment. In some patients, traction may be used to achieve closed reduction.

Immobilization

Explain that once the fracture has been reduced, the doctor will use a sling, cast, brace, splint, or other external support to immobilize and stabilize the fracture while the bone heals.

Surgery

If closed reduction isn't possible or advisable, tell the patient that he'll undergo surgery so the doctor can perform open reduction to restore normal alignment of bone fragments. Open reduction may be achieved by internal fixation or external fixation.

Open reduction with internal fixation

Tell the patient scheduled for this procedure that it involves inserting internal fixation devices — pins, nails, screws, rods, wires, or plates — into the affected bone to maintain its position and promote an early return to normal limb function. Assure him that the body tolerates internal fixation devices well.

Teach the patient about postoperative activity restrictions. Advise him to report signs and symptoms of possible complications, such as redness, tenderness, swelling, drainage, or increasing pain in the affected limb.

Open reduction with external fixation

If the patient has a severe open fracture and extensive soft-tissue injuries, he may require an external fixation device. Explain that metal pins will be surgically inserted above and below the fracture to hold the bones together. The pins are then attached firmly to the device's frame.

Assure the patient than once in place, an external fixation device won't hurt. Instruct him to clean his external pins daily using a solution of normal saline solution and peroxide. Tell him to watch for and report loose pins as well as signs or symptoms of infection, such as redness, swelling, warmth, fever, or drainage at the surgical site.

Other care measures

Encourage the patient to comply with his rehabilitation program, which may include physical and occupational therapy. Because most fractures result from trauma, be sure to address safety issues. For example, teach an elderly patient how to prevent falls at home, such as by installing safety rails around the shower or bath. If the patient needs crutches or other ambulatory devices, make sure he knows how to use this equipment safely.

 TIPS AND TIMESAVERS: To help prevent fractures, recommend wearing nonskid, flat-soled supportive shoes. Advise the patient to remove throw rugs and avoid walking on slippery, wet, or irregular flooring.

Finally, refer the patient to an appropriate resource if he needs further information and support.

Lyme disease

Initially identified in a group of children in Lyme, Connecticut, Lyme disease has now been reported in at least 43 states and 20 other countries. It's endemic to three parts of the United States — the northeast, from Massachusetts to Maryland; the midwest, in Wisconsin and Minnesota; and the west, in California and Oregon.

Before teaching a patient about Lyme disease, make sure you are familiar with the following topics:
• how Lyme disease is transmitted
• signs and symptoms of Lyme disease
• ways to prevent Lyme disease
• how to remove a deer tick
• drug therapy such as antibiotics
• importance of balancing rest and activity
• signs and symptoms of recurrence and complications that should be reported
• sources of information and support.

ABOUT THE DISORDER

Explain that Lyme disease may affect many body systems. Inform the patient that it's caused by the spirochete *Borrelia burgdorferi,* which is carried by the tiny tick *Ixodes dammini* or another tick in the Ixodidae family. No bigger than a poppy seed, the tick typically feeds on mice, dogs, cats, cows, horses, raccoons, deer and, of course, humans. Once it attaches to a host, it swells to five to seven times its original size. The peak season for human infection is during the summer months.

Point out that Lyme disease occurs when a tick injects spirochete-laden saliva into the patient's bloodstream or deposits fecal matter on the skin. After incubating for 3 to 32 days, the spirochetes migrate out to the skin, causing the classic skin lesion called erythema chronicum migrans (ECM), which resembles a bull's-eye.

The spirochetes then spread to other skin sites or organs by the bloodstream or lymph system. Weeks or months later, cardiac or neurologic abnormalities may develop, possibly followed by arthritis. The spirochete's life cycle isn't completely clear: it may survive for years in the joints or it may trigger an inflammatory response in the host and then die.

Disease stages

Inform the patient that Lyme disease typically progresses in three stages. In *stage 1,* heralded by ECM, a red macule or papule may form at the site of a tick bite. The lesion often feels hot and itchy and may grow to more than 20″ (50 cm) in diameter. Within a few days, more skin lesions may erupt, along with a malar rash, conjunctivitis, or diffuse urticaria. In 3 to 4 weeks, lesions are replaced by small red blotches, which last several more weeks.

Malaise and fatigue are constant, but other signs and symptoms are intermittent: headache, fever, chills, achiness, and regional lymphadenopathy. Less common effects are meningeal irritation, mild encephalopathy, migrating musculoskeletal pain, and hepatitis.

Weeks to months later, *stage 2* begins with neurologic abnormalities that usually resolve after days or months. Facial palsy is especially noticeable. Cardiac abnormalities also may develop.

Stage 3 begins weeks or years later. Musculoskeletal pain leads to arthritis with marked swelling, especially in large joints. Recurrent attacks may precede chronic arthritis with severe cartilage and bone erosion.

Removing a tick

Removing a tick from the skin the right way may prevent Lyme disease. Tell the patient who finds a tick on his skin to first cover the tick and surrounding skin with heavy mineral oil and wait for 30 minutes. Typically, the mineral oil will suffocate the tick, which responds by backing out of the skin.

If that doesn't work, instruct the patient to firmly grasp the tick at its head with tweezers placed as close to the skin as possible, and then slowly and gently pull the tick straight out. Caution him not to turn, twist, or jerk as he pulls the tweezers out. Tell him to place the tick in a container of alcohol and then flush it down the toilet. After disposing of the tick, the patient should clean the wound with an antiseptic or rubbing alcohol and then wash his hands thoroughly.

If the tick's head remains embedded in the skin, the patient should go to the doctor to have it removed. Also tell him to call the doctor if he experiences flu-like symptoms or notices a bull's-eye rash developing over the next few weeks.

DIAGNOSTIC WORKUP
Tell the patient that the doctor may diagnose Lyme disease based on the characteristic ECM lesion and related clinical findings. This is because isolation of *B. burgdorferi* is unusual in humans and because indirect immunofluorescent antibody tests are only marginally sensitive. To help determine whether the patient may have been exposed to ticks, the doctor will ask if he has recently traveled to areas where Lyme disease is endemic.

Mild anemia and elevations in the erythrocyte sedimentation rate, leukocyte count, serum immunoglobulin M level, and aspartate aminotransferase level support the diagnosis.

TREATMENTS
Treatment for Lyme disease typically involves antibiotics and, possibly, range-of-motion (ROM) and strengthening exercises. Be sure, also, to teach the patient how to avoid a recurrence.

Activity guidelines
Depending on the patient's disease stage and his signs and symptoms, the doctor may prescribe bed rest to allow inflamed joints to heal, or may prescribe ROM exercises to prevent muscle weakness and strengthen joints. Review with the patient how to perform these exercises. Caution him to avoid overexertion.

Medication
Inform the patient that the doctor usually prescribes a 10- to 20-day course of oral tetracycline for adults; penicillin and erythromycin are alternative drugs. A child usually receives oral penicillin. When given early in Lyme disease, these drugs can minimize later complications. For late stages, high-dose penicillin I.V. may be effective.

Preventing a recurrence
Reassure the patient that preventing a recurrence of Lyme disease doesn't mean he must give up walking in the woods or enjoying nature. But he should take certain precautions when going outdoors.

First, advise him to avoid areas with large deer populations. Also tell him to stay out of long grass because it's more likely to harbor hungry ticks. Stress the need to keep to trails when hiking.

Dressing properly is also crucial. Instruct the patient to wear light-colored, long-sleeved shirts and light-colored long pants when walking in a wooded area, meadow, or high grass. Emphasize that he should tuck his pants into his socks to make it harder for the ticks to reach him and make it easier for him to see the ticks on his clothing. Stress the importance of wearing socks and closed shoes outdoors; tell him *never* to go barefoot.

Before going walking in potentially tick-laden areas, the patient may want to spray a diethyltoluamide-containing insect repellent on his skin and clothes. But advise him to consult his doctor about this first.

After returning from a hike, the patient should brush or comb his hair. Recommend brushing his hiking companions with a broom or towel, and having them brush him.

Also instruct him to check for ticks before bathing. Remind him that deer ticks are tiny and easy to overlook on inspection, but that if he sees what looks like a speck of dirt on his skin, he should try to brush it off gently. If it's truly dirt, this action will remove it; if it's a tick that's already bitten, it won't brush off. (See *Removing a tick*.)

To prevent disease transmission by way of pets, advise the patient to place tick collars on pets and inspect them each time they return from a walk. Stress that pets shouldn't be allowed on furniture or beds. If the patient has a woodpile or birdfeeder, tell him to move these away from the house.

Finally, don't overlook everyday exposure to deer ticks. Even a lovely, tree-lined yard can harbor ticks. If the patient's backyard has signs of deer visitors, tell him to be especially diligent about checking himself and his family for ticks every day.

Osteoarthritis

Osteoarthritis (also called degenerative joint disease) is a chronic, progressive disorder affecting about 20 million Americans. Occurring in any age-group, it may follow trauma or arise as a complication of congenital malformations. Although osteoarthritis sometimes causes few symptoms, more often it affects the patient's ability to perform activities of daily living.

Because the chronic joint pain of osteoarthritis has no cure, your teaching will emphasize compliance with a program designed to manage pain, restore or maintain joint mobility, and preserve independence.

Occasionally, the effects of osteoarthritis require surgery to correct deformity or to improve function. Then, you'll need to teach the patient about his specific surgical procedure. As appropriate after surgery, you'll show him how to care for his brace, cast, or other device and how to resume safe exercise.

Before teaching a patient with osteoarthritis, make sure you are familiar with the following topics:
• osteoarthritis disease process
• types of osteoarthritis: primary and secondary
• how exercise preserves joint function
• preparation for tests, such as blood and urine studies, X-rays, joint aspiration, magnetic resonance imaging (MRI), and radionuclide bone scan
• range-of-motion (ROM), extension, flexion, and isometric exercises
• medications and their administration
• surgery, such as osteotomy, arthrodesis, or joint replacement
• appropriate postoperative exercises and activity restrictions
• other pain-relief measures, including heat or cold therapy and massage
• use of protective and assistive devices to avoid joint fatigue
• sources of information and support.

ABOUT THE DISORDER
Tell the patient that osteoarthritis is a degenerative disorder in which the smooth, elastic cartilage of the joint gradually wears down or erodes. The bones underneath the worn cartilage stiffen, and bony spurs develop around the joint, narrowing the space between the joints. During movement, the bones rub together, causing pain and loss of joint function. (See *What happens in osteoarthritis,* page 182.)

Tell the patient that, of the primary and secondary forms of osteoarthritis, *primary osteoarthritis* seems to be related to aging, although researchers don't understand why. This form of the disorder isn't attributable to pre-

INSIGHT INTO ILLNESSES

What happens in osteoarthritis

Explain to the patient that osteoarthritis doesn't happen suddenly. The characteristic breakdown of articular cartilage is a gradual response to aging or predisposing factors, such as joint abnormalities or traumatic injury. Use the illustrations below to help describe the disease process to your patient.

Normal anatomy
Begin with normal joint anatomy: Show the patient how the bones fit together and how cartilage — a smooth, fibrous tissue — cushions the end of each bone. Point out that synovial fluid fills each joint space. Explain that this fluid lubricates the joint to ease movement, much as brake fluid functions in a car.

uses the affected joints, but rest relieves the discomfort. Or he may feel stiffness in the affected joint, especially in the morning. The stiffness usually lasts 15 minutes or less.

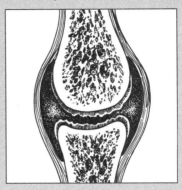

Later stage
As the disease progresses, whole sections of cartilage may disintegrate; osteophytes (bony spurs) form, and fragments of cartilage and bone float freely in the joint. Pain, more common now, may arise even during rest and typically worsens throughout the day. Movement becomes increasingly limited and stiffness may persist even after limbering exercises.

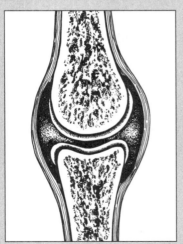

Early osteoarthritis stage
Usually, cartilage begins to break down long before symptoms surface. Typically, in early osteoarthritis the patient either has no symptoms or has a mild, dull ache when he

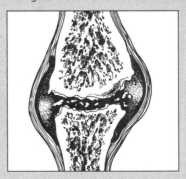

disposing factors; however, in some cases, it appears to be hereditary. Mention that primary osteoarthritis may be localized or generalized; generalized osteoarthritis involves 3 or more joints. Primary osteoarthritis may occur in the distal interphalangeal (DIP), proximal interphalangeal (PIP), metacarpophalangeal, and carpometacarpal joints of the thumb, hip, knee, and the cervical and lumbosacral spine.

Tell the patient that *secondary osteoarthritis* results from a predisposing factor such as traumatic injury, or a congenital abnormality such as hip dysplasia. Endocrine disorders (for example, diabetes mellitus), developmental processes (such as scoliosis), and calcium deposition disease can also lead to secondary osteoarthritis. Inform the patient that secondary osteoarthritis can affect any joint.

Point out that osteoarthritis usually comes on gradually, beginning with joint stiffness lasting less than 15 minutes. The soreness progresses to joint pain, which worsens with activity and is relieved with rest.

Reassure the patient that osteoarthritis doesn't cause systemic signs or symptoms; its effects are limited to joints. Characteristic signs and symptoms include limited joint movement, Heberden's nodes (DIP enlargement), Bouchard's nodes (PIP enlargement), varus or valgus deformity of the knee, bony enlargement of the joint, and flexion contracture of the knee, sometimes associated with crepitation.

DIAGNOSTIC WORKUP

Tell the patient that to confirm osteoarthritis, the doctor may order blood and urine tests, X-rays, MRI, and a radionuclide bone scan. X-rays may reveal narrowing of the joint space, osteophytosis (bony projections) of the joint margins, bone cysts, sharpened articular margins and dense subchondral bone. Joint aspiration may also be done to rule out rheumatoid arthritis. (See *Teaching patients about musculoskeletal tests,* pages 165 to 170.)

Blood and urine tests

Explain that the doctor may order routine laboratory tests, such as a complete blood cell count, a blood chemistry profile, erythrocyte sedimentation rate, and a urinalysis to rule out other arthropathic conditions (such as rheumatoid arthritis or infection) or to detect an underlying metabolic disorder.

TREATMENTS

Adequate rest, an appropriate exercise program, and medication to relieve pain and improve functioning are the mainstays of osteoarthritis treatment. To decrease stiffness and promote comfort, the doctor may recommend massage and application of moist heat and cold. To compensate for decreased mobility, the patient may need to use assistive devices.

Treatment measures also may include activity recommendations, weight reduction through dietary changes, medication, and surgery.

Activity guidelines

Emphasize that a balanced exercise program is the key to restoring, maintaining, and improving joint function and assuring a maximum level of independence. Assure the patient that he and the health care team will work together to plan a program that meets his needs. The program will alternate activity and rest. Explain that exercise maintains joint mobility and muscle strength, whereas rest prevents undue joint fatigue. For this reason, also urge the patient to achieve a balance between exercise and rest in his daily activities. The amount and type of activity and rest will depend on the severity of his disease, which joints are affected, and his lifestyle.

Demonstrate how to perform full, active ROM exercises daily (as prescribed), and give the patient a copy of the teaching aid *Performing active range-of-motion exercises,* pages 184 and 185.) Emphasize that these exer-

(Text continues on page 186.)

Performing active range-of-motion exercises

Dear Patient:
Review the following guidelines before you begin active range-of-motion exercises

Some guidelines
● Do your exercises daily to get the most benefit from them.
● Repeat each exercise three to five times or as often as your doctor recommends.
● Move slowly and gently so you don't injure yourself. If an exercise hurts, stop doing it. Then ask your doctor if you should keep doing that particular exercise.
● Consider spacing your exercises over the day if you prefer not to do them in a single session.

Neck exercise
Slowly tilt your head as far back as possible. Next, move it to the right, toward your shoulder.

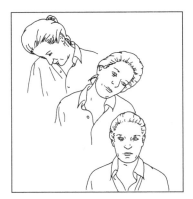

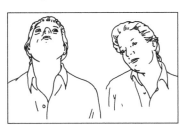

Next, lower your chin as far as it will go toward your chest. Then move your head toward your left shoulder. Complete a full circle by moving your head back to its normal position. (See illustrations at the top of the right column.)

After you do the recommended number of counterclockwise circles, reverse the exercise, doing an equal number of clockwise circles.

Shoulder exercise
Raise your shoulders as if you were going to shrug. Next, move them forward, down, back, then up in a single circular motion. Now move them backward, down, forward, then up again in a single circular motion.

Alternate forward and backward circles throughout the exercise.

Elbow exercise
Extend your arm straight out to your side. Open you hand, palm up, as if to catch a raindrop. Now, slowly reach back with your forearm so that you touch your shoulder with your fingers. Then slowly return your arm to its straight position. Now repeat with your other arm.

Continue to alternate arms throughout the exercise.

Wrist and hand exercise
Extend your arms, palms down and fingers straight. Keeping your palms flat, slowly raise your fingers and "point" them back toward you. Then slowly lower your fingers and "point" them as far downward as you comfortably can.

Performing active range-of-motion exercises *(continued)*

Finger exercise
Spread the fingers and thumb on each hand as wide apart as possible without causing discomfort. Then bring the fingers back together in a fist.

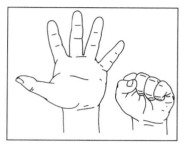

Leg and knee exercise
Lie on your bed on or the floor. Bend one leg so the knee is straight up and the foot is flat on the bed or floor.

Now bend the other leg, raise your foot, and slowly bring your knee as far toward your chest as you can without discomfort. Then straighten this leg slowly while you lower it. Repeat this exercise with your other leg. (See illustrations below.)

Ankle and foot exercise
Raise one foot and point your toes away from you. Move this foot in a circular motion — first to the right, then to the left.

Point your toes back toward you. With your foot in this position, make a circle with it — first right, then left.

Now do the same exercise with your other foot.

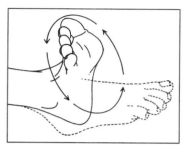

Toe exercise
Sit in a chair or lie on your bed. Stretch your legs out in front of you, with your heels resting on the floor or the bed. Slowly bend your toes down and away from you. Next, bend your toes up and back toward you. Finally, spread out your toes so that they're totally separated. Then squeeze your toes together.

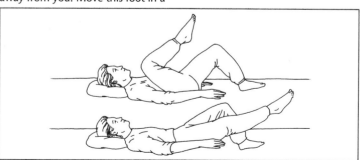

cises will improve his flexibility. To help him maintain muscle strength, show him how to perform isometric exercises. (See *Teaching about isometric exercises*.)

Caution the patient to avoid excessive exercise, which may increase joint inflammation. For instance, advise him to adjust his exercise program if he notices increased pain or swelling or decreased ROM. To reduce pain and swelling, advise him to cut down on the number of repetitions; to improve ROM, recommend that he increase the number of repetitions. If these changes don't help or if new joints become involved, instruct him to consult the doctor. Generally, pain that lasts until the next exercise period (or several hours) indicates that the exercise was too strenuous.

Dietary modifications
Because excess weight adds stress to already painful joints, advise the patient to follow a weight-reduction program, if ordered by the doctor.

Medication
Drugs of choice for treating osteoarthritis include aspirin and other salicylates and nonsteroidal anti-inflammatory drugs. Teach the patient the name, purpose, and dosage of each drug. Tell him to report such adverse effects as abdominal pain, breathing problems, unusual bleeding, bloody or tarry stools, bloody urine, rash, sore throat, yellowing of the skin and eyes, chest tightness, confusion, hallucinations, hearing loss, seizures, severe diarrhea, severe drowsiness, tinnitus, unusual sweating or thirst, visual disturbances, or vomiting.

Surgery
Let the patient know that the doctor may recommend orthopedic surgery to correct underlying congenital anomalies or defects caused by trauma. Typical surgical procedures include debridement, osteotomy, arthrodesis, and partial or total joint replacement.

Debridement
Inform the patient scheduled for joint debridement that this procedure is usually done to smooth irregular joint surfaces and to remove loose bone or cartilage particles and inflamed synovium. Tell him that after surgery, the affected joint will be immobilized for a few days.

Osteotomy
The doctor may recommend an osteotomy to correct joint misalignment. Usually performed on the knee, this procedure involves cutting the bone to remold the weight-bearing surfaces. Reassure the patient that osteotomy usually relieves joint pain and improves joint mobility and stability.

Arthrodesis
Also called fusion, arthrodesis involves fusing a joint to relieve pain or to provide support. Although typically performed on the spine, this surgery also can treat other joints. Forewarn the patient that after the procedure, the affected joint must be immobilized until X-rays confirm healing (which usually takes 3 to 6 months). Accordingly, prepare him to wear a halo vest or cervical collar (for cervical vertebrae); a brace or body cast (for other spinal vertebrae), or other mechanical device.

Joint replacement
Inform the patient with severe joint pain and disability that the doctor may recommend partial or total joint replacement. Hip and knee replacements are most common. Explain that this surgery involves replacing some or all of the joint with a prosthesis. Results usually include pain relief and greatly improved joint function.

Describe postoperative care, which may involve continuous passive motion for a total knee replacement or hip abduction after a total hip replacement.

Teaching about isometric exercises

Tell the patient that to perform iso-metric exercises properly, he must exercise against a resistive force. Explain that this increases the mus-cle-strengthening effect of the exer-cise. Remind him to repeat each ex-ercise as many times (typically three) as the doctor directs.

General guidelines

Emphasize that when doing isomet-ric exercise, the patient doesn't move his joints. Instead, he con-tracts his muscles against the resis-tance of a stationary object, such as a bed, a wall, or another body part. Explain that when he presses his palms together (pushing with one, resisting with the other) until he feels a tightness in his chest and up-per-arm muscles, he's doing a basic isometric exercise.

The patient doesn't have to be in any special position for most iso-metric exercises, so he can do them anytime and anywhere. Tell him to hold each contraction from 3 to 5 seconds, and to repeat the entire se-ries at least five times a day.

For the first week, tell him not to contract his muscles fully; this will give them a chance to get used to the exercises. After that, he should contract them fully.

Neck exercises

Instruct the patient to place the heel of his right hand above his right ear.

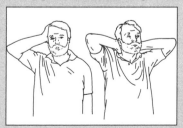

Without moving his head, neck, or arm, have him push his head to-ward his hand. Then instruct him to duplicate this exercise with his left hand above his left ear. Next, tell him to clasp his fingers behind his head. Without moving his neck or hands, he pushes his head back against his hands.

Shoulder and chest exercise

First, tell the patient to hold his right arm straight down at his side. Then have him grasp his right wrist with his left hand. Instruct him to try to shrug his right shoulder — but to prevent this by keeping a firm grip on his right wrist. Next, tell him to do a reverse version of this exercise with his left arm and shoul-der.

Arm exercise

Have the patient hold his right arm straight down at his side and then bend his elbow at a 90-degree an-gle. Tell him to turn his right palm up and place his left fist in it, and then try to bend his right arm up-ward while resisting this force with his left fist. Instruct him to do a re-verse version of this exercise with his left arm and right fist.

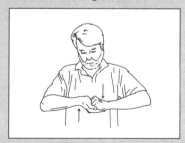

Abdominal exercise

Have the patient start by sitting on the floor or on a bed with his legs

(continued)

Teaching about isometric exercises *(continued)*

out in front of him. Then instruct him to bend forward and place his hands palm down on the midfront of his thighs. Urge him to try to bend farther forward, but to resist this movement by pressing his palms against his thighs.

Buttocks exercise
Instruct the patient to stand and squeeze his inner thighs and buttocks together as tightly as possible. If he's doing this exercise in bed, he should place a pillow between his knees to make it more effective.

Thigh exercise
For leg support, tell the patient to sit on the floor or on a bed. With his legs completely straight, have him vigorously tighten the muscles above his knees so that his kneecaps move upward.

Calf exercises
Tell the patient to sit up in bed and then bend down and grasp his toes. Then instruct him to pull gently

backward and hold this position briefly. Still touching his toes, he should push them forward and down as far as possible, holding this position briefly.

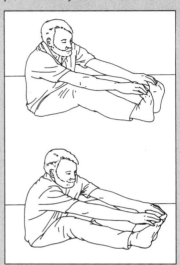

Other care measures
Teach the patient other measures to relieve discomfort, including massage and heat or cold therapy. Emphasize the importance of safety measures and correct use of assistive devices to compensate for restricted mobility. Tell the patient where he can obtain aids for personal care, such as for eating, driving, and walking. Suggest that he consider adapting his home, if necessary. Finally, refer him to appropriate organizations for additional information and support. (See Appendix 2.)

Osteoporosis
Osteoporosis is a major health problem affecting as many as 15 to 20 million Americans and causing more than 1 million fractures each year.

Sometimes called the "silent disease," osteoporosis often goes undetected until the patient sustains a fracture.

This makes your first opportunity for patient teaching more complicated than usual. You'll have to help ensure that the fracture heals properly and, at the same time, teach the patient how to avoid new fractures. Meanwhile, because osteoporosis has long been viewed as an inevitable part of aging, you may have to overcome the belief that little can be done to slow or prevent the disorder. Accordingly, you'll emphasize the roles played by proper diet, vitamin and mineral supplements, and regular exercise in controlling osteoporosis. You'll also emphasize proper body mechanics and new ways to perform daily activities safely.

Before teaching a patient about osteoporosis, make sure you are familiar with the following topics:

• how an imbalance between bone formation and resorption leads to osteoporosis

• explanation of osteoporosis types: type I and type II

• risk factors for osteoporosis

• diagnostic studies, such as X-rays, single- or dual-photon absorptiometry, transiliac bone biopsy, and blood and urine tests

• exercise program based on weight-bearing activities

• adequate dietary calcium and vitamin D intake

• drug therapy, including vitamin and mineral supplements, estrogen, and calcitonin

• observing safety practices and proper body mechanics to prevent fractures

• sources of information and support.

ABOUT THE DISORDER

Tell your patient that osteoporosis causes a gradual loss of bone mass while the size of the bones remains constant. This leaves bones brittle and prone to fractures. Explain that until age 35, bone formation and resorption occur at about the same rate. After age 35, the rate of bone resorption begins to exceed that of bone formation. The result is gradual bone loss.

Inform the patient that osteoporosis occurs in two forms: type I (post-menopausal) and type II (senile). Type I, which is related to estrogen loss, affects postmenopausal women between ages 55 and 75. (See *How menopause intensifies osteoporosis*, page 190.) In this disease form, trabecular bone loss exceeds cortical bone loss, with fractures of the vertebrae and wrist most common.

Explain that type II osteoporosis most commonly occurs between ages 70 and 85 and affects both men and women. Point out that it's characterized by both trabecular and cortical bone loss, which leads to fractures of the vertebrae, hip, and long bones. Mention that a calcium-poor diet may contribute to type II osteoporosis. (See *Risk factors for osteoporosis*, page 191.)

Complications

Explain to your patient with type II osteoporosis that failure to observe safety measures, proper body mechanics, and other treatment measures increases the risk of fractures. Stress that a fracture may result even from a simple activity, such as rising from a chair, raising a window, or bending over. Urge the patient to report even minor injuries to the doctor, particularly if pain or swelling persists.

DIAGNOSTIC WORKUP

Inform the patient that to confirm osteoporosis and to differentiate type I and type II, the doctor may order blood studies, X-rays, a transiliac bone biopsy, or a quantitative computed tomography scan. (See *Teaching patients about musculoskeletal tests,* pages 165 to 170.)

Blood and urine studies

Routine studies include serum protein electrophoresis; blood urea nitrogen; serum calcium, phosphorus, and thyroid hormone levels; and urine tests.

X-rays

X-rays can identify fractures and advanced bone loss. Advise the patient that special X-ray studies, such as single- or dual-photon absorptiometry, may also be performed. Point out that single-photon studies measure the mineral content of long bones, whereas dual-photon studies measure bone mass (density).

TREATMENTS

Treatments for osteoporosis aim to control bone loss and prevent fractures. The doctor may recommend moderate daily activities, a diet that boosts the body's calcium supply, vitamin and mineral supplements, and hormone therapy.

Activity guidelines

To help prevent further bone loss, urge the patient to follow a weight-

INSIGHT INTO ILLNESSES

How menopause intensifies osteoporosis

Explain to your patient that as a woman goes through menopause, circulating estrogen levels fall. As estrogen decreases, the bone's sensitivity to parathyroid hormone (PTH) increases. PTH stimulates resorption of calcium from the bone by activating the bone-resorbing cells and depressing bone-forming cells.

The subsequent increase in circulating calcium then depresses PTH secretion. In turn, the intestines absorb less dietary calcium, and the kidneys excrete more circulating calcium.

Eventually, the bones become so weak that they can't withstand force, and fractures result from minimal traumatic injury.

To help your patient understand the physiologic sequence that accelerates osteoporosis, show her the flow chart at right.

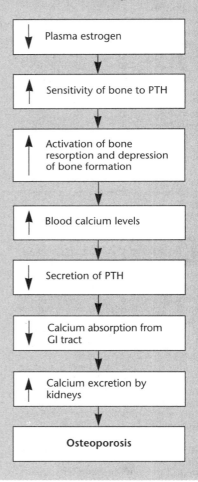

↓ Plasma estrogen

↑ Sensitivity of bone to PTH

↑ Activation of bone resorption and depression of bone formation

↑ Blood calcium levels

↓ Secretion of PTH

↓ Calcium absorption from GI tract

↑ Calcium excretion by kidneys

Osteoporosis

bearing exercise program. Emphasize that moderate weight-bearing activities, such as walking, jogging, bicycling, and low-impact aerobic exercises, activate osteoblastic bone formation and thus improve muscle strength, promote circulation, and enhance intestinal absorption of cal-

cium. For an elderly patient, the doctor may recommend swimming if weight-bearing exercise is not feasible.

WARNING: Instruct the patient to be cautious while exercising. Advise her to avoid activities that involve twisting, jumping, or straining the back (such as golf, tennis, and bowling) because these may cause fractures.

Make sure the patient understands the importance of incorporating safety practices and proper body mechanics into everyday activities.

Dietary modifications

Point out that although daily dietary calcium can't replace lost bone, it may slow or prevent further bone loss. Daily calcium requirements vary: children and young adults need about 800 mg, pregnant women need about 1,200 mg, and men and premenopausal women need about 1,000 mg. With menopause, a woman needs 1,000 to 1,500 mg/day.

To help achieve these requirements, encourage the patient to consume calcium-rich foods, such as milk and dairy products; milk provides about 275 to 300 mg/8-oz glass. Help the patient plan her menu selections to ensure adequate calcium intake.

 TIPS AND TIMESAVERS: Advise the patient to keep a supply of calcium-rich foods on hand. These include milk, cheese, yogurt, ice-cream, collards, turnip greens, broccoli, oysters, salmon, sardines, and tofu. For a patient who can't consume dairy products (such as a lactose-intolerant patient), recommend calcium supplements or calcium-containing antacids such as Tums.

A patient who smokes or consumes much dietary sugar and meat may have a higher calcium requirement. Advise her to follow her doctor's recommendations closely.

Medication

Inform the patient that calcium and vitamin D supplements, calcitonin, or estrogen (for menopausal women) may be prescribed to prevent or slow bone loss. Review how to take these medications, and discuss possible adverse effects. If appropriate, mention that certain new drugs may improve the long-term prospects for successful osteoporosis treatment.

Risk factors for osteoporosis

Everyone loses some bone tissue with age. However, some people are more likely to experience extensive bone loss. The following factors increase a person's risk for osteoporosis:

• sex — osteoporosis affects four times as many women as men
• age — after age 50, the osteoporosis risk increases
• race — Whites and Asians are at greater risk than Blacks
• body frame — osteoporosis affects more petite, small-framed persons than average-sized, large-framed persons
• onset of menopause in women; the earlier the onset (whether natural or surgically induced), the higher the risk
• a calcium-deficient diet
• a sedentary lifestyle
• a family history of osteoporosis
• regular alcohol and tobacco use or excessive caffeine consumption
• long-term corticosteroid, heparin, or certain antibiotic and anticonvulsant drug use
• multiparity or breast-feeding more than one nontwin infant
• medical conditions such as chronic renal failure, Cushing's syndrome, eating disorders such as anorexia, hyperparathyroidism, hyperthyroidism, intestinal absorption disorders requiring special therapy (such as intestinal bypass or gastrectomy), liver disease, or rheumatoid arthritis.

Vitamin and mineral supplements
Inform the patient who's not getting enough calcium in her diet that the doctor may recommend an over-the-counter calcium supplement. Remind her that the different calcium supplements contain differing amounts of

calcium. Calcium carbonate preparations, such as Cal-Sup, Os-Cal, Bio-Cal, Oyster Shell calcium, and some antacids (such as Tums), contain about 40% elemental calcium (the calcium form that the body is able to use). Calcium lactate and calcium gluconate contain much lower amounts of elemental calcium — 3% and 9%, respectively.

 WARNING: Caution the patient to avoid calcium supplements with dolomite and bone meal because these contain lead.

Instruct the patient to take the calcium supplement 1 hour before meals to ensure maximum absorption. However, if this decreases digestive acid production, advise her to take the supplement with meals. Recommend that she avoid laxatives and multivitamins containing zinc; these preparations decrease calcium absorption.

Mention that the doctor may recommend taking a vitamin D supplement along with the calcium to maximize intestinal absorption. Warn the patient never to exceed the recommended daily intake of vitamin D.

To ease adverse effects of calcium supplements (gas and constipation) suggest increasing fluid intake and increasing fiber *between* meals. However, point out that consuming extra fiber *during* a meal may impede calcium absorption.

Calcitonin
Explain to the patient that calcitonin is a hormone normally produced by the body that prevents bone loss by inhibiting bone resorption. Recommended to slow the progression of osteoporosis, calcitonin (salmon) is used to treat postmenopausal osteoporosis. Preferably, the drug is administered intranasally, although it's also available as an intramuscular or subcutaneous injection.

Teach the patient to administer the nasal spray into the nostril, alternating nostrils daily. Also instruct her to keep calcitonin refrigerated. Emphasize that she must use it in combination with calcium and vita-min D supplements as prescribed to prevent further bone loss.

Estrogen
The doctor may recommend estrogen replacement therapy for a postmenopausal patient or for a menopausal patient at high risk for osteoporosis. Estrogen doses as low as 0.625 mg have proven effective in preventing osteoporosis in postmenopausal women.

Because estrogen replacement therapy may increase the risk of endometrial and breast cancer, advise the patient to thoroughly discuss the pros and cons of this treatment option with her doctor before beginning therapy.

Etidronate
Etidronate (Didronel) is the first agent proven to restore lost bone. Already approved for treating Paget's disease, etidronate has been used safely and effectively in two clinical trials. Results indicate that just 2 weeks of use every 4 months increases bone mass. However, as a treatment for osteoporosis, the drug is still experimental.

Other care measures
In osteoporosis, safety practices and proper body mechanics go hand in hand in preventing fractures. Advise the patient to wear comfortable, well-fitting shoes with rubber heels to help cushion and protect the spine during walking. Discourage high heels.

To prevent falls, suggest removing throw rugs, placing a nonskid mat in the bathtub, and installing handrails on stairs. Advise the patient not to walk in dimly lit rooms. Also caution against lifting heavy objects, twisting suddenly, or bending from the waist.

Describe devices that may make daily activities easier — for example, a shoe horn, long-handled sponge, or a reacher-grabber. If appropriate, suggest a cane or walker to help the patient maintain balance and decrease lower back pain.

Finally, refer the patient to an appropriate resource for further information and support. (See Appendix 2.)

Sprains and strains

A sprain or a strain may seem like a minor injury to many patients. Left untreated, however, either of these injuries may seriously compromise the patient's ability to regain normal strength and function. And failure to rehabilitate the injured extremity may lead to more serious reinjury.

Therefore, you'll need to emphasize the importance of immobilizing or protecting the injured body part while it heals. Athletes, in particular, may pose special challenges if they're eager to resume training or competition before the injury has healed.

Regardless of the patient's attitude about his injury, you'll need to define a sprain or a strain and point out possible complications if the patient doesn't protect and rehabilitate the injured part. You'll also describe diagnostic tests and treatments.

Before teaching a patient about a sprain or a strain, make sure you are familiar with the following topics:
• explanation of the injury
• possible complications, including impaired circulation, nerve damage, and loss of function in the affected area
• diagnostic tests, such as X-rays
• the importance of protecting the limb from further injury
• anti-inflammatory and analgesic drugs to relieve swelling and pain
• treatments, such as rest, ice, compression, and elevation
• physical therapy for rehabilitation
• immobilization devices, such as elastic bandages, casts, and crutches
• surgery for severe sprains
• sources of information and support.

ABOUT THE DISORDER

Tell the patient that a *sprain* refers to stretching or tearing of the capsule or ligament surrounding a joint, resulting in acute pain and swelling. (See *Sprains and strains: An inside view*, page 194.) An ankle sprain, for instance, may occur from twisting the ankle during a fall or stepping on an uneven surface. Inform the patient that a *strain* is a partial, microscopic tear in a muscle or tendon or both. An *acute* strain results from a sudden forced movement that overstretches the muscle or tendon. The patient may not feel pain until sometime after the initial injury, during continued activity. A *chronic* strain stems from the cumulative effect of repeated muscle overuse. Such strains commonly result from injury during sports, such as tennis, golf, or basketball. A strain also can occur when a person uses poor body mechanics in lifting or carrying.

Mention that sprains and strains are classified by the extent of tissue damage, from grade I (mild damage) to grade III (severe damage).

DIAGNOSTIC WORKUP

Tell the patient that the doctor will perform a physical examination of the injured area to evaluate joint stability. He may also order an X-ray or a computed tomography scan to evaluate the severity and determine the location of the injury. (See *Teaching patients about musculoskeletal tests,* pages 165 to 170.) Inform the patient that to visualize the injured part, the technician may need to maneuver and reposition the injured part, which may cause pain.

TREATMENTS

When discussing activity restrictions and rehabilitation goals, emphasize the patient's contribution to recovery. Discuss medications his doctor may prescribe for pain and inflammation. Describe procedures to treat a sprain or a strain, including application of ice and heat, elevation of the affected area, and use of an elastic bandage. Also discuss immobilization devices and crutches and, if appropriate, surgery for a severe sprain.

Activity guidelines

Instruct the patient to rest the injured part for at least 24 hours — or longer, if the doctor directs him to withhold activities until all diagnostic studies are complete. After that, he may resume some activities using a sling, wrap, cast, or crutches.

INSIGHT INTO ILLNESSES

Sprains and strains: An inside view

Except for possible swelling and discomfort, your patient can't actually see a strain or a sprain. But he can surely feel it because a *sprain* is the stretching or tearing of a ligament, the fibrous tissue that binds joints together. A *strain*, whether acute or chronic, is a partial muscle tear. A strain can also affect tendons, the fibrous tissue that connects muscle to bone. Here's what sprains and strains look like "inside."

Knee sprain

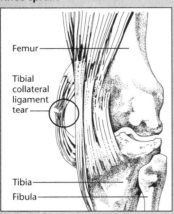

Femur
Tibial collateral ligament tear
Tibia
Fibula

Calf strain

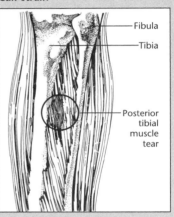

Fibula
Tibia
Posterior tibial muscle tear

Medication

Tell the patient that the doctor may prescribe analgesics to relieve pain and nonsteroidal anti-inflammatory drugs (NSAIDs) to decrease inflammation. Review the prescribed dosages and possible side effects of these drugs. Advise the patient with a history of ulcers or sensitivity to salicylates to take NSAIDs with meals to help prevent stomach upset.

 WARNING: Instruct the patient to stop taking pain medication and notify the doctor if nausea, vomiting, abdominal pain, or dark stools occur.

Procedures

Advise your patient to think of the mnemonic RICE (*R*est, *I*ce, *C*ompression, and *E*levation) to help him remember what to do during the first few days after a sprain or strain. Then instruct him about any immobilization device the doctor prescribes.

RICE

Emphasize that rest and ice reduce pain and swelling. Tell the patient to place an ice pack over the most tender part of the injury. Instruct him to use it for 48 hours, applying it at 30-minute intervals and moving it every 5 minutes to avoid frostbite.

 TIPS AND TIMESAVERS: If the patient doesn't have an ice pack, instruct him to place ice in a plastic bag, wrap the bag in a towel, and then apply it as described above.

To reduce swelling, advise the patient to elevate the injured extremity

How to apply an elastic bandage

An elastic bandage compresses the tissue around a sprain or a strain to help prevent swelling and provide support. Use the following instructions when teaching the patient how to wrap an elastic bandage around his ankle. (He can modify these instructions for wrapping his knee, wrist, elbow, or hand.)

1. To begin, tell the patient to hold the loose end of the elastic bandage on the top of his foot between his instep and toes. With his other hand, have him wrap the bandage twice around his foot, gradually moving toward his ankle. Make sure he overlaps the bandage in spiral fashion.

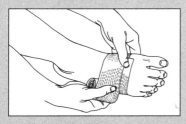

2. After he wraps his foot twice, tell him to move his hand to support his heel. Then instruct him to use his other hand to wrap the bandage in figure-eight fashion, leaving his heel uncovered.

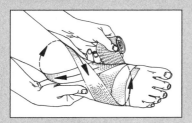

To do this, he should angle the bandage down, cross it over the top of his foot, and pass it under his foot to complete the figure-eight turn. Tell him to do this step twice.

3. Now, have him circle the bandage around his calf, moving toward his knee. Make sure he overlaps the elastic as he wraps. Tell him to stop just below the knee. Caution him not wrap downward.

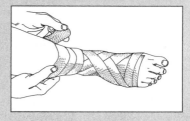

4. Finally, have him secure the end of the bandage with a metal clip or adhesive tape.

Comfort and safety tips

Instruct the patient to aim for a snug, not tight, fit. Warn him never to wrap the bandage so tightly that it restricts or cuts off his circulation. If he's stretching the bandage material, chances are he's wrapping too tightly.

To promote circulation, tell the patient to remove and rewrap his bandage at least twice daily. Instruct him to remove the bandage immediately if he has any numbness or tingling. When these symptoms disappear, he should reapply the bandage. If numbness or tingling doesn't stop, he should call the doctor.

above heart level for the first 24 hours after the injury. To further ease swelling, recommend wrapping the injured part in an elastic bandage to compress the tissue. Provide instruc-

tions on wrapping. (See *How to apply an elastic bandage.*)

Immobilization

Inform the patient that the doctor

may order an immobilization device to relieve pain and promote healing. Explain that this device supports or immobilizes the injured body part. The type of device used depends on the severity of his injury and the degree of disability.

If the patient has a moderate sprain, the doctor may order an air cast — an inflatable device with an adjustable, rigid, lightweight shell. Reassure him that the cast is easy to remove and promotes an early return to his previous level of mobility.

If the patient has a severe sprain, the doctor may recommend a plaster or fiberglass cast for more rigid support. Explain that he'll wear it for 3 to 4 weeks. A plaster cast may take up to 24 hours to dry; a fiberglass cast dries in only a few minutes. Tell the patient that the cast will feel warm as it dries.

 WARNING: Caution the patient not to bear weight on the injured limb until the cast is completely dry. Otherwise, he may reshape the cast and produce pressure points.

Surgery
Surgical intervention — usually arthroscopy — may be necessary for a sprain that causes joint instability or doesn't respond adequately to conventional measures. Tell the patient that after surgery, he will wear an immobilization device for several weeks, depending on the location and severity of the injury.

Other measures
The doctor may recommend an appropriate rehabilitation program. If the patient has a sprain, tell him that treatment may begin with range-of-motion exercises, followed by isometric exercises in the injured limb. As healing progresses, conditioning and strengthening exercises may be added. Stress the importance of exercising uninjured extremities as well as the injured one because this helps prevent loss of muscle tone and vascular problems.

Instruct the patient to check pulses, warmth, mobility, and sensory function around the injury site and to report any changes to the doctor right away.

Finally, encourage the patient to express his concerns about his condition. If appropriate, refer him to appropriate resources for information and support. (See Appendix 2.)

7

Skin conditions

Dermatitis

With dermatitis, patients are usually so uncomfortable that they seek medical attention right away — only to learn that relief from this skin inflammation may become a life-long struggle. Your goals, then, are to teach the patient how to recognize dermatitis and relieve pruritus, and thus promote healing.

To accomplish these goals, you'll help the patient identify aggravating factors by exploring his occupation, lifestyle, hobbies, and stressors. Most important, you'll teach him a meticulous skin care regimen that includes medications, baths, and dressings. You'll also discuss the disease process, how to identify the disorder, and the role of activity and diet.

Before teaching the patient about dermatitis, make sure you are familiar with the following topics:
• explanation of the type of dermatitis — atopic or contact — including causes and signs and symptoms
• preventing complications (permanent skin damage and skin infections) by complying with treatment
• diagnosis by appearance and by patch testing to identify allergens
• role of diet and activity restrictions in treatment
• medications, including antihistamines, topical corticosteroids, and emollients
• how to take a therapeutic bath and how to care for the skin
• how to apply a total body wrap
• how to apply wet-to-dry dressings
• importance of identifying and avoiding known allergens and aggravating factors
• sources of information and support.

ABOUT THE DISORDER

Because dermatitis has many names, your patient may be confused about exactly what he has. Tell him that the popular term for dermatitis is *eczema*. Then, as appropriate, explain that the most common types of dermatitis are *atopic dermatitis*, caused by an inherited immunologic response, and *contact dermatitis,* an acquired immunologic response. Atopic dermatitis may last through a lifetime of exacerbations and remissions; contact dermatitis usually is incidental. In both disorders, itchy skin causes the patient to scratch, which produces a rash and lesions. The rash and lesions, in turn, cause pruritus and perpetuate the cycle.

Inform the patient that in *atopic dermatitis,* skin hypersensitivity occurs with increased sweating. Lipids and water are carried away from the skin, leaving it dry and itchy. Older patients with atopic dermatitis usually have a history of asthma, allergic rhinitis, or a genetic predisposition to allergies.

Typically beginning between ages 2 and 6 months, atopic dermatitis affects about 9 of every 1,000 persons. In infants, red, blisterlike, exudative lesions appear on the face, arms, and legs. Explain to the infant's parents that remission sometimes occurs spontaneously around age 2 or 3; however, dermatitis may recur when the patient experiences aggravating factors.

Tell the patient that the *acute form* of atopic dermatitis is a red, bumpy, swollen rash that causes intense itching. Scratching the rash produces oozing, crusted lesions. The *chronic form,* in contrast, is characterized by barklike skin with thickened lesions and hypopigmented (white) and hyperpigmented (brown) areas.

Teach the patient with *contact dermatitis* that this disorder results from prolonged, repeated contact with an allergen. It causes intense itching and, depending on the severity, may progress to a rash like that of atopic dermatitis. Although usually localized, the rash may generalize in severe cases. Repeated exposure can lead to chronic dermatitis.

Complications

Let the patient know that uncontrolled atopic dermatitis increases his susceptibility to viral infections, such as vaccinia and herpes simplex, which can lead to the potentially fatal Kaposi's varicelliform eruption. Also tell him that without proper treatment, dermatitis can cause permanent skin damage, including lichenification (skin thickening and hardening, with exaggerated normal markings), altered pigmentation, and scarring.

Tell the patient with severe, chronic contact dermatitis that the disorder can progress to *exfoliative dermatitis* — a medical emergency. In this disorder, peeling disrupts the skin's integrity and barrier function, causing thermoregulatory problems, electrolyte imbalances, protein and iron losses, and secondary infections.

 WARNING: Urge the patient to seek immediate medical attention if chronic dermatitis progresses — especially if he has heart disease. Left untreated, chronic dermatitis can progress to heart failure in the presence of heart disease.

DIAGNOSTIC WORKUP

Inform the patient that the doctor diagnoses dermatitis from patient and family health histories and the lesions' appearance. Differentiating atopic and contact dermatitis requires skin and blood tests, skin cultures, and allergy tests.

Tests for atopic dermatitis

Describe a simple test for atopic dermatitis: The doctor will firmly stroke the affected area with a blunt instrument and observe for a white — not reddened — reaction. This skin response commonly occurs in patients with atopic dermatitis.

Explain that blood tests can detect increased amounts of immunoglobulin E and eosinophils — indicators of atopic dermatitis. Add that tissue cultures can help rule out fungal, bacterial, or viral superinfections. (Patients with atopic dermatitis are prone to *Staphylococcus aureus* infections.)

If the patient with atopic dermatitis has asthma or allergic rhinitis, the doctor may order allergy testing to detect other possible allergy sources that may aggravate atopic dermatitis.

Tests for contact dermatitis

Tell the patient that the doctor diagnoses contact dermatitis in the same way as atopic dermatitis but will also examine lesion distribution, which may help pinpoint allergens. For example, if the lesions appear only on the ear, wrist, and finger, the allergen may be a metal found in jewelry. (See *Identifying allergens by affected body part*.)

The doctor may then proceed with a *patch test*, applying small amounts of the suspected allergens to disks of filter paper attached to aluminum and coated with plastic. The disks are taped to clear, hairless skin on the patient's back or forearm and then observed for reactions (typically hives, redness, and pruritus if the patch contains an allergen). Tell the patient not to touch the patches for 48 hours. However, if pain, itching, redness, or warmth occurs, he should remove the patches immediately.

Inform the patient that a skin reaction confirms contact sensitivity to an allergen but doesn't necessarily confirm that the specific allergen in the patch caused the dermatitis.

TREATMENTS

Explain that the best treatment for dermatitis is prevention — avoiding known allergens and other aggravating factors. When this fails, adhering to the prescribed skin care regimen

Identifying allergens by affected body part

Different allergens produce reactions on different parts of the body. Use this diagram to target contact points and identify possible allergens.

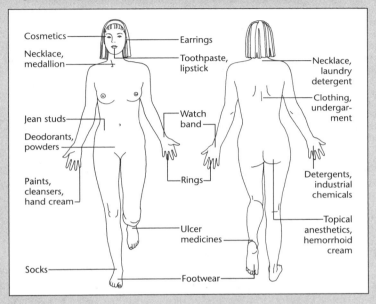

Cosmetics

Necklace, medallion

Jean studs

Deodorants, powders

Paints, cleansers, hand cream

Socks

Earrings

Toothpaste, lipstick

Watch band

Rings

Ulcer medicines

Footwear

Necklace, laundry detergent

Clothing, undergarment

Detergents, industrial chemicals

Topical anesthetics, hemorrhoid cream

becomes all-important. Treatment measures for dermatitis may involve temporary activity restrictions, dietary changes, medications, tepid baths, and wet wraps or wet-to-dry dressings.

Activity guidelines

Tell the patient with *atopic dermatitis* that he'll have to curtail his activities temporarily for treatment when his disorder flares up. However, encourage him (especially if he's a child) to pursue moderate activity. Teach him how to clean and moisturize his skin after exercise.

Inform the patient with *contact dermatitis* that he needn't restrict his activities unless they involve contact with an allergen.

Dietary modifications

Explain that the value of dietary changes in dermatitis treatment remains controversial. Although patch tests and elimination diets may be used to identify food allergies, test results aren't always reliable. Besides, elimination diets are tedious and difficult to follow, especially for children.

 TIPS AND TIMESAVERS: Inform the patient that his best bet is to avoid any food that he knows triggers his dermatitis. Common food allergens include eggs, cow's milk, shellfish, and foods containing soybeans, nuts, and wheat.

Medication

Point out that prescribed medications will help reduce inflammation, relieve pruritus, and promote healing. Then describe a typical medication

regimen that includes a systemic antihistamine, a topical corticosteroid,
and a bland emollient. Inform the patient that if severe dermatitis doesn't
respond to topical treatment, the doctor may order systemic corticosteroids.

Antihistamines
Discuss how systemic antihistamines,
such as hydroxyzine hydrochloride
(Atarax) and diphenhydramine hydrochloride (Benadryl), relieve pruritus. Tell the patient he may have to
take antihistamines around the clock
until the scratch-itch-scratch cycle
breaks. Suggest that he drink water or
use ice chips if the drug causes dry
mouth. Warn him that he'll feel
drowsy at first, so he should approach physical activity with extra
caution. Reassure him that drowsiness will decrease with continued
drug use.

Corticosteroids
Topical corticosteroids reduce pruritus
and inflammation and act as skin barriers. They also act as vasoconstrictors
to counteract vasodilation and inflammation associated with erythroderma.
Mention that corticosteroids are available as creams or ointments, but that
ointments are preferred for dermatitis
because they're more occlusive. Then
explain that corticosteroids come in
varying strengths.

Explain that percutaneous absorption can increase with long-term use,
occlusion, or application to broken
skin. Inform the patient that systemic effects occur only after years of
use. If he develops any adverse reaction or if his dermatitis doesn't seem
to be responding, instruct him to discontinue the medication and notify
his doctor.

Emollients
The doctor may recommend using a
bland emollient such as petrolatum
along with a topical corticosteroid.
Tell the patient that this creates a better skin barrier to maintain home-
ostasis and skin hydration.

Procedures
Describe self-care procedures that
may help reduce dermatitis, including therapeutic baths, wet wraps,
wet-to-dry dressings and, for severe
dermatitis, occlusive dressings.

Therapeutic baths
Although some doctors restrict
bathing because of its drying effect,
others suggest soaking in tepid water
containing nonperfumed bath oil or
colloidal oatmeal. This soothes the
skin by helping it remain moist, thus
reducing pruritus.

Caution the patient to avoid hot
baths because heat induces pruritus
by increasing vasodilation. Instruct
him to use a soft towel to pat excess
moisture from his skin (rubbing induces pruritus) and to immediately
apply the recommended hydropho-
bic occlusive preparations to help
seal in moisture.

For daily cleanliness, advise the patient to use mild, nonperfumed soap
with minimal defatting (detergent)
activity and a neutral pH — or a prescribed nonsoap cleaning agent.

Wet wraps
For severe or persistent dermatitis in
children or adults, the doctor may recommend wet wraps to optimize hydration and topical therapy. To do a
total body wrap, tell the patient to
first soak a pair of pajamas or long underwear in water and wring out the
excess moisture. Then instruct him to
apply his medication and step into
the wet pajamas or long underwear.
Next, tell him to cover the wet clothes
with dry pajamas, dry clothes, or a dry
or plastic sweatsuit. He should cover
his hands and feet with wet gauze followed by dry elastic bandages. Caution
him to keep the room warm so that
he doesn't become chilled.

Wet-to-dry dressings
Show the patient with oozing lesions
how to apply a wet-to-dry dressing.
(See *How to apply wet-to-dry dressings.*)

How to apply wet-to-dry dressings

If the doctor recommends wet-to-dry dressings, teach your patient that these dressings can help relieve flare-ups of dermatitis; soothe inflammation, itching, and burning; remove crusts and scales from dry lesions; and help dry up oozing lesions. What's more, using these dressings may prevent complications, such as bacterial or fungal infections.

Explain that these dressings are applied in four steps. Then provide the following instructions.

For an acute flare-up

1. Tell the patient to moisten a piece of gauze or a soft, clean cloth with warm tap water, normal saline solution, or Burow's solution. Have him squeeze out the excess moisture, but stress that he shouldn't squeeze the gauze or cloth completely dry; it should still make a squishy sound when gently squeezed.
2. Instruct the patient to apply the wet dressing to the affected skin area, making sure he covers all of the rash.

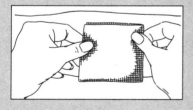

3. Now tell the patient to use dry roller gauze or pin a towel to hold the dressing in place. Instruct him to let the dressing air-dry for about 20 minutes. Caution him not to hold the dressing in place with tape because the adhesive may irritate his skin.

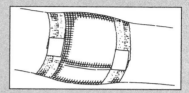

4. Tell the patient to remove the dressing without remoistening it and then to apply the topical preparations as prescribed by the doctor.

Have him repeat the entire procedure every 4 to 6 hours, changing the dressing material every 24 hours.

For a generalized flare-up

Advise the patient to follow the steps above. At step 2, he should first apply the prescribed ointment or cream, and then apply the wet dressing as directed. This will make the blood vessels constrict, leaving the skin feeling cool. It also will help his sore, irritated skin absorb the medicine and decrease inflammation and itching.

Occlusive dressings
In severe dermatitis, show the patient how to use an occlusive dressing. For example, hands with severe contact dermatitis may require a topical corticosteroid and occlusion with gloves to increase drug absorption and skin hydration.

Other care measures
For patients with *atopic dermatitis*, stress the importance of identifying

and avoiding aggravating factors and allergens. If the patient's symptoms are exacerbated by stress, refer him to a counselor or encourage him to find a local stress management support group. (See Appendix 2.)

 TIPS AND TIMESAVERS: Advise the patient to wear rubber gloves when cleaning and to rinse his laundry twice to ensure that all detergent washes away. Suggest that he remain mindful of other possible irritants in his daily life, such as cosmetics, drugs, or home remedies.

For a patient with *contact dermatitis,* discuss the importance of finding the source of the inflammation and then avoiding it. Tell him to think carefully about substances he comes into contact with regularly — chances are he's allergic to one or more of them.

Herpes simplex virus

The physical discomfort and social stigma associated with herpes simplex virus (HSV) present a formidable teaching challenge. Besides educating the patient about the disease process, you'll be called on to help him cope with the emotional distress that having HSV creates.

Your teaching will help the patient understand how he contracted the disease, learn to use medication and other measures to relieve symptoms, recognize factors that trigger recurrent disease, and avoid transmitting HSV.

Before teaching a patient about HSV, make sure you are familiar with the following topics:
• recognizing signs and symptoms of HSV infections
• how HSV infection spreads
• recurrence and trigger factors
• complications, such as ocular herpes and increased cancer risks
• drug therapy, such as acyclovir and vidarabine
• comfort measures, such as bed rest and sitz baths
• preventing HSV transmission
• sources of information and support.

ABOUT THE DISORDER
Inform the patient that an estimated 20 million people suffer from genital herpes. Explain that HSV — also called *Herpesvirus hominis* — occurs in two strains: Type 1 (HSV-1), and Type 2 (HSV-2). Both strains are highly contagious.

HSV-1 usually produces lesions on the skin and the mucous membranes of the lips and mouth (gingivostomatitis). HSV-2 is a sexually transmitted viral infection of the urogenital tract. Emphasize that both HSV-1 and

HSV-2 may remain contagious whether the carrier has active lesions or no signs and symptoms at all.

HSV-1
If your patient has an HSV-1 infection, explain that initial symptoms usually include a sore throat or oral lesions (on the skin and the mucous membranes of the lips and mouth) or both. The virus also may involve the eye, specifically the conjunctiva and cornea (keratoconjunctivitis). Other signs and symptoms may include fever, chills, muscle aches, and swollen lymph nodes (especially common if the patient has tonsillitis).

The lesions associated with HSV-1 — commonly called cold sores or fever blisters — ulcerate, and in about 2 days form a yellow crust over the area. The sores begin to heal without scarring in 10 days. Recurrence is usually preceded by a tiny burning or itchy sensation before eruption of lesions (called the *prodrome*).

HSV-2
If your patient has genital herpes caused by HSV-2, explain that the initial infection usually occurs 2 to 20 days after exposure. (See *Genital herpes cycle.*) Add that a tingling or burning sensation may precede the cluster of small, fluid-filled or pus-filled blisters that erupt on the vulva, rectum, penis, buttocks, thighs, or legs. (If the lesions persist longer than 1 month, this may indicate an opportunistic viral infection associated with acquired immunodeficiency syndrome.)

Explain that recurring episodes of genital herpes usually cause less pain than the initial infection and last between 7 and 10 days. Discuss possible trigger factors, such as physical or emotional stress, sunlight, menstrual cycle changes, and sexual intercourse.

Complications
Inform the patient that inadequate measures to contain herpes simplex may lead to its spread and to disease complications. For example, accidental self-inoculation by HSV-1 or HSV-2 can cause infection of the fingers,

INSIGHT INTO ILLNESSES

Genital herpes cycle

Inform the patient that after the initial herpes infection, a latency period follows. During this time, the virus enters nerves surrounding the lesions and remains there. Intermittent viral shedding may take place.

Explain that repeated herpetic outbreaks may develop at any time, again followed by a latent stage when healing's complete. The frequency of these outbreaks varies; in some patients, they recur as often as three to eight times yearly. Although the cycle continues indefinitely, some people remain symptom-free for years.

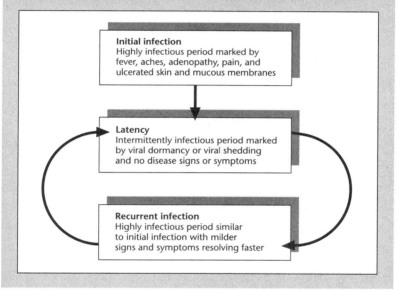

Initial infection
Highly infectious period marked by fever, aches, adenopathy, pain, and ulcerated skin and mucous membranes

Latency
Intermittently infectious period marked by viral dormancy or viral shedding and no disease signs or symptoms

Recurrent infection
Highly infectious period similar to initial infection with milder signs and symptoms resolving faster

called herpetic whitlow. When spread to the eyes, herpes simplex can cause keratitis and visual impairment.

If your patient is a woman with genital herpes, tell her that urine retention is a common complication that results from difficult and painful urination. Also explain that genital herpes is associated with an increased risk of cervical cancer and of neonatal infection in infants whose mothers transmitted herpes during vaginal birth. Because neonatal infection carries a 90% mortality, vaginal delivery is permitted only if the mother has

been free of herpes symptoms throughout pregnancy, is experiencing no herpes symptoms at the time of expected delivery, is free of vulvar and vaginal lesions, and has had two recent negative cervical cultures and no more than one positive culture throughout her pregnancy.

HSV may also pass to the fetus transplacentally and, in early pregnancy, may cause spontaneous abortion, premature birth, microcephaly, chorioretinitis, and mental retardation.

Sex and genital herpes

Genital herpes can cause long-term sexual problems. The person with herpes may fear that he's a source of danger to his partner. He may retreat from revealing his condition to his partner, or he may hesitate to initiate a relationship.

To compound the problem, the patient's herpes-free partner always runs the risk of acquiring the disease through sexual intercourse.

Offer the patient acceptance and support as he deals with his dilemma: how to have a meaningful sex life without transmitting a lifelong disease. Here are a few guidelines.

• Tell the patient to avoid having sexual intercourse from the disease's prodromal stage until 10 days after the lesions heal. Though herpes can be transmitted at any time, it appears that transmission occurs less frequently during symptom-free periods.

• Make sure the patient understands that using condoms does not guarantee protection against herpes, but it does increase safety.

• Advise the patient to approach relationships with honesty, but to avoid shocking revelations like, "I have something terrible to tell you." Rather, he should broach the subject of herpes with discretion at a convenient time, using neutral words and terms. For instance, recommend that he think of herpes as intermittently self-limiting rather than incurable.

DIAGNOSTIC WORKUP
Before the diagnostic workup begins, ensure the patient that all results will be strictly confidential. Because pa-

tients with herpes commonly experience feelings of anger, shame, and depression, be sure to maintain a nonjudgmental attitude and allow time for the patient to express his feelings. (See *Sex and genital herpes*.)

Tell the patient that HSV is usually diagnosed from the health history and physical examination. Inform him that a Tzanck test may confirm the diagnosis. In this test, the doctor scrapes some material from a blister, smears it on a slide, and stains it for microscopic examination. Point out that although the test can confirm the presence of HSV, it can't distinguish among HSV-1, HSV-2, and herpes zoster (shingles).

A blood sample may reveal the HSV antibody but, like the Tzanck test, doesn't provide a differential diagnosis. The doctor may also order a viral culture of material scraped from a blister. This aids confirmation of HSV infection and differentiates HSV-1 and HSV-2.

TREATMENTS
Although HSV infections are incurable, drug therapy and other measures — such as bed rest and fluid intake — can reduce pain, prevent the spread of lesions, and possibly decrease symptom recurrence. Besides discussing treatments and comfort measures, familiarize the patient with measures to prevent disease transmission.

Activity guidelines
If the patient has a severe case of HSV with many painful lesions, reinforce the doctor's recommendation of bed rest for 1 or 2 days.

Dietary modifications
If urination causes pain, the patient may want to avoid consuming fluids. However, encourage him to drink 10 to 12 glasses of water or other fluids daily. Explain that avoiding fluids and urinating less frequently can place him at risk for urinary tract infection.

Medication

Make sure the patient understands how to take prescribed medications. These may include antiviral agents, analgesics, and lysine. Teach the patient that medications don't cure herpes but may relieve some symptoms.

Antiviral agents

Acyclovir (Zovirax) is the drug of choice for treating genital herpes. Tell the patient that although acyclovir won't speed healing or prevent recurrences, it may decrease the severity of outbreaks and the duration of viral shedding. For safety and effectiveness, advise the patient to take acyclovir exactly as the doctor directs. If he's taking tablets or capsules, tell him to take them with food to avoid stomach upset, to try not to miss any doses, and not to take them longer or more often than directed.

 WARNING: Remind the patient that acyclovir won't keep him from passing herpes to others. If he has genital herpes, he should avoid sex until he's symptom-free.

If the patient's taking topical *vidarabine* (Vira-A Ophthalmic) for ocular herpes, explain that this eye ointment may relieve symptoms of recurrent keratitis. Instruct him to follow the application directions exactly and not to exceed the recommended dosage. Caution him to wash his hands before using the drug and to avoid touching the tube to his eye or surrounding areas. Teach him to store the ointment according to label directions. Forewarn him that this drug may increase tearing or make him feel as if something is in his eye. Suggest that he wear sunglasses if light bothers his eyes during treatment. Remind him to discard the ointment after treatment is complete. If burning, increased sensitivity to light, itching, pain, redness, or new eye problems occur after using vidarabine, tell the patient to contact the doctor promptly.

Analgesics

Explain that the doctor may recommend aspirin or acetaminophen (Tylenol) to relieve pain and reduce fever. Review typical adverse effects (such as GI upset) associated with these drugs.

 WARNING: To reduce the risk of Reye's syndrome, caution parents not to give aspirin to a child with cold sores.

The doctor may prescribe a topical anesthetic such as lidocaine (Stanacaine, Xylocaine Jelly) for painful skin lesions or a lidocaine mouthwash for mouth and throat ulcers. This drug, which gives temporary relief, may make eating and drinking less painful, promoting adequate hydration.

Lysine

Advise the patient that the amino acid lysine may offer effective prophylaxis against recurrent herpes outbreaks. Explain that taking lysine in response to prodromal symptoms, such as burning, itching, or tingling, may limit or prevent lesions.

Encourage the patient with recurrent infections to drink milk and to eat lysine-rich foods, such as chicken, fish, pork, and legumes (beans and peas).

Other care measures

Suggest washing herpetic lesions several times a day with mild, unscented soap and warm water. Tell the patient to pat the lesions dry and to avoid scratching them.

To obtain additional pain relief for genital lesions, suggest that the patient apply compresses soaked in a drying substance such as Burow's solution. Suggest that a woman pour warm water over the vulva or urinate in a portable sitz bath.

Explain that keeping the lesions clean and dry will help prevent them from spreading. Advise the patient to wear cotton underpants to help absorb excess moisture.

Point out other ways to avoid transmitting infection. For instance, encourage the patient to wash bed linens, clothes, and eating utensils separately from those of other family members. Demonstrate proper hand-washing techniques, and caution him not to let others use his personal items, such as his towel, washcloth, soap, toothbrush, or drinking cup.

Discuss how genital herpes affects sexual relationships, and offer guidelines on preventing its spread during intercourse. Because genital herpes increases the risk of cervical cancer, recommend that women with herpes have Pap smears every 6 to 12 months.

Keep in mind that HSV infections may exact a high emotional toll. Feelings of loneliness, anger, and self-pity are common among patients with genital herpes. Invite the patient to share his concerns with you, the doctor, or a support group. To help him adjust to living with this disease, provide information on support groups. (See Appendix 2.)

Herpes zoster

Commonly called shingles, herpes zoster will test your teaching skills. Because this disorder can cause extreme pain, you may need to spend extra time teaching about analgesic measures and reassuring the patient that herpetic pain usually goes away.

If you care for elderly patients or those with serious immunosuppressive illnesses, you're likely to have many opportunities for teaching about the disease. That's because herpes zoster has become increasingly common with the growing numbers of elderly and immunocompromised patients — cancer survivors, transplant recipients, and those with acquired immunodeficiency syndrome.

Initially, you'll discuss the cause of herpes zoster and its course and inform the patient about drug therapy. Because the disorder may be associated with inadequate immune defenses, you'll need to emphasize the importance of recognizing and avoiding infection.

Before teaching a patient about herpes zoster, make sure you are familiar with the following topics:
• what causes herpes zoster

• signs and symptoms of herpes zoster infection
• complications such as postherpetic neuralgia
• tests such as the Tzanck test to confirm diagnosis
• drug therapy with acyclovir, analgesics, antihistamines, and other agents
• other care measures, including infection prevention.

ABOUT THE DISORDER
Tell the patient that herpes zoster is an acute viral infection marked by painful skin eruptions. It's caused by the varicella zoster virus — the same virus that causes chickenpox. Explain that during the course of chickenpox, the virus invades the peripheral nerves and remains dormant in the nervous system. As long as the immune system functions properly, the virus stays suppressed. However, it may become reactivated if the immune system deteriorates with age, disease, drug therapy, radiation treatment, or trauma.

Initially, shingles causes mild fever, pain, and tingling or burning along the course of the affected nerve pathway. A rash may appear at the same time or within 5 to 6 days. The fever subsides when the rash appears as red patches. Within 1 to 2 days, the rash develops into blisters, which may coalesce into large eruptions. The blisters fill with pus, eventually crust and scab, and usually heal within a month. Characteristically, the rash is confined to one or two lumbar dermatomes; the virus spreads in a bandlike manner along the dermatome. (See *Herpes zoster sites.*)

Tell the patient that herpes zoster can affect the eyes (herpes zoster ophthalmicus), causing conjunctivitis, scleritis, keratitis, or iridocyclitis. If it involves the 8th cranial nerve (Ramsay Hunt syndrome), the patient will experience ear pain (often severe) and blisters on the eardrum, along with tinnitus, hearing loss, loss of taste, and facial paralysis. Facial paralysis and loss of taste may be permanent.

INSIGHT INTO ILLNESSES

Herpes zoster sites

The herpes zoster virus infects the nerves that innervate the skin, eyes, and ears. Each nerve (tagged for its corresponding vertebral source) emanates from the spine, banding and branching to innervate a skin area called a dermatome.

Show your patient how the herpes zoster rash erupts along the course of the affected nerve fibers, covering the skin of one or more of the dermatomes shown below.

Explain that the thoracic (T) and lumbar (L) dermatomes are most commonly affected, but that other dermatomes, such as those covering the cervical (C) and the sacral (S) areas can be affected, too. In fact, the herpes zoster rash can occur anywhere on the face or body.

Keep in mind that dermatomes are variable and overlap.

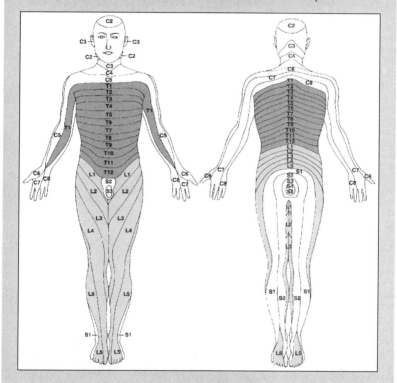

Complications

Inform the patient that despite excellent medical care, long-lasting or serious complications of herpes zoster sometimes occur. The most common complication is persistent pain in the area of the skin lesions or the affected dermatome, known as *postherpetic neuralgia.* Some patients may continue to experience aching, burning, or itching sensations for more than a month after the initial rash clears up. In some, pain may persist for about 15 years.

In severely immunocompromised patients, the zoster rash may spread over the entire body. This form of the disease, called *disseminated herpes zoster,* is usually accompanied by fever and malaise. Ultimately, it may infect the central nervous system and lungs.

DIAGNOSTIC WORKUP

Tell the patient that the doctor can diagnose herpes zoster from a thorough health history and physical examination. Once the rash develops, he can confirm the diagnosis. Before the rash appears, however, accompanying pain may mimic that of other disorders, such as appendicitis, peptic ulcer, herniated disk, and pleurisy.

Explain that the doctor may use the cutaneous Papanicolaou smear or the Tzanck test to confirm the diagnosis. These tests involve scraping material from an open vesicle, smearing it on a slide, and staining the smear for microscopic examination. Although they can confirm a herpes infection, they don't distinguish herpes zoster from herpes simplex. Therefore, the doctor may order other tests — a culture of the scraping, for example.

TREATMENTS

Inform the patient that treatment consists primarily of drug therapy to relieve pain and promote healing of skin lesions. Also emphasize measures to prevent infection, especially in immunocompromised patients.

Medication

Teach the patient about medications used to treat herpes zoster, including acyclovir, aspirin and other analgesics, silver sulfadiazine, tricyclic antidepressants, and capsaicin.

Acyclovir

Tell the patient that acyclovir (Zovirax), the drug of choice, inhibits the herpes zoster virus. Inform him that although it can't cure the disease, it can relieve pain and promote healing.

Aspirin and other analgesics

Aspirin or, in severe or unresponsive cases, narcotic analgesics may control the pain associated with herpes zoster. Alert the patient receiving high-dose aspirin therapy to signs of GI bleeding, such as vomit or stools that obviously contain blood, and vomit or stools that look like coffee grounds. Advise him to report these signs to the doctor immediately.

Silver sulfadiazine

Explain that silver sulfadiazine (Silvadene), an anti-infective cream commonly used to treat burns, seems to relieve pain and dry herpes zoster blisters. Reassure the patient that this cream won't stain his skin. Instruct him to wash his hands before applying it, or suggest that he apply it with a disposable finger cot or glove.

Tricyclic antidepressants

Inform the patient that a tricyclic antidepressant such as amitriptyline (Elavil, Endep) may be prescribed to relieve pain, especially that of postherpetic neuralgia. The medication also alleviates the insomnia and depression that may accompany severe pain.

Capsaicin

Tell the patient that capsaicin (Axsain, Zostrix) relieves the pain of peripheral neuropathy and postherpetic neuralgia. Point out that topical application three to four times a day should provide pain relief in 2 to 4 weeks. Advise him to rub enough cream into his skin to cover the painful area but not enough to form a cake residue. Forewarn him that he may experience a temporary burning sensation and reddening of the skin during the first several days of use.

Other care measures

Instruct the patient to apply cool compresses to the lesions to soothe burning and itching. To promote healing and avoid infection, warn him to avoid scratching. Tell him to notify the doctor if pain persists more than 2 months after the rash disappears or if he experiences sleep disturbances, appetite loss, or malaise.

Discuss his increased risk of infection. Explain that because his immune system is impaired or suppressed, he is more vulnerable to infection. Teach him ways to recognize and prevent infection. Review the classic signs and symptoms of infection — warmth, redness, swelling, tenderness, or pain in any body area; fever; persistent or productive cough; and drainage from any opening or wound.

Then discuss what the patient can do to prevent infection. For instance, recommend that he get adequate sleep, eat a well-balanced diet, and exercise regularly. Tell him to avoid crowds and anyone with a known infection. Show him proper handwashing technique, and instruct him to wash his hands before eating and after using the toilet, blowing his nose, stroking a pet, or handling money.

Explain that infants and young children who have not been immunized and persons who are immunocompromised can develop chicken pox from contact with the herpes zoster virus. Therefore, the patient should avoid contact with these individuals whenever possible.

Latex allergy

As the use of latex gloves and condoms has increased over the last 15 years, latex allergy — a potentially lethal disorder — has become a major public health problem. About 1 in every 64 Americans now has latex sensitivity. However, among people frequently exposed to latex, the incidence is much higher.

Latex sensitization may result from direct exposure to the proteins in latex or from indirect exposure, as when the protein adheres to the powder in a glove, becomes airborne, and is inhaled. The latex-sensitive person is particularly vulnerable in environments such as hospitals where there is a high level of airborne latex.

Although some reactions to latex are relatively minor, causing hay fever–like symptoms (such as sneezing and runny nose), others are life-threatening. What's more, some people who experience mild reactions eventually progress to more serious ones such as anaphylactic shock.

Latex isn't found only in gloves and condoms. It's used in many other medical products as well as in thousands of industrial and household items ranging from toys and clothing to adhesive tape and sports equipment. To make matters worse, some polypeptides found in latex are also present in various plants and fruits and can cause cross-sensitivity in some people.

Understandably, fear of latex exposure can cause a high level of stress in latex-sensitive patients. And because latex products are abundant in hospitals and doctors' offices, some patients are afraid to seek medical help for fear of further latex exposure. Thus, besides teaching your patient how to prevent such exposure and how to treat it if it occurs, you must provide a great deal of emotional support to help him cope with stress.

Before teaching a patient about latex allergy, make sure you're familiar with the following topics:
• cause of latex allergy
• substances and products that may contain latex
• possible routes of exposure to latex
• types of latex reactions — type I (immediate reaction), type IV (delayed reaction), and chemical irritation dermatitis
• individuals at high risk for latex allergy
• diagnosis, including patient history, physical examination, skin prick and intradermal testing, and radioallergosorbent (RAST) blood test
• importance of avoiding exposure to latex, informing all health care provi-

Latex allergy: Identifying those at high risk

Some patients are more likely than others to develop latex sensitivity. Those at highest risk include women, rubber industry workers, health care professionals who are exposed to latex products every day, and those with any of the following conditions:
● history of allergies and asthma
● allergy to bananas, avocados, tropical fruits, or chestnuts
● allergy to poinsettia plants
● history of multiple intra-abdominal or genitourinary surgeries, especially starting in infancy
● spina bifida
● chronic condition that requires continuous or intermittent catheterization.

ders of latex allergy, carrying epinephrine to administer in case of exposure, and wearing a medical identification tag
● sources of information and support.

ABOUT THE DISORDER
Explain that latex allergy is caused by sensitivity to the proteins in natural latex rubber or to additives used in manufacturing latex. Tell the patient that latex is the milky sap of the rubber tree, *Hevea brasiliensis,* and is used in more than 40,000 industrial, household, and medical products. Natural latex is about 2% to 3% protein and contains more than 240 polypeptides. Many of these polypeptides are found in fruits and plants, which may explain why persons with latex allergy have experienced cross-reactions with such foods as bananas, cherries, peaches, plums, figs, papayas, chestnuts, tomatoes, celery, avocados, and kiwi.

Point out that latex allergy can take one of three forms. *Type I* is an immediate antibody-antigen reaction that occurs within minutes or 1 to 2 hours after latex proteins enter the body through the skin, respiratory tract, or mucosal or serosal membranes. Some experts classify type I reactions into four categories based on severity:
● localized urticaria (hives) in the area of contact
● generalized urticaria with angioedema
● urticaria with asthma, watery eyes, runny nose, and orolaryngeal and GI symptoms
● urticaria with anaphylaxis.

The overall prevalence of type I latex allergy in the general population is about 1%, but is much higher in health care providers (roughly 10% to 15%) and in children with spina bifida (roughly 65%). (See *Latex allergy: Identifying those at high risk.*)

Tell the patient that *type IV* reactions are delayed reactions localized to the skin or mucous membranes. They are thought to be triggered by the chemicals added to latex during its manufacture.

Chemical irritation dermatitis — the most common adverse reaction to latex — also is thought to result from the chemicals used in latex manufacturing. It usually takes the form of a mild chemical dermatitis or skin inflammation. Although this reaction doesn't involve the immune system, it may contribute to later development of immunologic reactions to latex. Chemical irritation dermatitis is especially common among people who wear latex gloves continually at work.

DIAGNOSTIC WORKUP
Explain that no single test for latex allergy is widely accepted. To evaluate a patient for a suspected latex allergy, the doctor will take a thorough patient history. History findings that suggest latex allergy include other known allergies (especially to certain foods), hand dermatitis or development of hives after using latex gloves, allergic conjunctivitis after touching

the eye with a recently degloved hand, swelling around the mouth after blowing up a balloon or undergoing a dental procedure, vaginal burning after contact with a condom, occupational asthma related to latex exposure, or undiagnosed reactions or complications during surgery, dental work, or anesthesia.

As a further means of diagnosis, the patient may undergo an immunologic evaluation involving a skin prick test, intradermal testing, patch contact skin testing, or the RAST blood test.

Skin prick test
In the skin prick test, a drop of liquid latex is diluted with normal saline solution and placed on the skin. The skin is then pricked at that site and observed for a reaction. Because of the high potential risk for anaphylaxis, this test is rarely performed.

Intradermal testing
In intradermal testing, diluted latex is injected under the skin and the patient is observed closely for a reaction. Like the skin prick test, intradermal testing carries a high risk of anaphylaxis.

RAST blood test
The RAST *in vitro* blood test is much safer than the skin prick test and intradermal testing. However, it is still plagued with a high number of false-positive results. Also, it's quite expensive.

Spirometric flow measurements
A patient with occupational asthma may undergo spirometric flow measurements to evaluate for changes in lung function caused by latex exposure at work. Within an hour of entering a latex-contaminated workplace, some persons with latex allergy show a 20% to 30% reduction in peak flow.

TREATMENTS
Tell the patient that he must take all possible measures to avoid latex exposure. Mention that once a reaction

occurs, he may receive such medications as antihistamines, steroids, and epinephrine, depending on the severity of his reaction.

Medication
If the patient has a mild reaction, he'll probably receive antihistamines. A patient with hives may also receive antihistamines, although if the hives become generalized, he may require oral or systemic steroids.

A more serious reaction, with such signs and symptoms as laryngeal edema, bronchospasm, wheezing, and shortness of breath, calls for antihistamines, steroids, histamine$_2$ blockers, bronchodilators and, possibly, epinephrine.

Anaphylaxis warrants immediate administration of epinephrine and airway maintenance, along with steroids, antihistamine, and histamine$_2$ blockers. A patient with angioedema (swelling of the face, mouth, and airway) may require endotracheal intubation.

If anaphylaxis progresses to cardiac arrest, the patient is treated as for cardiac arrest but will also receive epinephrine, high-dose steroids, and histamine$_1$ and histamine$_2$ blockers.

 WARNING: If you work in a health care facility, be aware that a patient may react to the latex found in latex gloves and such medical devices as plastic syringes with latex-tipped plungers, drug vials with latex rubber stoppers, I.V. tubing with latex injection ports, latex hand-held resuscitation bags, anesthesia ventilator bellows, black latex rubber face masks, and certain nasopharyngeal tubes. If you're caring for a latex-sensitive patient, keep known latex products away from him. Ask your nurse-manager to obtain latex product substitutes.

Preventing latex allergy
Prevention is the cornerstone of treatment for latex allergy. Provide the patient with a list of known household items containing latex, and emphasize the importance of avoiding these. Inform him about nonlatex product

substitutes. Also teach him about the foods and plants associated with cross-sensitivity to latex.

Underscore the crucial need for him to notify all health care providers about his latex sensitivity. Stress the importance of wearing a medical identification tag that specifies latex sensitivity.

Teach the patient how to use medications such as diphenhydramine (Benadryl) to manage allergic reactions. Provide instruction in using autoinjectable epinephrine (EpiPen) in case a severe reaction occurs. Instruct him to always carry these medications with him, and advise him to keep nonlatex (vinyl or neoprene) gloves on hand for emergencies.

 WARNING: Inform the patient that "hypoallergenic" latex gloves are *not* safe for persons with latex allergy.

Be sure, also, to teach family members what to do in case the patient has a reaction to latex. Make sure the patient and family members know the warning signs of latex exposure — hives, wheezing, coughing, shortness of breath, palpitations, hives, and redness, swelling, and itching of the skin. Tell them to call for emergency medical assistance if these symptoms occur, and to inform emergency rescuers of the patient's latex sensitivity.

If your patient has a documented latex allergy, advise him to enter only those health care facilities with a latex-free policy, including a latex allergy cart. If he needs surgery, advise him to request the first operating room available for that day to help avoid airborne latex exposure that may occur later in the day. Inform him that, before a medical or surgical procedure, he can expect to be premedicated with diphenhydramine, methylprednisolone (Prednisone), and ranitidine (Zantac) to reduce the severity of any reaction that develops.

Finally, to help the latex-sensitive patient cope with the disorder and its implications, refer him to appropriate resources for further information and support. (See Appendix 2.)

Psoriasis

Although psoriasis isn't contagious or life-threatening, its unsightly skin lesions can cause discomfort and embarrassment. You'll be challenged to teach the patient to cope with this incurable and frustrating skin condition.

Initially, your teaching may focus on describing the remissions and recurrences that characterize psoriasis. Then you'll point out factors that cause flare-ups. You'll also review treatment options, such as skin care, medications, ultraviolet (UV) light therapy, support groups, and psoriasis treatment centers.

Before teaching a patient with psoriasis, make sure you're familiar with the following topics:
● explanation of psoriasis and its course, including alternating remissions and recurrences
● types of psoriasis
● factors that trigger flare-ups, such as stress, sunburn, and skin injury
● drug treatment, including tar preparations, topical corticosteroids, anthralin, methotrexate, and etretinate
● UV light therapy
● skin care, including cleaning, dressings, and measures to relieve itching
● managing psoriasis of the scalp and nails
● preventing flare-ups
● coping with the psychological effects of psoriasis
● sources of information and support.

ABOUT THE DISORDER

Inform the patient that psoriasis is a chronic skin condition characterized by abnormally accelerated growth and multiplication of the epidermal cells. Explain that whereas normal skin cells reproduce every 28 days, skin cells affected by psoriasis may reproduce as frequently as every 4 days. Consequently, dead skin cells accumulate rapidly, emerging as dry, silvery scales atop patchy erythematosus lesions. Called *plaques,* these lesions usually affect the elbows, knees, and scalp, but they can appear anywhere. Removal of the scales typically reveals tiny punctate bleeding spots known as Auspitz sign.

Inform the patient that psoriatic plaques affect the scalp of about half of the patients with psoriasis. The disease usually spares the face, but the plaques may appear behind the ears. In a few patients, psoriasis may affect the nails, producing pitting, discoloration, hyperkeratosis, and separation of the nail from the nail bed.

Describe the acute phase, which involves general skin reddening, usually with itching. The itching may intensify at night as dead cells accumulate during sleep. As the rash progresses, the cracked, encrusted plaques may cause pain. Furthermore, the rash may mimic other diseases, such as seborrhea, allergic skin reactions, and secondary syphilis. This can lead to misunderstanding and social isolation.

Tell the patient that psoriasis typically alternates between recurrences and remissions. During remission, symptoms disappear. The patient may express frustration and hopelessness during recurrences — responses that may intensify his symptoms and decrease the effectiveness of treatment.

Outline the types of psoriasis. (See *Identifying the types of psoriasis*, page 214.) As appropriate, distinguish among mild, moderate, and severe disease forms. Most patients have mild to moderate psoriasis, which doesn't affect their general health.

Explain that the cause of psoriasis is unknown, although research continues to point to a biochemical malfunction that triggers a defect in cell division. Mention, too, that psoriasis tends to run in families, suggesting a genetic predisposition to the disease. Alcohol, endocrine imbalance, infection, pregnancy, skin injuries, emotional stress, and environmental factors (such as cold and sunburn) may trigger recurrences. (See *Stress and psoriasis — a vicious cycle*, page 215.)

Complications
Stress that compliance with the prescribed treatment regimen reduces the patient's risk for infection. Point out that infection increases discom-

fort and retards healing. Also emphasize that compliance may speed remission, thereby helping the patient to avoid the social isolation and depression that may accompany and complicate psoriasis.

DIAGNOSTIC WORKUP
Explain that a health history and physical examination usually are all that's needed to confirm the diagnosis. For some patients, though, a skin biopsy may be done along with chest X-rays, a blood test, and urinalysis to confirm the disorder and rule out other diseases.

TREATMENTS
Describe the treatment regimen for psoriasis, which may include activity and dietary recommendations, medication, and procedures such as UV light therapy (alone and combined with various medications). Explain that these measures help control abnormal skin cell proliferation, heal plaques, and prevent new lesions. Reinforce the patient's coping skills to boost his self-esteem. Remember to discuss ways to reduce flare-ups — for example, by practicing stress-reduction techniques.

Activity guidelines
Tell the patient that he probably doesn't need to limit his activities. If fatigue or severe pain accompanies flare-ups, however, advise him to rest. If he has psoriatic arthritis, recommend regular rest periods.

Dietary modifications
Caution the patient to avoid certain foods and beverages that may aggravate psoriasis, such as meat, seafood, and alcohol. Suggest that he keep a record of his intake and eliminate any foods that seem to trigger flare-ups.

Medication
Teach the patient to use psoriasis medications properly. For example, if he's using special shampoos for scalp psoriasis, advise him that he may need to change or alternate products

INSIGHT INTO ILLNESSES

Identifying the types of psoriasis

Psoriasis occurs in various forms, ranging from one or two localized plaques to widespread lesions with crippling arthritis.

Erythrodermic psoriasis
Erythrodermic psoriasis is marked by extensive flushing all over the body, which may or may not result in scaling. The rash may begin rapidly, signaling new psoriasis; it may develop gradually in chronic psoriasis; or it may occur as an adverse reaction to a drug.

Guttate psoriasis
Guttate psoriasis typically affects children and young adults. Erupting in drop-sized plaques over the trunk, arms, legs, and sometimes the scalp, the plaques generalize in several days. This disease form is commonly associated with upper respiratory tract streptococcal infections.

Inverse psoriasis
Plaques that are smooth, dry, and bright red typify inverse psoriasis. Located in skin folds (the armpits and groin, for example), these plaques fissure easily.

Psoriasis vulgaris
The most common psoriasis form, psoriasis vulgaris begins with red, dotlike lesions that gradually enlarge and produce dry, silvery scales. The plaques usually appear symmetrically on the knees, elbows, extremities, genitals, scalp, and nails.

Pustular psoriasis
Pustular psoriasis is an eruption of local or extensive small, raised, pus-filled plaques. Precursors include emotional stress, sweat, infections, and adverse drug reactions.

Psoriatic arthritis
Psoriatic arthritis develops in about 10% of psoriasis patients. Commonly affecting the terminal joints of the fingers and toes, the disease also attacks the lower back, wrist, knees, or ankles, causing pain and swelling. It can be crippling. Blood tests indicate no rheumatoid factor — the key to distinguishing psoriatic arthritis from rheumatoid arthritis. Family history, nail malformation, and distal interphalangeal joint involvement also characterize this disorder.

---

if he develops tolerance. As appropriate, discuss such medications as coal tar preparations, topical corticosteroids, anthralin, methotrexate, and etretinate.

Coal tar preparations
Explain that coal tar products (Aquatar, Estar Gel, Fototar, Psorigel, T/Derm, and others) retard skin cell growth and relieve inflammation, itching, and scaling. Most can be purchased without a prescription.

Instruct the patient to use a coal tar preparation daily at bedtime. To prevent folliculitis, advise him to apply the medicine in the direction of hair growth. Caution him, though, not to apply it to his face or the armpits, groin, and other skin folds. The preparation may cause redness and burning in these sensitive areas. Forewarn him that coal tar will stain sheets, towels, and night clothes. To prevent this, advise him to let the medicine air-dry before dressing.

 WARNING: Tell the patient using coal tar preparations to avoid too much sun because these preparations increase photosensitivity.

Stress and psoriasis — a vicious cycle

Stress exacerbates psoriasis, and the discomfort and disfigurement of psoriasis cause stress. Help the patient break this vicious cycle by explaining how stress and psoriasis interact (either singly or simultaneously) on three levels.

Physical effects

The effects of psoriasis on the body (scaling, itching, and bleeding plaques) cause discomfort, which can lead to anxiety and fatigue. Worry over the progress of the disease can create additional stress, which may lead to appetite loss and sleep disturbances. Furthermore, inadequate nutrition and rest intensify physical stress.

Emotional effects

Psoriasis can lead to an altered self-image. Anger, frustration, and hopelessness can cause the patient to withdraw from personal and professional relationships. This isolation adds to the patient's emotional burden and low self-esteem and creates more stress.

Social effects

Without a support system, the patient may be devastated by negative experiences in daily life. For example, if psoriasis affects his scalp, he may complain that the barber refuses to cut his hair. The patient may conclude that he's all alone in his struggle with psoriasis.

Topical corticosteroids

Inform the patient that topical corticosteroids are the treatment of choice for mild to moderate psoriasis of the trunk, arms, and legs. Explain that these drugs decrease epidermal cell growth and reduce inflammation.

Demonstrate the downward stroke he should use to apply a topical corticosteroid. Instruct him to wash his hands thoroughly before and after using the medicine. Caution him to avoid touching his eyes; repeated eye exposure to these drugs has been associated with cataract formation.

Anthralin

Inform the patient that anthralin (Anthra-Derm, Drithocreme, or Lasan) may help heal large plaques that don't respond to coal tar or topical corticosteroid preparations. This topical psoriatic agent inhibits skin cell proliferation without being absorbed systemically.

Explain that the patient's tolerance of the drug and the severity of his psoriasis determine the drug strength that the doctor will prescribe.

Mention that he'll use a less concentrated preparation as his skin heals.

Methotrexate

A drug that inhibits cell replication, methotrexate (Folex, Mexate) may relieve severe, unresponsive psoriasis. Instruct the patient who's taking this drug to immediately tell the doctor if he experiences chills, diarrhea, fever, mouth or lip sores, reddened skin, stomach pain, or unusual bleeding or bruising. Warn him to avoid drinking alcoholic beverages while taking methotrexate. Advise him to check with the doctor before taking any medication, and tell him to avoid over-the-counter analgesics, such as aspirin and ibuprofen (Advil, Nuprin). Explain that these drugs may raise plasma concentrations of methotrexate to toxic levels. Also caution him to avoid people with contagious diseases, if possible, because the drug can lower his white blood cell count.

Because methotrexate may cause photosensitivity reactions, instruct the patient to take precautions to avoid excessive exposure to sunlight.

For example, suggest that he wear a wide-brimmed hat and sunglasses. Finally, because methotrexate increases the bleeding risk by lowering platelet counts, instruct him to consult the doctor before undergoing surgery or dental work. Also advise him to use a soft toothbrush and to exercise care when using dental floss.

Etretinate

Inform the patient taking this potent retinoic acid derivative that it's used to treat severe psoriasis that's resistant to other drugs or treatments. Etretinate (Tegison) may also relieve extensive plaque-type psoriasis — although recurrences within 2 months after therapy ends are common.

Emphasize that this teratogen may remain in the body for up to 3 years after treatment ends. That's why it shouldn't be used by women who are pregnant, who intend to become pregnant, or who use unreliable contraception.

Instruct the patient to report these reactions immediately: dark-colored urine, flulike symptoms, vision changes, and yellowing of the eyes or skin. Other drug-related effects include abdominal pain, bone or joint pain, chapped lips, dry nose and mouth, eye irritation, fatigue, hair thinning, muscle aches, photosensitivity, and unusual bleeding.

Inform the patient that his psoriasis may seem to worsen during the first month of treatment. Reassure him that this is common and that 2 to 3 months may pass before he notices an improvement. Advise him to contact the doctor if skin irritation or other psoriatic symptoms grow severe.

To relieve dry mouth, suggest using sugarless hard candy, chewing gum, or ice chips. If dry mouth persists after 2 weeks, advise the patient to consult the doctor or dentist because this condition increases the risk of gum disease.

Procedures

In controlled amounts, UV light — from either artificial sources or natural sunlight — suppresses skin cell replication and controls psoriatic symptoms. Caution the patient, however, that too much UV light can exacerbate his disease, probably because normal skin cells reproduce more quickly to repair the damage. Of the three UV light wavelengths — UVA (short wave), UVB (middle wave), and UVC (long wave) — UVB is most commonly used to treat psoriasis.

If appropriate, discuss procedures that combine UV light with medications, such as coal tar preparations or psoralen, to increase the effectiveness of treatment.

UVB light therapy

UVB therapy is considered the most effective and least risky treatment for moderate to severe psoriasis. Explain that such therapy may be used daily during a flare-up. Once the flare-up resolves, the treatments may taper off. If the patient's skin turns severely red or burns, however, treatment may stop temporarily for 1 to 2 days. After the treatment course, maintenance UVB light therapy may prolong remission.

Goeckerman therapy

Inform the patient that this procedure combines topical coal tar treatment with UVA or UVB light therapy to increase the effectiveness of each. Used mostly during flare-ups, Goeckerman therapy also may be effective for extended periods to treat chronic, resistant plaques.

Review instructions for applying a ⅛"-thick layer of 1% or 5% crude coal tar ointment to the plaques. Instruct the patient to leave the ointment on his skin for 12 to 14 hours. Then, before he bathes, advise him to remove the ointment with clean towels or sheets saturated in olive or mineral oil. Next, he'll receive a UV light treatment equivalent to between 20 and 30 minutes of sunlight. Inform him that his skin will turn slightly red or pink 12 hours later. Symptoms should begin subsiding within 5 days. Caution him that this treatment may produce a burn much like sunburn. Also point out that long-term, continued treatment increases his risk of skin cancer.

Modified Goeckerman therapy
Tell the patient that using UVB light therapy after applying topical drugs, such as coal tar preparations (for example, Estar Gel), corticosteroids, or kerolytic agents, rather than crude coal tar ointment constitutes modified Goeckerman therapy. Although this treatment may relieve psoriasis faster than standard Goeckerman therapy, remission may be briefer.

Ingram therapy
Explain that this procedure uses anthralin rather than a tar preparation. Instruct the patient to apply anthralin to his plaques and to leave it on as directed (usually between 8 and 12 hours). Next, he should remove the anthralin with mineral oil. Then, after bathing, he'll receive a UVB light treatment. With Ingram therapy, normal skin surrounding the plaques is protected by a layer of zinc oxide or petrolatum. Tell the patient that his symptoms should improve within 4 weeks.

Photochemotherapy
Inform the patient that photochemotherapy (PUVA) combines UVA light treatment with psoralen — either orally or topically. Explain that psoralen, a photosensitizing agent, increases sensitivity to UVA light. Point out that UVA light alone does not relieve psoriasis. Combined with psoralen, however, UVA light treatments block skin cell replication. Psoriasis vulgaris, which responds poorly to topical corticosteroids, anthralin, or coal tar treatments, may respond to PUVA therapy. Tell the patient that he may need about 30 treatments before symptoms clear totally.

Instruct the patient either to take psoralen tablets or to apply topical psoralen 2 to 3 hours before his UVA light treatment. Tell him that his initial exposure may last only a few minutes. Explain that the exposure time will lengthen incrementally, based on how much melanin his skin contains, his usual response to sunlight, and his sunburn history. Point out that because skin redness may peak from 48 to 72 hours after the treatment, he'll receive PUVA treatments every other day or twice weekly.

Mention that he'll wear special glasses, or goggles, to protect his eyes during the light treatment. Instruct him also to keep his eyes closed during the treatment. Because psoralen remains active for at least 24 hours, remind him to protect his skin and eyes from sunlight and artificial UVA light sources for at least a day after the PUVA session. Recommend wearing long-sleeved clothing (to avoid sunburn) and sunglasses (to prevent corneal and retinal damage) that filter out UV light (both indoors and outdoors).

List the possible adverse effects of PUVA treatment, including short-term nausea, itching, and skin redness. Advise the patient to take the psoralen with milk or food to minimize nausea. Other risks are the same as those associated with overexposure to sunlight, including cataracts, freckling, premature skin aging, and an increased risk of skin cancer.

Other care measures
Instruct the patient to avoid scratching the plaques. Suggest that he divert his attention from his discomfort by reading, playing a game, watching television, talking on the phone, or listening to music. To avoid scratching, recommend that he wear gloves or a special plastic suit. Applying ice cubes or mentholated shaving cream may also provide relief. Advise him to use a room humidifier in the winter; this may help prevent skin dryness, which increases itching.

Preventive measures
Discuss measures to prevent flare-ups. For example, caution the patient to avoid activities that could injure his skin, and emphasize meticulous compliance with his daily skin care regimen.

Promoting coping and self-esteem

The patient may need your help in dealing with social and professional problems. For example, he may lose interest in sex because he feels embarrassed about his appearance. You may suggest the use of a scented emollient (such as Alpha Keri Lotion or bath oil) to soften and smooth the skin before intimacy. If his appearance inhibits his drive or responses, suggest that he undress after turning out the lights, or to have sex in a dimly lit or dark room.

Finally, refer him to appropriate resources for further information and support. (See Appendix 2.)

8

Endocrine conditions

Diabetes mellitus

About 8 million Americans have been diagnosed with diabetes mellitus. Another 8 to 10 million are thought to have the disease without knowing it. To control the disease and avoid complications, the patient must strictly comply with treatment. And because such treatment usually involves major and permanent lifestyle changes, the patient must be highly motivated to comply. In fact, diabetes mellitus probably requires greater compliance than any other medical condition.

Obviously, what a diabetic patient must learn can't be taught in a few hours. You'll need to encourage him and his family to ask questions, and then watch as they demonstrate the techniques they've learned — for example, testing blood for glucose and urine for ketones and drawing up, mixing, and injecting insulin, if appropriate. You'll also need to discuss complications, diagnostic tests, and treatments, such as exercise, diet, and medication. What's more, you'll stress preventive health care, such as managing illness and practicing eye and foot care.

Before teaching a patient about diabetes mellitus, make sure you're familiar with the following topics:
• pathology underlying type I and type II diabetes
• complications from untreated or poorly controlled diabetes
• preparation for diagnostic tests
• role of exercise, including exercise precautions
• role of diet, including meal planning and timing, exchange lists, and insulin injections

• medications, such as insulin, oral antidiabetics, and glucagon, and how to administer them properly
• obtaining and testing blood for glucose levels
• testing urine ketone levels
• ways to prevent or reduce long-term complications, such as proper foot and eye care, sick-day precautions, and travel tips
• sources of information and support.

ABOUT THE DISORDER

Tell the patient that diabetes mellitus is a chronic disorder in which the pancreas fails to produce enough insulin to control blood glucose levels or the body's cells don't make efficient use of the insulin produced.

Although diabetes occasionally results from malnutrition or certain syndromes, two common forms are type I, or insulin-dependent diabetes mellitus, and type II, or non-insulin-dependent diabetes mellitus. Type II diabetes accounts for more than 90% of all cases of diabetes mellitus, and is the predominant disease form in the elderly.

Inform the patient with type I diabetes that it can develop at any age but typically appears before age 30. Usually, its onset is sudden. Mention that this form of diabetes may result from a genetically determined autoimmune disease or from a viral infection that destroys the insulin-producing pancreatic beta cells. Point out that because his pancreas doesn't produce sufficient insulin in response to elevated blood glucose levels, he needs daily insulin injections to control diabetes and prevent ketoacidosis.

Tell the patient with type II diabetes that this disease form can occur at any age, but is more likely to appear in middle age or later. Because its onset is gradual and symptoms are often vague, many cases go undiagnosed and untreated. Inform him that his body is producing insulin, but that a defect in insulin synthesis and release from beta cells, or insulin resistance in the peripheral tissues causes his blood sugar level to rise. Mention that type II diabetes has a strong genetic component and is often associated with being overweight.

Complications
No matter which diabetes form your patient has, emphasize that complying with treatment can help prevent severe complications. Several complications can be fatal — for instance, diabetic ketoacidosis (DKA), seen primarily with type I diabetes, and hyperglycemic hyperosmolar nonketotic syndrome, which can occur with type II diabetes.

Inform the patient at risk for DKA that this condition is triggered by extremely high blood glucose levels (hyperglycemia). Although life-threatening, it's reversible. Explain that buildup of ketones causes metabolic acidosis, and severe hyperglycemia leads to dehydration. Point out that DKA commonly results from failure to increase the insulin dosage during times of stress (such as illness, infection, or surgery).

Emphasize that hypoglycemia, another acute complication, usually results from an error in diabetic management — for example, excessive exercise or insulin, or insufficient food intake. Untreated, it can cause seizures, brain damage, coma, and death.

Explain that chronic complications of diabetes include retinopathy, neuropathy, kidney disease, cardiovascular disease, and infections. Stress that by testing his blood glucose levels daily, the patient may be able to stabilize the disease and prevent complications.

DIAGNOSTIC WORKUP
The diagnostic tests ordered for a patient with suspected diabetes will depend on his signs and symptoms. However, tell the patient that he can count on having tests to measure blood glucose levels. Describe what he can expect from venipuncture, and discuss such typical tests as the fasting plasma glucose test, random plasma glucose test, oral glucose tolerance test, and glycosylated hemoglobin test.

Inform the patient that in 1997 the American Diabetes Association (ADA) published new guidelines for diagnosing diabetes. These guidelines define a diabetic as anyone with a fasting blood glucose level of 126 mg/dl or more, measured on at least two occasions. (The previous threshold was 140 mg/dl.) The ADA has also added a new category of impaired glucose metabolism to describe persons with blood glucose levels between 110 and 125 mg/dl, and recommends that those in this danger zone get tested more often and be counseled about ways to lower their blood glucose.

The ADA advises testing every 3 years for all healthy persons aged 45 and older. Tell the patient that federal health authorities have endorsed the new guidelines.

Fasting plasma glucose test
Instruct the patient not to eat or drink anything except water for 12 hours before the test. Explain that glucose levels exceeding 126 mg/dl on two or more occasions confirm diabetes.

Random plasma glucose test
Advise the patient that fasting isn't necessary for this test, which measures his glucose level at the time of the test.

Oral glucose tolerance test
Inform the patient that because the ADA now considers the fasting plasma glucose test sufficient to diagnose diabetes, the doctor may not order the oral glucose tolerance test. If he does order it, however, tell the patient that this test evaluates his body's response to ingested glucose. Explain that for 3 days before the test, he'll follow a diet that ensures a daily intake of 150 to 300 grams of carbohy-

drates. Then he won't be allowed food or fluids for 12 hours before the test. Tell him to avoid caffeine, alcohol, strenuous exercise, and smoking during the fasting and testing periods because these factors can cause misleading test results. Discuss any medications that must be withheld during the test period.

Inform him that he'll be given a sweet solution to drink at the start of the test; urge him to drink it all. Mention that this test can take up to 5 hours.

Glycosylated hemoglobin test

Performed about every 3 months, this test monitors the patient's blood glucose control during the previous 2 months. Explain that persistently elevated glycosylated hemoglobin levels predict a greater risk for developing chronic complications.

TREATMENTS

Emphasize the importance of strict compliance with all treatment measures, including medication, controlled activity and diet, blood and urine testing, and other self-care measures.

Activity guidelines

Teach the patient that a balanced program of exercise and rest will help stabilize his blood glucose levels and reduce his insulin requirements.

 WARNING: Caution the patient to gear the amount of exercise to his food consumption and medication use and to follow his doctor's exercise guidelines to the letter.

Recommend participating in aerobic exercises, such as walking, running, cycling, and swimming, to help decrease blood glucose levels.

Caution the patient to avoid anaerobic exercise such as weight-lifting because it can increase blood glucose levels.

Exercise in phases

To achieve maximum benefits, instruct the patient to exercise regularly, every other day, for 40 to 60 min-

utes at a time. During the warm-up phase, he should stretch his muscles and slowly increase his heart rate for 5 to 10 minutes. During the conditioning phase, he should reach his target heart rate and maintain it for 20 to 30 minutes. Tell him to ask the doctor how high his heart rate can safely go during this most intense part of the workout.

During cool-down, the patient should walk slowly or do other activities for 10 to 15 minutes to gradually return his body systems to normal. Instruct him to monitor his heart rate by taking his pulse before, during, and after exercise.

Exercise precautions

Warn the patient always to carry a source of simple carbohydrates and an identification tag that gives his name, medical condition, and medications — just in case he becomes hypoglycemic while exercising. Also advise him to eat a snack before exercising, if appropriate.

If the patient is taking insulin, advise him not to inject it into a part of his body that he'll use during exercise. Instruct him to avoid exercising at the peak of insulin activity or before meals, and caution him to refrain from drinking alcohol before exercise. Also instruct him never to exercise alone.

Instruct the patient to stop exercising immediately if he experiences chest pain, severe dyspnea, palpitations, dizziness, weakness, or nausea. If any of these symptoms persist, he should see his doctor at once.

Dietary modifications

Because diabetes affects metabolism, diet therapy is a key component of the treatment plan. Stress the importance of carefully following the prescribed diet to prevent rapid blood glucose changes. Make sure the patient understands his specific meal plan, and urge him to stick to it. Advise him to eat about the same number of calories each day and to spread out his meals and snacks evenly.

What's new in diabetes treatment

After you discuss conventional diabetes treatment with your patient, give him encouraging news about investigative treatments that aim to refine the monitoring and control of blood glucose levels.

Glycemic index

Explain that this diet therapy links blood glucose fluctuations with specific foods and identifies low-fat, starchy foods that diabetic patients can eat to increase carbohydrate intake without triggering high postprandial blood glucose levels. Emphasize that the patient must comply with therapy by determining his blood glucose level after every meal and snack.

Pancreas islet cell grafts

Inform the patient that grafted islet cells may help control blood glucose metabolism and prevent or resolve microangiopathic complications. However, this therapy requires pure, undamaged pancreas islet cells for grafting, and they're hard to obtain. Another obstacle: Isolated islet cells are more likely to be rejected than islet-cell grafts in an intact pancreas.

Pancreas transplants

Tell the patient that a pancreas transplant carries a high rejection risk, so patients receiving pancreas transplants need immunosuppres-

sive drug therapy. Unfortunately, long-term immunosuppression can cause more problems, including hepatotoxicity, nephrotoxicity, and infection.

Consequently, most patients currently selected for a pancreas transplant are already receiving immunosuppressive drugs for a previous transplant; they also face a greater risk to life from diabetic complications than from long-term immunosuppression.

Implantable probes and pumps

Tell the patient that implantable probes and pumps are designed to monitor blood glucose levels and automatically deliver the correct insulin dose. Point out that these devices offer the potential for more exact blood glucose control. However, problems with clogging and unreliable insulin secretion remain unresolved.

Cyclosporine therapy

A promising treatment for type I diabetes, cyclosporine therapy aims to prevent islet beta-cell destruction. Explain that cyclosporine's immunosuppressive action may prevent circulating serum islet-cell antibodies from attacking islet cells. However, the drug can also cause nephrotoxicity and hepatotoxicity.

Encourage the patient to consult a nutritionist to help adapt the meal plan to his lifestyle, preferences, and income. If appropriate, discuss investigative diet therapy to help control blood glucose levels. (See *What's new in diabetes treatment.*)

If the patient has type II diabetes, explain that diet alone may control his blood glucose levels. Simply eating less will lower the amount of glucose he produces and thus the

amount of insulin he needs to control his blood glucose levels.

If he's overweight, however, emphasize the importance of weight reduction. Explain that an obese person must produce more insulin to control his glucose levels than does a person of normal weight. Discuss ways to help the overweight type II diabetic decrease his calorie intake.

Medication

Depending on your patient's condition, he may be taking insulin or an oral antidiabetic agent. The doctor may also prescribe glucagon for emergencies. Teach the patient about the purpose, administration, and possible adverse effects of all his medications. Encourage him to ask for drug information sheets on each medication.

Insulin

If the patient will be taking insulin, explain that this drug helps control blood glucose levels — but that it's not meant to replace a proper diet. Then outline the types of insulin available — rapid-acting, intermediate-acting, and long-acting. Caution the patient not to change the insulin type or brand without first consulting the doctor.

Next, reinforce the doctor's instructions on how to administer insulin. If the patient must take two different kinds of insulin, reinforce instruction on mixing insulins together in a syringe.

Then show the patient how to draw up insulin in a syringe and how to give himself a subcutaneous injection. Identify the best insulin injection sites — the abdomen (except around the navel and at the waistline), outer area of the upper arm, front and sides of the upper thighs, and buttocks. Tell the patient that the abdomen is preferred because it has the fastest absorption rate and is least affected by exercise (which can cause insulin to work faster and peak early). In descending order of preference, he may use the upper arm, thigh, and buttocks.

Regardless of the specific injection site he uses, stress that the patient should rotate injections *within* that area rather than between areas to ensure consistent absorption. (See *Rotating insulin injection sites*, page 224.)

Also impress upon him the importance of adhering to the prescribed medication regimen. Tell him always to take his insulin on schedule and never to adjust the dosage or stop taking the drug without his doctor's

approval — his blood glucose level could rise rapidly. Also caution him to always use the same brand of insulin, syringe, and needle and to be sure that the syringe corresponds with his insulin concentration. For instance, syringes for U-100 insulin should say U-100 on the package.

 WARNING: Stress the need to avoid alcohol by explaining that alcohol increases insulin's hypoglycemic effect.

Point out that changing food or fluid intake or taking over-the-counter drugs can affect insulin requirements. Advise the patient to keep extra bottles of insulin in the refrigerator and never to let his insulin freeze. If refrigeration isn't possible, tell him to keep the insulin as cool as possible (below 86° F [30° C]) and to shield it from heat and light. Warn him not to shake the insulin excessively.

Finally, tell the patient to report the following adverse reactions to the doctor: difficulty breathing, frequent or severe hypoglycemic or hyperglycemic symptoms, generalized itching, or redness, swelling, stinging, or itching at injection sites.

Oral antidiabetic agents

If the patient's taking an oral antidiabetic agent, explain that the drug will help regulate his blood glucose levels by increasing insulin secretion and decreasing cellular insulin resistance. Emphasize that oral antidiabetics *augment* diet therapy and don't replace it. Then caution him never to adjust the dosage or stop taking the drug without his doctor's approval.

Until recently, sulfonylureas (such as glipizide, glyburide, and tolazamide) were the only oral antidiabetic agents approved for use in the United States. However, two new oral agents, metformin (Glucophage) and acarbose (Precose) are now available. These agents may be administered alone or given in combination with sulfonylurea therapy.

Metformin, a biguanide, suppresses glucose absorption by the liver, decreases intestinal glucose absorption,

Rotating insulin injection sites

Whether the patient administers his insulin by needle or by insulin pump, he'll need to rotate the injection sites.

Why rotate sites?

Explain that rotating the site for injecting insulin reduces injury to the skin and underlying fatty tissue and prevents a buildup of scar tissue and swelling and lumps.

It can also minimize a slow insulin absorption rate. This can result from repeated injections in one spot, which can cause fibrous tissue growth and decreased blood supply in that area.

Point out that site rotation can also offset changes that exercise causes in insulin absorption. Exercise increases blood flow to the body part being exercised, thereby increasing the insulin absorption rate. That's why the patient should not inject himself in an area about to be exercised. (For example, he shouldn't inject himself in the thigh before walking or riding a bike.)

Where should the patient inject insulin?

Tell the patient that he can inject insulin into these areas:
- outer part of both upper arms
- right and left parts of the stomach, just above and below the waist (except for a 2" [5–cm] circle around the navel)
- right and left parts of the back below the waist, just behind the hip bone

- front and outsides of both thighs, from 4" (10 cm) inches below the top of the thigh to 4" above the knee.

Remind the patient that different parts of the body absorb insulin at different rates. The stomach absorbs insulin best, then the upper arm, and last, the thighs. Advise him to use this approach:
- Inject into the same body area for 1 to 2 weeks, depending on the number of injections needed daily. For example, if he needs four injections a day, he should use one area for about 5 days only.
- Cover the entire area within an injection site, but don't inject into the same spot.
- Don't inject into spots where you can't easily grasp fatty tissue.
- Have a family member give injections in hard-to-reach areas.
- Check with the doctor if a site becomes especially painful, or if swelling or lumps appear.

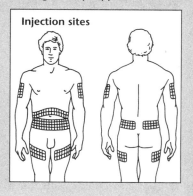

Injection sites

---

and increases tissue response to insulin. Unlike sulfonylureas, metformin doesn't stimulate insulin secretion and thus won't trigger hypoglycemia. However, it may cause other adverse effects, so make sure your patient receives a drug informa-

tion sheet from his doctor or pharmacist.

Acarbose is an oligosaccharide that works in the digestive tract, delaying carbohydrate absorption and thus preventing blood glucose levels from rising sharply after meals. Like metformin, acarbose doesn't precipitate hypoglycemia because it doesn't stimulate insulin secretion. However, if used in combination with a sulfonylurea, it may increase the hypoglycemic potential of the sulfonylurea. If your patient is taking this combination, teach him how to recognize signs and symptoms of hypoglycemia. Instruct the patient to take acarbose daily with the first bite of each of his three main meals.

WARNING: If the patient is taking acarbose, emphasize that he must treat a hypoglycemic reaction by ingesting glucose tablets or milk instead of table sugar because the drug prevents digestion of simple sugars (sucrose).

Warn the patient taking oral antidiabetic agents to avoid alcohol because it may cause a disulfiram reaction (severe nausea, vomiting, and sweating) or a hypoglycemic reaction. Advise him to take the oral antidiabetic before meals to avoid possible GI upset and to call the doctor if he has any other adverse reactions, such as stomach fullness, facial flushing, headache, heartburn, nausea, rash, vomiting, and jaundice. He should also notify the doctor if he's ill or under increased stress because these conditions may increase his insulin needs. The doctor may adjust the dosage accordingly or prescribe insulin.

If the patient takes both insulin and an oral antidiabetic, make sure he understands the purpose of combining these agents. (See *Helping the patient understand insulin and oral antidiabetic therapy*, page 226.)

Glucagon
Explain to the patient and his family that glucagon, a drug administered to treat hypoglycemic crisis, raises the blood glucose level when the patient cannot take oral glucose. Teach the family how to administer glucagon subcutaneously. Tell them that once glucagon has been reconstituted, it may be stored in the refrigerator for up to 3 months. Advise them to check the expiration date regularly and to keep the correct type of syringes available.

Forewarn the family that nausea and vomiting may occur after taking this drug. Instruct them to call the doctor immediately if the patient has difficulty breathing, develops a rash, or doesn't respond to glucagon.

PROCEDURES
Stress that checking blood glucose levels every day is crucial to diabetes management. If your patient or a family member can learn the technique, blood glucose self-monitoring can be a valuable management tool. If appropriate, teach the patient how to use a blood glucose meter. Also teach him to test his urine for ketones when he's hyperglycemic or ill. Besides explaining how to interpret the results, describe what he should do if results are abnormal.

Encourage him to keep a diary of his meals, exercise, medications, self-monitored blood glucose levels, and any hypoglycemia symptoms. Reviewing this daily record helps him understand how meals and activities affect his blood glucose levels.

Other care measures
Educate the patient about preventive health care measures and ways to deal with special problems.

Hypoglycemia
Make sure the patient knows the signs and symptoms of hypoglycemia (weakness, headache, anxiety, sweating, and vision changes) and how to prevent it by avoiding overexertion, inadequate food, and excessive insulin.

Infection
Point out that breaks in the skin can increase the risk of infection. Instruct the patient to check his skin daily for cuts and irritated areas, and to see his doctor, if necessary. Advise him to bathe daily with warm water and a mild soap, and to apply a lanolin-based lotion afterward to prevent dryness. He should pat his skin dry thoroughly, taking extra care be-

Helping the patient understand insulin and oral antidiabetic therapy

The better your patient understands how insulin and oral antidiabetic agents work, the better he'll comply with his prescribed regimen. Explain that oral antidiabetic agents were first used nearly 50 years ago to treat type II diabetes. They were found to lower blood glucose levels, presumably by stimulating the pancreas to produce more insulin.

Recent findings
Recent research shows that these agents act principally by enhancing peripheral cell sensitivity to insulin; their stimulating effect on the pancreas declines within a few months. This explains why, after initial success, these drugs often fail to sustain blood glucose control in patients with Type II diabetes.

Combined therapy
Today, some doctors prescribe both oral antidiabetics and insulin to regulate blood glucose levels and to combat the insulin deficiency and peripheral resistance to insulin common in type II diabetics.

Patients take a daily supplemental dose, usually of an intermediate or long-acting insulin, to correct their insulin deficiency. Then they take an oral antidiabetic agent to correct peripheral insulin resistance.

Usually, they take the oral antidiabetic agent 30 minutes before meals and the insulin as a small dose at bedtime. This timing takes advantage of increased peripheral cell receptivity resulting from the effects of the oral antidiabetic agent used during the day.

Who benefits most?
Combined therapy works best for type II diabetics who don't respond to oral agents alone or who require large doses of insulin (more than 100 units a day). Because the oral antidiabetic agent increases cellular sensitivity to insulin, the insulin dosage can then be reduced. This therapy doesn't help type I diabetics, who characteristically have total insulin deficiency, not insulin resistance.

tween the toes and in any other areas where skin surfaces touch. Tell him to always wear cotton underwear to allow moisture to evaporate and help prevent skin breakdown.

Advise the patient to avoid extreme temperature changes and thus reduce the risk of infection (especially in the respiratory tract). Also teach him to perform meticulous foot care. Warn him that some diabetics develop neuropathies, typically in the legs. To prevent such problems, tell him not to use a hot-water bottle or heating pad; he may burn himself because of reduced sensation. Also teach him the signs and symptoms of impaired circulation, such as dependent ede-

ma, pallor, numbness and tingling (paresthesia), and hair loss on the affected limb.

Instruct the patient to be especially careful to avoid accidents. If he works, discuss possible job hazards. If he's likely to cut or bruise himself on the job, advise him to wear sturdy clothing and shoes and to be extremely cautious. Teach him how to treat cuts or bruises if they do occur. Even a relatively minor injury such as a stubbed toe can be serious for a diabetic; he could develop an infection from impaired circulation. Also recommend using a night-light or a flashlight if he habitually goes to the bathroom in the middle of the night.

Taking care of your feet in diabetes

Dear Patient:
Because you have diabetes, your feet require meticulous daily care. Why? Diabetes can reduce blood supply to your feet, so normally minor foot injuries, such as an ingrown toenail or a blister, can lead to dangerous infection. Because diabetes also reduces sensation in your feet, you can burn or chill them without feeling it. To prevent foot problems, follow these instructions.

Routine care
• Wash your feet in warm, soapy water every day. To prevent burns, use a thermometer to check the water temperature before immersing your feet.
• Dry your feet thoroughly by blotting them with a towel. Be sure to dry between the toes.
• Apply oil or lotion to your feet immediately after drying, to prevent evaporating water from drying your skin. Lotion will keep your skin soft. But don't put lotion between your toes.
• If your feet perspire heavily, use a mild foot powder. Sprinkle it lightly between your toes and in your socks and shoes.
• File your nails even with the end of your toes. Don't cut them. And don't corner nails or file them shorter than the ends of your toes. If your nails are too thick, tough, or misshapen to file, consult a podiatrist. Also, don't dig under toenails or around cuticles.
• Exercise your feet daily to improve circulation. Sitting on the edge of the bed, point your toes upward, then downward, 10 times. Then make a circle with each foot 10 times.

Special precautions
• Make sure your shoes fit properly. Buy only leather shoes (because

only leather allows air in and out), and break in new shoes gradually, increasing wearing time by half an hour each day. Check worn shoes frequently for rough spots in the lining.
• Wear clean cotton socks daily. Don't wear socks with holes or darns that have rough, irritating seams.
• Consult a podiatrist for treatment of corns and calluses. Self-treatment or application of caustic agents may be harmful.
• If your feet are cold, wear warm socks or slippers and use extra blankets in bed. Avoid using heating pads and hot-water bottles. These devices may cause burns.
• Check the skin of your feet daily for cuts, cracks, blisters, or red, swollen areas.
• If you cut your foot, no matter how slightly, contact the doctor. Meanwhile, wash the cut thoroughly and apply a mild antiseptic. Avoid harsh antiseptics, such as iodine, which can cause tissue damage.
• Don't wear tight-fitting garments or engage in activities that can decrease circulation. Especially avoid wearing elastic garters, sitting with knees crossed, picking at sores or rough spots on your feet, walking barefoot, or applying adhesive tape to the skin of your feet.

Managing diabetes during illness

Minor illnesses — a cold, flu, infection, or an upset stomach — can drastically alter a diabetic patient's ability to control his blood glucose level. As his body attempts to compensate for the stress of an illness, his blood glucose level may rise.

To help prevent this increase, advise the patient to prepare a personal sick-day plan with his doctor before he becomes ill. Provide him with these general guidelines to follow when he's ill.
● Be sure to take prescribed diabetes medicine even if you're not able to eat.
● Rest and drink plenty of fluids.
● Even if you're not eating regularly, replace solid foods containing starch and sugar (such as bread and fruit) with liquids containing sugar (such as fruit juices and soft drinks).
● Test your blood glucose level at least every 4 hours.
● Test your urine for ketones.

When to call the doctor

Call the doctor promptly if:
● your blood glucose level is consistently higher than 250 mg/dl
● your urine ketone test result is moderate or high
● you think you might have an infection.

Cardiovascular problems
Inform the patient that diabetes raises his risk of heart disease. Recommend that he take care of his heart by maintaining normal weight, exercising regularly (based on the doctor's recommendations), and eating a low-fat, high-fiber diet to help control his blood pressure and cholesterol levels.

Vision problems
Instruct the patient to have his eyes examined by an ophthalmologist at least once a year. He may detect any damage, which can cause blindness, before symptoms appear. Stress that early treatment may prevent further damage.

If your patient has diabetic retinopathy with vision loss, be sure the booklets and other teaching aids you give him have large type. Urge him to read with a strong light behind him.

Dental problems
Tell the patient to schedule regular dental checkups and follow good home care to minimize dental problems, such as gum disease and abscesses, that may occur with diabetes. If he experiences bleeding, pain, or soreness in his gums or teeth, he should report this to the dentist immediately.

Tell him to brush his teeth after every meal and to floss daily. If he wears dentures, he should clean them thoroughly every day, and be sure they fit properly.

Foot care
Inform the patient that diabetes can reduce blood flow to the feet, dulling their ability to feel heat, cold, and pain. Instruct him to follow his doctor's or nurse's instructions on daily foot care and necessary precautions to prevent foot problems. Give the patient a copy of the teaching aid *Taking care of your feet in diabetes,* page 227.)

Checking the urine
Tell the patient that the doctor will check his urine routinely for protein, which can signal kidney disease. Urge him not to delay telling his doctor if he has symptoms of a urinary tract infection (burning, painful, or difficult urination, or blood or pus in the urine).

Getting regular checkups
Tell the patient to see his doctor regularly so that he can detect early signs

of complications and start treatment promptly.

Managing illness
Advise the patient of measures to take during illness. (See *Managing diabetes during illness*.)

Sexual concerns and pregnancy
Mention that diabetic patients, particularly men, may experience sexual dysfunction such as impotence. Encourage the patient to discuss any sexual problems he may be having.

Discuss problems of pregnancy with female diabetics. If your patient is already pregnant, refer her to a specialist who cares for diabetic women of childbearing age.

Travel precautions
Tell the patient who travels for business or vacation to make plans for meals and medication beforehand. He should also pack his insulin and syringes separately, and adjust his insulin schedule accordingly.

Advise him to carry his diabetes supplies with him so they don't get lost. When flying, for instance, he should pack his insulin and syringes in a carry-on bag, not in checked luggage. Also instruct him to carry extra insulin and syringes and to protect insulin from excessive heat and cold. When traveling by car, caution him not to leave his insulin in a parked car.

Living alone
If the patient lives alone, spend a little extra time with him; he may find it more difficult to comply with therapy than someone who has a spouse or other family member to encourage him. Ask him how he deals with stress. Many people overeat when they're frustrated or anxious. A diabetic who tries to cope with stress in this way won't be able to control his blood glucose levels. Encourage him to develop a buddy system to keep in touch with others through regular phone calls or visits.

Preventing complications
Emphasize that controlling diabetes means checking blood glucose levels daily and making good health habits a way of life.

Help your patient prevent DKA by teaching him to recognize its early signs and symptoms and taking immediate and appropriate action. Tell him to test regularly for urine ketones and perform home glucose monitoring, and to call the doctor right away if he has any of the following danger signals: cramping, nausea, vomiting, headache, dizziness, rapid breathing, shortness of breath, muscle and joint aches, increased urination, thirst, dizziness, or visual disturbances.

To help the patient cope with all aspects of diabetes management, provide the names and phone numbers of appropriate resources. (See Appendix 2.)

Hyperthyroidism
Although chronic, hyperthyroidism can be a relatively benign condition if the patient complies with therapy. To encourage compliance, you'll need to explain that thyroid hormone overproduction can be curbed by medication or other treatments. You'll want to emphasize that such measures will allow the patient to lead a nearly normal life.

Before teaching a patient about hyperthyroidism, make sure you are familiar with the following topics:
• explanation of hyperthyroidism
• complications such as thyroid storm
• blood tests and X-ray studies to evaluate thyroid function
• activity restrictions to help counteract an increased metabolic rate
• dietary measures to ensure sufficient caloric intake
• medications and their administration
• radioactive iodine therapy, if indicated
• subtotal thyroidectomy, if indicated, and possible need for lifelong hormonal replacement therapy

- relationship between stress and hormonal balance
- eye care, if exophthalmos or visual changes occur
- sources of information and support.

ABOUT THE DISORDER
Explain that hyperthyroidism results from excessive production of thyroid hormone. Point out that this hormone is produced by the thyroid, a butterfly-shaped gland in the anterior portion of the lower neck. Tell the patient that overproduction of thyroid hormone accelerates all bodily functions and activities. The condition is more common in women than men.

Point out that hyperthyroidism's exact cause is unknown. Mention that the condition has several forms. The most common, Graves' disease, may be related to an immune defect that causes formation of abnormal antibodies; it may follow an emotional shock, stress, or infection.

In toxic nodular goiter, one or more thyroid nodules become hyperproductive. This condition is more common in older women with preexisting goiter. Autoimmune thyroiditis (Hashimoto's disease) may cause initial hyperthyroidism before developing into hypothyroidism. Factitious hyperthyroidism results from excessive amounts of thyroid hormone medications.

Inform the patient that elevated thyroid hormone levels increase the rate at which the body uses energy. This can lead to signs and symptoms that affect all body systems. (See *Reviewing clinical features of hyperthyroidism.*)

Cardiovascular effects, for instance, include hypertension and tachycardia, which can lead to flushing, palpitations, and heart failure. Central nervous system effects include emotional instability, irritability, difficulty concentrating, and insomnia. Other signs and symptoms are fine hand tremors, weight loss, and fatigue.

Encourage compliance with the treatment regimen by pointing out

that untreated or poorly managed hyperthyroidism can lead to severe complications. For example, thyroid storm, an acute complication, can be fatal without prompt treatment. In thyroid storm, the patient's metabolic rate rapidly accelerates, severely taxing the functions of all body systems. Body temperature may rise as high as 106° F (41° C); heart and respiratory rates increase dramatically. Total systemic collapse becomes imminent.

Explain that compliance can also forestall common chronic complications of hyperthyroidism, such as cardiac dysfunction, weight loss, and GI problems.

DIAGNOSTIC WORKUP
Tell the patient that tests commonly used to evaluate thyroid function include blood tests, thyroid scan, ultrasonography, and a radioactive iodine uptake test. (See *Teaching patients about endocrine tests,* page 232.)

Blood tests
Explain that blood tests require a small blood sample drawn by venipuncture at regular intervals. Studies will be done on the thyroid hormone itself or on its by-products found in the blood.

Serum thyroxine (T_4)
Levels of circulating T_4 are used to screen for hyperthyroidism. Elevated levels confirm the disease.

Serum long-acting thyroid stimulator
This test may be ordered to check for the abnormal antibody thought to be responsible for Graves' disease. If this hormone is present, hyperthyroidism is attributed to Graves' disease.

T_3 (triiodothyronine) resin uptake
Occasionally, this test is ordered to further evaluate thyroid function. An elevated T_3 level strengthens a diagnosis of hyperthyroidism. A thyroid scan may also be ordered to aid diagnosis.

Reviewing clinical features of hyperthyroidism

When discussing the signs and symptoms of hyperthyroidism with the patient and her family, tell them to be alert for the following:
- weight loss
- muscle wasting
- muscle weakness and tremors
- fatigue
- dyspnea
- breast enlargement
- palpitations
- increased appetite
- irritability and nervousness
- exophthalmos, lid lag
- sweating, heat intolerance
- localized edema
- fine, straight hair.

Graves' disease — a common form of hyperthyroidism — produces three characteristic signs:
- uniformly enlarged thyroid gland (goiter)
- infiltrative ophthalmopathy
- infiltrative dermopathy.

(*Note:* All three signs may not appear in every patient.)

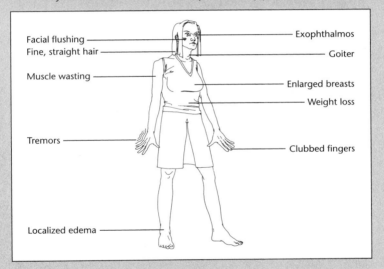

Facial flushing — Exophthalmos
Fine, straight hair — Goiter
Muscle wasting — Enlarged breasts
— Weight loss
Tremors — Clubbed fingers
Localized edema

Thyrotropin-releasing hormone (TRH) stimulation
This test may be ordered if only an eye abnormality, such as exophthalmos, suggests Graves' disease. It involves TRH injection followed by a series of blood samples drawn periodically over the next hour.

TREATMENTS
Tell your patient that he'll probably be able to live a nearly normal life if he follows the treatment plan. Explain that treatment aims to restore the basal metabolic rate to normal as soon as possible and then to maintain the normal rate. Encourage the patient to eat a well-balanced diet to prevent vitamin deficiencies. Point out the benefits and risks of major treatments, including drugs, radioactive iodine therapy, and thyroidectomy.

The specific treatment approach depends on the cause, the patient's age, disease severity, and any existing complications.

Teaching patients about endocrine tests

TEST AND PURPOSE	TEACHING POINTS
Radioactive iodine uptake test • To assess thyroid function • To aid diagnosis of hyperthyroidism or hypothyroidism • In conjunction with other studies, to help distinguish between primary and secondary thyroid disorders	• Explain to the patient that this painless test evaluates thyroid function. Instruct him to fast after midnight before the test. • Discuss what happens during the test: The patient will be given a radioactive iodine capsule or liquid. After 2, 6, and 24 hours, his thyroid will be scanned in the X-ray department to determine how much of the substance is present in the thyroid. Reassure him that the amount of radioactivity involved is extremely small and is harmless.
Thyroid scan (radionuclide thyroid imaging) • To evaluate the size, structure, and position of the thyroid gland • To evaluate thyroid function, in conjunction with thyroid uptake studies	• Tell the patient that this test assesses the thyroid gland for abnormalities. Reassure him it is painless and will not expose him to dangerous radiation levels. • Advise him to follow his doctor's guidelines for discontinuing medications before the test. Also instruct him to avoid iodized salt, iodinated salt substitutes, and seafood for 3 days before the test. • Before the X-ray, instruct him to remove dentures and jewelry. Explain that he will be placed in a supine position with his neck extended. A special X-ray machine called a gamma camera will then be placed over his throat to visualize the thyroid gland. • Describe what will happen during the test: The patient will be given a radioisotope orally or intravenously. If he's given the drug orally, tell him that his thyroid gland will be X-rayed 24 hours later. If he's given the drug intravenously, it will be X-rayed within 20 to 30 minutes.
Ultrasonography of the pancreas, or the parathyroid, thyroid, or adrenal glands • To evaluate the size and structure of the endocrine gland • To distinguish between a cyst and a solid tumor • To monitor response to therapy	• Explain to the patient that this test reveals the size and shape of the gland. Tell him that it takes about 30 minutes and is painless. • For ultrasonography of the pancreas, instruct the patient to fast for 12 hours before the test. This reduces bowel gas, which hinders transmission of ultrasound. • Explain what happens during the test: The patient will be placed in a supine position. For ultrasonography of the thyroid or parathyroid gland, a pillow will be tucked under his shoulder blades to hyperextend his neck. Tell the patient that the skin over the gland will be coated with a water-soluble gel. Next, the technician will move the transducer over the area to study the gland.

Activity guidelines
Inform the patient that excessive exertion will worsen his symptoms. Encourage him to engage instead in less strenuous activities and to rest frequently. Keep in mind that this may be difficult because of the patient's accelerated metabolic rate.

Dietary modifications
Stress the importance of following the prescribed diet to prevent nutritional deficiencies, such as vitamin A and B deficiencies. Advise the patient to eat well-balanced meals each day, plus snacks, so that his caloric intake can keep pace with his rapid caloric expenditures. If appropriate, arrange for nutritional counseling.

 WARNING: Caution the patient to avoid caffeine, food with yellow and red dyes, and artificial preservatives because these substances may make him more irritable.

Medication
Teach the patient about thyroid hormone antagonists and propranolol, if prescribed, to control cardiac effects. Also teach about other prescribed drugs such as tranquilizers to control irritability and hyperactivity. Warn him to avoid taking aspirin and any aspirin-containing drugs because they increase the metabolic rate.

Procedures
The doctor may recommend radioactive iodine therapy if thyroid hormone antagonists prove ineffective. If the patient is scheduled for this treatment, explain that it reduces thyroid hormone production by destroying thyroid tissue. Reassure him that the procedure is painless and won't harm other body tissues. Be sure he understands the risk of hypothyroidism, which can result from excessive destruction of thyroid tissue and may occur several months to 1 year after treatment. Assure him that exposure to this small amount of radioactivity doesn't cause cancer. (See *Precautions after radioactive iodine therapy,* page 234.)

Inform the patient that symptoms of hyperthyroidism should subside after radioactive iodine therapy. If they don't, he may need a second round of therapy.

Surgery
Surgery may be recommended if the patient has a very large goiter or can't receive thioamides or radioiodine. In subtotal thyroidectomy, more than 80% of the thyroid is removed, significantly reducing the gland's ability to produce thyroid hormone. If the patient is scheduled for subtotal thyroidectomy, instruct him to increase his caloric intake before surgery to regain weight. (Surgery may have to be delayed until the patient gains back any weight he lost.) If a special preoperative diet (such as a high-protein diet) has been ordered, explain its purpose and urge strict compliance. Remind the patient to avoid caffeine and other stimulants, which will aggravate his condition.

Explain the purpose of preoperative thyroid medication — to suppress secretion of thyroid hormone so that an excessive amount isn't released during surgery. Iodine preparations may also be ordered to diminish blood flow to the thyroid, thereby minimizing bleeding during surgery.

Before surgery, review preoperative and postoperative procedures. Explain preoperative preparation of the incision site. Tell the patient that the incision will be made in the lower neck.

Show the patient how to avoid putting stress on his incision postoperatively by placing his hands behind his neck for support whenever he wants to turn his head. When rising to a sitting position, he should support his head with a pillow and put his hands together behind his head. If he has difficulty swallowing, he should report it immediately. This problem may indicate hemorrhage or swelling, which could interfere with breathing. Mention that cold drinks and ice will help relieve discomfort and that he'll be on a soft diet temporarily.

Precautions after radioactive iodine therapy

If the patient is scheduled for radioactive iodine to treat his thyroid condition, reassure him that this treatment won't affect his other body tissues. Tell him that, although it's a safe treatment, he'll need to follow some instructions to prevent any harm to himself or others.

Eating and drinking

Inform the patient that he can eat what he likes but must use disposable plates, cups, and utensils for 48 hours after the treatment. Urge him to drink plenty of fluids (about 2 quarts, or liters) for those 48 hours to help remove the radioactive iodine from his body.

Using the bathroom

The patient's urine, feces, saliva, and perspiration will be slightly radioactive for 48 hours after therapy. Although he may use the family bathroom to urinate or defecate, he should flush the toilet three times to make certain all waste is discarded. Tell him to wash his hands thoroughly afterward.

Bathing and laundering

If the patient takes a shower or bath within 48 hours after treatment, tell him to rinse the shower stall or tub after each use. Instruct him to wash his clothes, towels, and washcloths separately from those of his family.

He can brush his teeth and re-sume any other normal mouth care. Remind him, though, to make sure to rinse and drain the sink when he's finished.

Living arrangements

Caution the patient to avoid close contact with infants, children, and pregnant women for 1 week after therapy. For safety's sake, he should sleep alone and avoid kissing or sexual intimacy for 48 hours after the treatment. After that, he may resume his normal relationship unless the doctor gives other instructions.

If the patient is breast-feeding, she must stop. The doctor will tell her when she can start again.

When to call the doctor

Instruct the patient to call his doctor immediately if he vomits within 12 hours after therapy. Tell him to flush the vomit down the toilet and, if possible, wear gloves while cleaning up. (He should discard the gloves in a plastic bag after use.) Warn him to discourage other people from coming in contact with the vomit. If they do, however, they should wash their hands thoroughly.

If the patient gets a fever and feels restless or upset within 48 hours of therapy, he should call his doctor right away. Also tell him to call the doctor if his neck feels tender. The doctor may prescribe medicine to make him more comfortable.

Tell the patient that his voice will be checked periodically for hoarseness after surgery. Advise him to talk as little as possible during the first few days postoperatively. If he has difficulty breathing, he should report it at once; oxygen may have to be administered. Tell him he can expect to be out of bed on the first day after surgery.

Reassure the patient that he'll receive pain medication postoperative-ly. Inform him that sutures or surgical clips are usually removed on the second postoperative day, just before discharge.

To help prepare the patient for discharge, teach him how to take care of his incision at home. Make sure he understands the importance of getting adequate rest and nutrition during recovery. Tell him to promptly report signs or symptoms of infection and hypothyroidism to his doctor.

Other care measures

Advise the patient to avoid stressful situations, which can exacerbate his irritability. Recommend keeping environmental stimulation to a minimum. Reassure him and his family that behavioral changes, such as irritability, anxiety, lack of concentration, and fatigue, stem from hyperthyroidism and will subside with treatment.

If ophthalmopathy is present, teach the patient the essentials of good eye care. Advise him to wear sunglasses and to avoid irritating his eyes. If eyedrops are ordered, show him how to instill them. Instruct him to limit his fluid and salt intake to minimize fluid retention, because such retention will worsen exophthalmos.

Suggest that the patient sleep with his head elevated to prevent fluid accumulation behind the eyes. Instruct him to notify his doctor at once if he experiences visual changes such as blurring. Advise him to visit an ophthalmologist regularly. Refer him to sources of information and support. (See Appendix 2.)

Hypoglycemia

As with other chronic disorders, hypoglycemia management can pose a never-ending challenge to the patient. Besides learning how to recognize the telltale symptoms of a hypoglycemic episode, the patient must master its prompt treatment to prevent possibly irreversible tissue damage. What's more, because hypoglycemia can cause fatigue, difficulty concentrating, and considerable discomfort, he must comply with certain lifestyle changes.

To help the patient overcome these barriers, you'll need to support his efforts to comply with prescribed dietary changes, weight reduction (if necessary), drug regimens, and other prescribed treatment measures.

Before teaching the patient about hypoglycemia, make sure you are familiar with the following topics:
• explanation of the patient's type of hypoglycemia — fasting, pharmacologic, or reactive — along with its causes and signs and symptoms
• importance of preventing or promptly treating hypoglycemia
• emergency treatment of a hypoglycemic episode to avoid severe complications
• preparation for diagnostic tests, such as the fasting plasma glucose test and oral glucose tolerance test
• dietary modifications to prevent changes in the blood glucose level
• prescribed medications and their administration
• surgery for tumors, if necessary
• prevention of hypoglycemic episodes.

ABOUT THE DISORDER

Tell the patient that hypoglycemia occurs when glucose, the body's major energy source, isn't being produced fast enough or is being used too rapidly. Mention that a certain amount of glucose must always be present in the blood to meet the energy needs of vital tissues (such as brain cells).

How low the blood glucose level must fall before triggering a hypoglycemia reaction varies greatly among individuals. Typically, a blood glucose level below 70 mg/dl causes symptoms.

Tell the patient that the nature of his symptoms may reveal how rapidly his glucose level is falling. For example, nervousness, diaphoresis, and an elevated heart rate can result from a rapid decline in glucose levels. Changes in mental status can result from a slow decline.

Teach the patient about the type of hypoglycemia he has — fasting, pharmacologic, or reactive. Tell the patient with *fasting hypoglycemia* that in this disorder, the blood glucose level gradually falls until, 5 hours or more after a meal, he has a headache, dizziness, restlessness, mental status changes, and intense hunger. This rare type of hypoglycemia often occurs during the night. Untreated, it can cause severe symptoms — including seizures, unconsciousness, and coma — which resist even prompt treatment.

Fasting hypoglycemia may result from liver disease or a tumor. For example, a pancreatic tumor called an insulinoma causes excessive insulin secretion. An extrapancreatic tumor can also lead to hypoglycemia, although the mechanism isn't clear. Liver disease interferes with the liver's ability to raise the blood glucose level by gluconeogenesis and glycogenolysis. Other causes of fasting hypoglycemia include adrenocortical insufficiency, growth hormone deficiency, and severe chronic renal failure.

Tell the patient with *pharmacologic hypoglycemia* that his blood glucose level may fall slowly or rapidly in response to a drug that does one of three things:

• increases the amount of insulin circulating in the bloodstream

• enhances insulin action

• impairs the liver's glucose-producing capacity.

If the blood glucose level falls slowly, he'll have a headache, dizziness, restlessness, and decreased mental capacity. If untreated, he could experience seizures, unconsciousness, or coma. A rapid glucose fall causes hunger, weakness, diaphoresis, tachycardia, pallor, anxiety, tremors, nervousness, and rebound hyperglycemia.

Explain that the most common causes of pharmacologic hypoglycemia are insulin and oral sulfonylureas used to treat diabetes. Other causes include use of beta blockers and excessive ingestion of alcohol. Signs and symptoms depend on when the patient took the particular drug.

Tell the patient with *reactive hypoglycemia* that his blood glucose level will fall rapidly but won't drop drastically below normal. He'll experience hunger, weakness, diaphoresis, tachycardia, pallor, anxiety, tremors, and nervousness. These symptoms are usually mild, occurring within a few hours after a meal and resolving quickly with treatment.

Explain that three types of reactive hypoglycemia have been identified: alimentary hypoglycemia, hypoglycemia secondary to imminent onset of type II diabetes mellitus or impaired glucose tolerance, and idiopathic reactive hypoglycemia.

If the patient has *alimentary hypoglycemia,* explain that it reflects digestive dysfunction, usually from extensive gastric surgery. Teach him that food passes through the stomach and enters the small intestine more rapidly than normal, causing glucose to be absorbed quickly. This first produces hyperglycemia, which stimulates release of excessive insulin. The insulin, in turn, causes the blood glucose level to drop abruptly. Alimentary hypoglycemia usually occurs within 1 to 3 hours after eating.

Tell the patient with *reactive hypoglycemia secondary to type II diabetes mellitus or impaired glucose tolerance* that this rare condition produces an abrupt drop in blood glucose levels 3 to 5 hours after a meal, but just why this happens remains a mystery. One theory is that delayed and excessive insulin secretion, triggered by carbohydrate ingestion, causes the drop.

Inform the patient with *idiopathic reactive hypoglycemia* that this type of reactive hypoglycemia is the most common. Its hallmark is a rapid drop in the blood glucose level 2 to 4 hours after eating carbohydrates. The exact cause of idiopathic reactive hypoglycemia is unknown. Explain that signs and symptoms — diaphoresis, tremors, and dizziness — will subside with appropriate therapy within 20 minutes. Reassure the patient that his condition doesn't predispose him to diabetes mellitus, as is commonly believed.

Complications
Emphasize the importance of preventing or promptly treating hypoglycemic episodes to avoid severe complications. Make sure the patient understands that the key danger with hypoglycemia is that, once it occurs, he may quickly lose his ability to think clearly. If this should happen

while he's driving a car or operating machinery, it could cause a serious accident.

Explain that brain cells can't survive long without glucose. Prolonged or severe hypoglycemia (a blood glucose level of 20 mg/dl or lower) causes permanent brain damage and could be fatal.

DIAGNOSTIC WORKUP
Inform the patient that the diagnostic tests ordered depend on whether his symptoms are related to eating or fasting. Once the doctor determines this, he'll order serial blood glucose studies, such as a plasma glucose test. He may also order an oral glucose tolerance test, an I.V. glucose tolerance test, and a C-peptide assay.

Plasma glucose test
Inform the patient that this test confirms a low blood glucose level and determines how low his glucose level has fallen during a hypoglycemic episode. Review the signs and symptoms of hypoglycemia with the patient, and tell him to notify the doctor or nurse as soon as any of these occur, so that a blood sample can be drawn before treatment begins.

Instruct the patient not to eat or drink anything except water for 12 hours before the test. Inform him that test results may be inconclusive. If so, he'll need to be admitted to the hospital so that the fasting period can be extended another 24 to 72 hours. Explain that the liver can provide enough glucose to maintain adequate blood levels during a prolonged fast. But if his hypoglycemia results from an underlying disease such as an insulinoma, then test results will show it.

Tell the patient that a separate test will be done after the fasting plasma glucose test to measure his insulin levels and evaluate pancreatic function. If an insulinoma is present, his insulin levels will be elevated.

Oral glucose tolerance test
Tell the patient that this test helps diagnose reactive hypoglycemia. The doctor will prescribe a diet that ensures a daily intake of 150 to 300 g of carbohydrates for 3 days before the test. Then, for 12 hours before the test, the patient will need to fast. Tell him to avoid caffeine, alcohol, strenuous exercise, and smoking during the fasting and testing periods because these factors can cause misleading test results. Also discuss any medications that must be withheld during the test period.

Mention that the test itself lasts 5 hours and that he'll be given a sweet solution to drink at the start of the test. Urge him to drink the entire solution, and instruct him to notify the doctor or nurse immediately if symptoms of hypoglycemia occur. Make sure he understands that the interval between ingestion of the glucose solution and onset of symptoms can help determine his type of reactive hypoglycemia.

I.V. glucose tolerance test
Inform the patient that this test helps detect fasting hypoglycemia caused by insulinomas and other tumors that secrete insulin or an insulin-like substance. Help prepare him for the test in the same manner as for an oral glucose tolerance test. However, point out that instead of being given oral glucose, he'll receive an I.V. substance known to stimulate insulin secretion (such as tolbutamide, glucagon, or leucine). Teach him the importance of reporting hypoglycemic symptoms immediately. Tell him that the test will be stopped and he'll be treated promptly if such symptoms occur.

C-peptide assay
Explain that this test helps diagnose fasting hypoglycemia. It also differentiates fasting hypoglycemia caused by an insulinoma from fasting hypoglycemia caused by insulin injections. No preparation is needed.

TREATMENTS
Treatment for hypoglycemia combines diet to prevent the glucose level from dropping rapidly and medications to control anxiety, delay gastric

emptying, alleviate symptoms, and treat tumors. Surgery may also be used to remove tumors.

Dietary modifications

Emphasize to the patient the importance of carefully following his prescribed diet to prevent a rapid drop in the blood glucose level. Discuss his specific meal plan, and encourage him to comply with it.

Advise him to eat small meals throughout the day, and mention that bedtime snacks may be necessary to keep his blood glucose at an even level. Instruct him to avoid alcohol and caffeine because they may trigger severe hypoglycemic episodes.

Tell the patient with *reactive hypoglycemia* to avoid simple carbohydrates and other foods high in carbohydrates. Such foods load the body with glucose and may stimulate excessive insulin production, triggering a hypoglycemic episode. Help the patient plan low-carbohydrate, high-protein meals by reviewing with him the foods belonging to these food groups. Advise him to add fiber to his diet because it delays glucose absorption from the GI tract.

If the patient is obese and has impaired glucose tolerance, suggest that he can restrict his caloric intake and lose weight. If necessary, help him find a weight-loss support group.

Tell the patient with *fasting hypoglycemia* that he'll need to increase his caloric intake because his body needs more glucose to counteract excessive insulin secretion. Warn him not to postpone or skip meals and snacks because severe and possibly prolonged hypoglycemia may develop. Tell him to call his doctor for instructions if he doesn't feel well enough to eat.

Medication

Teach the patient about prescribed drug therapy. For example, if an antianxiety drug such as diazepam (Valium) is prescribed, warn him that it may cause drowsiness. Advise him to avoid potentially hazardous activities, such as driving a car or other ac-

tivities that require alertness, until this adverse reaction subsides.

If the doctor prescribes medication to delay gastric emptying in reactive hypoglycemia, teach the patient about possible adverse effects. Propranolol (Inderal) may also be ordered to alleviate symptoms of a hypoglycemic episode, such as hypertension, diaphoresis, tachycardia, and palpitations.

If the patient has an inoperable insulinoma, explain that diazoxide (Hyperstat) helps treat fasting hypoglycemia by inhibiting insulin release. Together with a high-calorie diet, it helps maintain adequate blood glucose levels.

If the patient will undergo chemotherapy to treat an inoperable tumor, explain the protocol to him and review possible adverse reactions to each drug.

Advise the patient not to take nonprescription medications such as antihistamines without his doctor's approval. Explain that many nonprescription medications contain ingredients that mask symptoms of decreased blood glucose levels or induce hypoglycemia.

Surgery

If your patient with fasting hypoglycemia is scheduled for surgery to remove an extrapancreatic tumor or an insulinoma, review standard preoperative and postoperative procedures. After surgery, instruct the patient to notify his doctor if symptoms of hypoglycemia recur. He should also know the symptoms of hyperglycemia, such as increased urine output and thirst. (See *Is it hypoglycemia or hyperglycemia?*) Hyperglycemia may occur postoperatively if surgery destroys more than 90% of the insulin-producing cells in the pancreas.

Other care measures

As with diabetes mellitus, a large part of the treatment plan for a hypoglycemic patient consists of careful teaching of the patient and his family. Teach them how to recognize signs and symptoms of hypoglycemia, such

Is it hypoglycemia or hyperglycemia?

Some signs and symptoms of hypoglycemia resemble those of hyperglycemia, and patients with hypoglycemia often suffer rebound hyperglycemia.

Review the chart below with your patient and his family to help them distinguish between these two disorders and take the correct actions.

HYPOGLYCEMIA	HYPERGLYCEMIA
Causes • High-carbohydrate meals • Delayed meals • Excessive amounts of certain medications • Excessive exercise • Alcohol or caffeine • Stress • Diabetes mellitus, liver disease, or tumors • Extensive gastric surgery	**Causes** • Insufficient insulin • Failure to follow prescribed diet • Infection, fever, emotional stress
Signs and symptoms • Diaphoresis • Faintness • Headache • Palpitations • Trembling • Impaired vision • Hunger • Difficulty awakening • Irritability • Personality changes	**Signs and symptoms** • Polydipsia and polyuria • Increased blood glucose and ketone levels • Weakness, abdominal pain, generalized aches • Deep, rapid breathing • Anorexia, nausea, vomiting
Actions • If the patient is conscious, give food or liquid containing sugar (for example, orange juice, cola, candy). • If the patient is unconscious, administer glucagon and call the doctor immediately.	**Actions** • Call the doctor immediately. • Give sugar-free fluids if the patient can swallow. • Instruct a diabetic patient to test blood for glucose and urine for ketones every 4 hours during a hyperglycemic episode.

as tremors, palpitations, confusion, and diaphoresis. Review the treatment measures they should take if the patient has a hypoglycemic episode, and make sure they understand the importance of getting immediate care. (See *Managing a hypoglycemic episode,* page 240.)

Also teach them how to administer glucagon. Advise them to notify the doctor if hypoglycemic episodes don't respond to treatment or if they

occur frequently. Help the patient and his family verbalize their feelings and concerns.

Preventing hypoglycemic episodes
Be sure to teach the patient how to prevent a hypoglycemic episode. Discuss his lifestyle and personal habits to help him identify possible precipitating factors, such as poor diet, stress, or mismanagement of diabetes mellitus. Explore ways that he

Managing a hypoglycemic episode

A sudden hypoglycemic episode may affect the patient's ability to recognize his symptoms and take appropriate action. It will be up to you, family members, or other caregivers to manage the crisis for him.

In such an emergency, the patient's blood glucose level *must* be raised immediately to prevent permanent brain damage and even death. So be sure to keep sources of glucose (sugar) available.

If the patient is conscious
Give a conscious patient any of the following:

FOODS AND FLUIDS	AMOUNT
Apple juice, orange juice, or ginger ale	4 to 6 oz
Regular cola or other soft drink	4 to 6 oz
Corn syrup, honey, or grape jelly	1 tablespoon
Hard candy	5 to 6 pieces
Jelly beans	6
Gumdrops	10

If the patient is unconscious or has trouble swallowing
Give him a subcutaneous injection of glucagon. Be sure to check the expiration date on the glucagon kit frequently and replenish the supply as needed.

How to inject glucagon
1. Prepare the glucagon following the manufacturer's instructions included in the kit.
2. Select an appropriate injection site.
3. Pull the skin taut; then clean it with an alcohol swab.
4. Using your thumb and forefinger, pinch the skin at the injection site; then quickly plunge the needle into the skin fold at a 90-degree angle, up to the needle hub. Push the plunger down to quickly inject the glucagon.
5. Withdraw the needle and rub the site with an alcohol swab.
6. Turn the patient onto his side. Because glucagon may cause vomiting, this position reduces the possibility of choking.
7. If the patient doesn't wake up in 5 to 20 minutes, give a second dose of glucagon and seek emergency help.

If he wakes up and can swallow, give him some sugar immediately. Do this because glucagon is effective for only about 90 minutes. Then call the doctor.

can change or avoid each factor. (See *Preventing hypoglycemic episodes*.)

If necessary, teach the patient stress-reduction techniques and encourage him to join a support group. For a patient with pharmacologic hypoglycemia caused by insulin or oral hypoglycemic agents, review the essentials of managing diabetes mellitus, if indicated.

Finally, because hypoglycemia is a chronic disorder, encourage the patient to see his doctor regularly.

Preventing hypoglycemic episodes

Although hypoglycemia is a chronic disorder, the patient can keep it under control and prevent most hypoglycemic episodes. Provide these simple guidelines.

Sticking to the diet
Tell the patient to eat all his meals and snacks at the prescribed time and in the prescribed amounts.

Also instruct him to avoid alcohol and caffeine — they can cause his blood glucose level to drop.

Taking prescribed medicine
If the doctor prescribes medicine to control the patient's hypoglycemia, advise him to strictly follow his schedule. Emphasize that he must take the right amount of medicine at the right time.

Tell him to always check with the doctor who is treating his hypoglycemia before taking any over-the-counter medicine or any other prescribed medicine. Also tell him to inform the doctor about any new treatments he is having for another condition.

Controlling stress
Encourage the patient to reduce stress by practicing relaxation techniques, such as deep breathing and guided imagery. Recommend that he change his lifestyle, if possible, by working less and taking more time for hobbies, traveling, and other leisure activities.

Exercising with caution
Instruct the patient to take some precautions when he exercises. For example, he should not exercise alone or when his blood glucose level is likely to drop. He should consume extra calories to make up for those burned.

For example, if he has *fasting hypoglycemia,* his blood glucose level is likely to drop 5 hours or more after a meal. If he has *reactive hypoglycemia,* his blood glucose level will fall 2 to 4 hours after a meal. If he has *pharmacologic hypoglycemia,* he should ask his doctor for guidelines.

If he's a *diabetic,* tell him not to inject insulin into a part of his body that he'll be exercising during the next few hours.

Carrying carbohydrates
Advise the patient to carry a source of fast-acting carbohydrate, such as hard candy or sugar packets, with him at all times.

Knowing the warning signs
Tell the patient to note what symptoms he typically has before an episode of hypoglycemia. Stress that he should make certain his family, friends, and coworkers know that he has hypoglycemia and that they can also recognize the warning signs. Early recognition can prevent an acute episode.

Alerting others
Instruct the patient to wear a medical identification tag or carry a medical identification card that describes his condition and what emergency actions to take.

Hypothyroidism

If left untreated or managed improperly, hypothyroidism can have devastating effects. Both acute and chronic complications may occur, affecting the quality of the patient's life and possibly even shortening his life span. That's why it's important for you to teach the patient about the chronic nature of his disorder.

Most important, you must stress the need to comply with lifelong thyroid hormone replacement therapy. Other areas to cover include dietary and activity precautions and possible adjunctive care measures.

Before teaching a patient about hypothyroidism, make sure you are familiar with the following topics:
• explanation of the patient's type of hypothyroidism: primary or secondary
• signs and symptoms of hypothyroidism
• complications
• preparation for diagnostic tests to evaluate thyroid function
• activity restrictions
• dietary guidelines for ensuring adequate nutrition
• importance of lifelong thyroid hormone replacement therapy
• signs and symptoms of hyperthyroidism (in accidental thyroid hormone overdose).

ABOUT THE DISORDER
Explain that hypothyroidism is a chronic disorder in which the thyroid gland fails to secrete sufficient thyroid hormone. Tell the patient about his specific type of hypothyroidism: primary or secondary.

Primary hypothyroidism results from gradual destruction of vital thyroid tissue. In the absence of goiter, its most common cause is radioactive iodine therapy or surgery. When goiter is present, its most common cause is Hashimoto's thyroiditis, in which lymphocytes mistake normal thyroid cells for foreign cells and destroy them.

Secondary hypothyroidism, which is rare, results from destruction of pituitary tissue responsible for producing thyroid-stimulating hormone (TSH), or thyrotropin. Without TSH stimulation, the thyroid gland cannot produce thyroid hormone.

Describe how hypothyroidism affects the body. For example, explain that thyroid hormone deficiency decreases the body's ability to use energy. As a result, cells don't function effectively and use up what little ener-

gy is available to them. This causes the patient to tire easily.

Besides fatigue, early symptoms include forgetfulness, sensitivity to cold, and constipation. The patient may also gain weight, even though his caloric intake is unchanged. (See *Reviewing clinical features of hypothyroidism.*)

Complications
To underscore the importance of complying with therapy, discuss the complications that might occur if hypothyroidism is poorly managed or left untreated. Myxedema, for example, may develop gradually. In early stages, it produces generalized symptoms, such as fatigue and lethargy. Later, it causes cool, dry skin along with decreased sweat and oil production, thinning of scalp hair, and loss of body hair.

The patient with myxedema may also develop menstrual irregularities, hearing loss, ataxia, dependent edema, and heart failure. Muscles may increase in bulk but decline in strength, and the patient may have muscle cramps.

Impaired muscle function from myxedema predisposes the patient to constipation and urinary tract infection. Decreased lung expansion heightens the risk of respiratory infection. As myxedema worsens, profound hypotension, bradycardia, hypoventilation, and hypothermia may develop. Stress that without prompt treatment, myxedema can be fatal or can lead to other life-threatening conditions such as coma.

Other chronic complications of uncontrolled hypothyroidism arise from the accumulation of fatty substances in interstitial tissues and decreased metabolism. Atherosclerosis is one such complication.

DIAGNOSTIC WORKUP
Explain that thyroid hormone deficiency is easily confirmed by measuring serum levels of thyroxine and protein-bound iodine.

The thyrotropin-releasing hormone (TRH) infusion test may be ordered to measure the pituitary's thyrotropin reserve if the patient's thyrotropin level is normal or borderline. Explain that this procedure requires insertion of an I.V. catheter and infusion of synthetic TRH through it. Tell the patient that several blood samples will be drawn over about an hour and that the catheter will be removed after the last sample has been collected. If the pituitary responds to the TRH infusion by releasing an excessive amount of TSH, primary hypothyroidism is indicated; a blunted response indicates secondary hypothyroidism.

Additional tests may include a thyroid scan or ultrasonography to evaluate the thyroid's size and structure and a radioactive iodine uptake test to assess gland function. (See *Teaching patients about endocrine tests,* page 232.)

TREATMENTS
Discuss treatments for hypothyroidism, including guidelines for safely increasing activity, dietary restrictions, and thyroid hormone replacement therapy. Also teach the patient how to recognize possible complications of this lifelong disorder.

Activity guidelines
Because hypothyroid patients have so little energy, they tend to be sedentary. As a result, you'll need to encourage the patient to increase his activity level. But caution him to do this gradually because he risks pain and impaired muscle function from myxedema. Discuss activities he enjoys and can fit into his lifestyle. (His doctor will have to provide guidelines for all such activities.)

 WARNING: Instruct the patient to stop any activity and to notify his doctor immediately if he feels chest pain or tightness or experiences severe dyspnea or palpitations.

Dietary modifications
Stress the importance of following dietary restrictions to minimize weight

---

Reviewing clinical features of hypothyroidism

To help the patient and her family understand hypothyroidism, describe its characteristic effects:
- lethargy and weight gain
- cold intolerance
- constipation
- muscle aches and weakness
- rough, thick, scaly skin
- dry, coarse, brittle hair
- facial edema, blank facial expression
- thick tongue, slow speech.

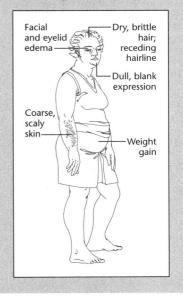

Facial and eyelid edema

Dry, brittle hair; receding hairline

Dull, blank expression

Coarse, scaly skin

Weight gain

---

gain, reduce cholesterol intake, and alleviate constipation. Remind the patient that thyroid hormone deficiency decreases his body's ability to use sugars and carbohydrates as energy sources. It will also cause him to store fats.

Advise the patient to avoid foods high in saturated fats and cholesterol. Suggest that he talk with his doctor about whether he can drink alcohol.

Explore ways to help him adhere to a calorie-restricted diet. If appropriate, encourage him to join a support group.

Also teach the patient how to increase the fiber content in his diet. If he has nonpitting edema, advise him to reduce fluid intake by one to two glasses daily, as prescribed.

Medication

Thyroid hormone replacement is the primary treatment for hypothyroidism and will help the patient achieve a normal metabolic rate and energy level. Explain that this therapy will be tailored to meet his individual requirements and that he'll need to continue thyroid hormone replacement for the rest of his life. The dosage will depend on the severity of his hypothyroidism.

Explain that finding just the right dosage for him is a gradual process. This will allow his body to adjust slowly to the changes resulting from the medication, thus helping to prevent complications.

Instruct the patient who is taking a thyroid hormone replacement, such as levothyroxine (Levothroid, Levoxine, or Synthroid), liothyronine (Cytomel), or thyroid USP to take the drug exactly as prescribed and not to adjust the dosage or discontinue the drug without his doctor's approval. Advise him to take the medication at the same time every day for uniform absorption. Tell him to store his medication in the original container.

Instruct him to watch for adverse reactions, including a change in appetite, abnormal bleeding or bruising, chest pain, diarrhea, fever, severe headache, heat intolerance, insomnia, leg cramps, nervousness, palpitations, shortness of breath, rash, sweating, tremors, and weight loss. Mention that constipation, drowsiness, dry skin, headache, menstrual irregularities, nausea, and temporary hair loss may occur.

WARNING: Caution the patient never to take nonprescription drugs without his doctor's approval. Explain that hypothyroidism slows down his metabolism and thus prolongs drug effects, creating the risk of drug toxicity. Advise him to inform all health care providers of his hypothyroidism so that any prescribed medications (especially narcotics, barbiturates, and digoxin) may be chosen carefully and the dosage reduced appropriately.

Other care measures

Review the signs and symptoms of hypothyroidism with the patient. Advise him to be especially alert for increased lethargy, sensitivity to cold, weight gain, facial and hand puffiness, changes in his skin or hair, and muscle cramps. Instruct him to report any of these changes immediately to his doctor.

At the same time, make sure he's familiar with the signs and symptoms of hyperthyroidism, which would develop if his thyroid hormone dosage were too high. These include heat intolerance, increased sweating, nervous activity, difficulty concentrating, frequent defecation, skin changes, apprehensiveness, and irritability.

Because hypothyroidism is a chronic disorder, encourage the patient to see his doctor regularly for blood tests and physical examinations. Tell him to report any signs or symptoms of infection, such as fever, malaise, diarrhea, and muscle pain. Remind him that hypothyroidism makes him vulnerable to infections. Finally, refer him to an appropriate source of information and support. (See Appendix 2.)

Immune and hematologic conditions

Acquired immunodeficiency syndrome

No disease in recent memory has generated more fear and publicity than acquired immunodeficiency syndrome (AIDS). The World Health Organization estimates that AIDS has infected 15 to 16 million adults and 1 to 2 million children, and has killed at least 2.7 million. The disease transmission mode and the absence of a cure make patient teaching vitally important.

Teaching a patient with AIDS requires patience, perseverance, and a sound knowledge of the disease. You can expect your patient to feel a myriad of emotions, including shock, anger, fear, despair, and isolation. In this state of mind, he won't be receptive to learning. As a result, you'll need to plan your teaching around times when he's most receptive, and you may have to repeat much of the information. You'll also need to keep up to date on AIDS research and treatments so you can answer questions knowledgeably. What's more, you must explore your own feelings and fears about AIDS before you can establish the trusting relationship that's so important for successful teaching.

Before teaching a patient with AIDS, make sure you are familiar with the following topics:
• how human immunodeficiency virus (HIV) affects the immune response
• opportunistic infections, cancer,

and neurologic effects associated with AIDS
• diagnostic criteria for AIDS
• diagnostic tests, such as HIV antibody tests and T-cell assays
• activity modifications, including adequate rest and moderate exercise
• adequate nutrition to help prevent opportunistic infections
• drug therapy
• safer sex practices
• providing home care for an AIDS patient
• caring for children with AIDS
• sources of information and support.

ABOUT THE DISORDER
Inform the patient that AIDS results from infection with HIV, which impairs immune function. This virus attaches to specialized white blood cells (WBCs) called T_4 or helper T cells, gradually depleting their number and hindering their response to infection. The crippled immune system leaves the patient vulnerable to opportunistic infections and cancers. (See *How HIV affects immunity*, page 246.)

Tell the patient that HIV occurs in body fluids, especially blood, semen, and vaginal secretions. Explain that the infection can be transmitted through unprotected vaginal or anal intercourse, needles contaminated with blood, blood transfusions, or (in infants) through transplacental contact or breast-feeding.

Point out that HIV-infected patients develop AIDS at a variable rate. Some remain asymptomatic until they abruptly develop an opportunistic infection such as *Pneumocystis*

INSIGHT INTO ILLNESSES

How HIV affects immunity

Briefly explain normal and impaired immune function to your patient, using clear language. Include the following information in your teaching.

Normal immune function
When viruses enter a healthy body, they're identified as antigens by macrophages. Then macrophages process the antigens and present them to T cells and B cells.

The antigen-activated T cells proliferate and form several kinds of T cells. For example, helper T cells stimulate B cells, whereas suppressor T cells control the extent of T-cell help for B cells. Lymphokine-producing T cells are involved in delayed hypersensitivity and other immune reactions. Cytotoxic, or killer, T cells directly destroy antigenic agents. Memory T cells are stored to recognize and attack the same antigen on subsequent invasions.

The B cells multiply, forming memory cells and plasma cells that produce antigen-specific antibodies, which then attack and kill the invading virus.

Impaired immune function
Human immunodeficiency virus (HIV) selectively infects the helper T cells, impairing their ability to recognize antigens. Now the virus is free to proliferate, causing abnormal immune system function and progressive destruction.

As immunity weakens, the patient becomes vulnerable to potentially fatal protozoal, viral, and fungal infections and to certain forms of cancer. Meanwhile, many more HIV particles are released and invade other T cells, further weakening the immune system and intensifying the problem.

---

carinii pneumonia (PCP) or cancer such as Kaposi's sarcoma. More often, though, they have a recent history of nonspecific signs and symptoms, such as fatigue, afternoon fevers, night sweats, weight loss, diarrhea, or cough. Soon afterward, they typically develop several concurrent infections.

Complications
Point out that, although no cure has been found for AIDS, recent scientific developments hold promise for the future. Emphasize the importance of recognizing symptoms, seeking medical help promptly, and following recommended treatment to limit the number of infections the patient incurs. Make sure he clearly understands that preventing further injury to his damaged immune system can help him preserve the quality of his life.

Inform the patient that the most common opportunistic infection associated with AIDS is PCP. It's caused by a one-celled protozoan that infects the lungs of immunosuppressed people. Numerous cysts composed of clumped organisms multiply in alveolar spaces and eventually cause obstructive disease. Signs and symptoms range from a dry cough, mild fever, and dyspnea on exertion to respiratory failure. Successful management depends on early detection of pulmonary involvement.

Tell the patient that Kaposi's sarcoma is a common form of cancer in AIDS patients. The disease aggressively compromises the blood vessels, then invades the deeper organs and tissues, especially in the GI tract. Small red or purple multicentric lesions develop over the entire body. In advanced stages, the disease obstructs the lymphatic system, causing edema of the leg, head, and neck.

DIAGNOSTIC WORKUP

Inform the patient about HIV antibody tests and other diagnostic studies that establish an initial diagnosis of HIV infection and detect associated opportunistic infections or cancer. (See *Diagnostic criteria for AIDS,* page 248.)

HIV antibody tests

Explain that two blood tests are commonly used to detect HIV antibodies: the enzyme-linked immunosorbent assay (ELISA) and the Western blot. In the ELISA, the patient's serum sample is incubated with live HIV. If HIV antibodies are present, they react with the test solution. If findings are positive, a Western blot assay is performed to confirm the results and identify specific HIV antibodies.

Tell the patient that positive results with both tests establish HIV infection. Stress that this doesn't mean that he has AIDS, only that he's been infected with the virus. On the other hand, a negative result doesn't necessarily mean that he's not infected. The patient may carry HIV for several weeks to months before developing detectable antibody levels and therefore should be tested again at a future date.

T-cell assay

Inform the patient that an absolute helper T-cell count may be performed to evaluate his immune status. When the count falls below 200, opportunistic infections occur, confirming the AIDS diagnosis. Normally, the ratio of helper T cells to suppressor T cells is 2:1. In AIDS, this ratio is reversed.

Direct tests

Tell the patient that direct tests can also be performed to detect HIV. These tests include antigen tests (p24 antigen), HIV cultures, nucleic acid probes of peripheral blood lymphocytes, and the polymerase chain reaction.

Other tests

Teach the patient about other ordered tests to support the diagnosis and help evaluate the severity of immunosuppression. To diagnose PCP, a bronchoscopy is done. Brushings or washings are necessary to obtain a specimen for silver stain to identify the *P. carinii* protozoa. Chest X-rays help detect pulmonary complications, such as diffuse bilateral interstitial infiltrates with PCP. Arterial blood gas studies and pulmonary function tests are routinely used to diagnose pulmonary complications and to monitor progress, especially in patients with PCP. A tissue biopsy confirms a diagnosis of Kaposi's sarcoma.

Discuss tests that confirm the diagnosis of AIDS-related disorders — for example, gallium scan, colonoscopy, bone marrow aspiration, computed tomography scan, or magnetic resonance imaging.

TREATMENTS

Although at this time AIDS is incurable, explain to the patient that various treatments can suppress HIV, control opportunistic infections, and improve his quality of life. These treatments include rest, exercise, diet, and medications.

Activity guidelines

Tell the patient that adequate rest is crucial to reduce the risk of infection. Explain that moderate exercise can help him maintain muscle mass, improve circulation, and achieve a feeling of well-being.

Advise the patient to exercise regularly, avoid overexertion, and alternate periods of activity and rest. If he's well enough to go outdoors, recommend walking as an ideal exercise. If he spends long hours in bed, suggest lifting light hand weights. Of course, he should modify his exercise program as his condition deteriorates. Suggest that he discuss an exercise program with his doctor or a physical therapist.

Diagnostic criteria for AIDS

Inform the patient that the Centers for Disease Control and Prevention defines acquired immunodeficiency syndrome (AIDS) as an illness characterized by one or more indicator diseases (opportunistic infections or cancers). The criteria for a diagnosis, listed below, are based on the presence or absence of laboratory evidence of human immunodeficiency virus (HIV) infection.

Without laboratory evidence of HIV infection

Patients with a definitive diagnosis of one or more of the following indicator diseases are diagnosed with AIDS even without laboratory evidence of HIV infection:
● bronchitis, pneumonitis, or esophagitis persisting longer than 1 month
● candidiasis of the esophagus, trachea, bronchi, or lungs
● extrapulmonary cryptococcosis
● cryptosporidiosis with diarrhea persisting more than 1 month
● cytomegalovirus (CMV) of an organ other than the liver, spleen, or lymph nodes
● herpes simplex virus ulcers persisting longer than 1 month
● Kaposi's sarcoma
● lymphoid interstitial pneumonia, pulmonary lymphoid hyperplasia, or both (LIP/PLH complex) in a patient under age 13
● disseminated *Mycobacterium avium* or *Mycobacterium kansasii* infection at a site other than or in addition to the lungs, skin, or cervical or hilar lymph nodes
● *Pneumocystis carinii* pneumonia (PCP)
● progressive multifocal leukoencephalopathy
● toxoplasmosis of the brain.

With laboratory evidence of HIV infection

Patients with a definitive diagnosis of one or more of the *preceding* indicator diseases or one or more of the *following* indicator diseases are diagnosed with AIDS if they test positive for HIV:
● disseminated coccidioidomycosis at a site other than or in addition to the lungs or cervical or hilar lymph nodes
● HIV encephalopathy
● disseminated histoplasmosis at a site other than the lungs
● isosporiasis with diarrhea persisting longer than 1 month
● Kaposi's sarcoma
● primary lymphoma of the brain
● other non-Hodgkin's lymphoma of B-cell or unknown immunologic phenotype
● disseminated mycobacterial disease caused by other than *Mycobacterium tuberculosis* at a site other than or in addition to the lungs, skin, or cervical or hilar lymph nodes
● extrapulmonary disease caused by *M. tuberculosis,* involving at least one site
● recurrent *Salmonella* (nontyphoid) septicemia
● HIV wasting syndrome (emaciation).

Patients with a *presumptive* diagnosis of one or more of the following indicator diseases are diagnosed with AIDS if they test positive for HIV:
● candidiasis of the esophagus
● CMV retinitis with vision loss
● Kaposi's sarcoma
● LIP/PLH complex in a patient under age 13
● disseminated mycobacterial disease (acid-fast bacilli with species not identified by culture) involving at least one site other than or in addition to the lungs, skin, or cervical or hilar lymph nodes
● PCP
● toxoplasmosis of the brain.

Dietary modifications

Teach the patient the importance of maintaining adequate nutrition to prevent infection and weight loss. Encourage him to eat small, frequent, high-calorie, high-protein meals, and emphasize the importance of drinking plenty of fluids. Discuss ways to stimulate the appetite, promote food preparation, and make mealtimes more pleasant. If he continues to lose weight, show him how to keep a calorie count, and teach him about commercial dietary supplements.

Medications

Educate the patient about drugs used to modify HIV infection, including antiviral agents such as zidovudine (Retrovir, AZT), saquinavir, didanosine, stavudine, and zalcitabine. To treat related infections and cancers, the patient may receive such drugs as pentamidine, co-trimoxazole, and chemotherapeutic agents.

Also teach about drugs and drug combinations currently under testing. Point out that the combination of protease inhibitors and reverse transcriptase inhibitors holds promise. Advise the patient to check with the doctor about the availability of investigative drugs.

Zidovudine

Tell the patient that no drug has been discovered to restore immune function, but zidovudine can limit the replication of HIV. This drug slows the progression of AIDS, relieving many of its incapacitating symptoms and decreasing the number of opportunistic infections. It's also used to prevent maternal transmission of HIV to infants.

Co-trimoxazole

Teach the patient that co-trimoxazole (sulfamethoxazole and trimethoprim [Bactrim, Septra]) is the drug of choice for PCP. Discuss how and when to take the drug and its possible adverse effects. Instruct the patient to complete the prescribed course of therapy and to take each dose as ordered.

Pentamidine

If the patient is allergic to sulfa drugs or if co-trimoxazole isn't effective in treating PCP, the doctor may order pentamidine isethionate (Pentacarinat, Pentam 300). Given by injection, this drug can cause severe hypotension. Instruct the patient to lie down while receiving it. Tell him that the nurse will take his blood pressure when the drug is being administered and several times afterward until blood pressure stabilizes.

 WARNING: Inform the patient that pentamidine may lower his WBC count, increasing his chance of infection. It may also lower his platelet count, increasing the risk of bleeding. Advise him to avoid people with colds or other infections and to check with the doctor immediately if he thinks he's getting a cold or other infection. He should also contact the doctor if he notices any unusual bleeding or bruising. Tell him to brush and floss his teeth carefully, to check with the dentist for other ways to clean his teeth and gums, and to contact the doctor before having any dental work done. Instruct him to use an electric shaver instead of a safety razor and to use fingernail and toenail clippers cautiously.

Chemotherapy

Inform the patient that vincristine and vinblastine are the cornerstone of Kaposi's sarcoma treatment, although etoposide, doxorubicin, and alpha-interferon also may be used. Provide advice on controlling the adverse effects of chemotherapy.

Other treatments

Two procedures are sometimes used to treat Kaposi's sarcoma. If the sarcoma affects only the skin, the lesions may be treated with electron beam therapy. If the sarcoma invades deeper tissues, radiation therapy or chemotherapy may be used. If the doctor orders radiation, explain the procedure to the patient.

Preventing and recognizing infection in AIDS

Dear Patient:

Because AIDS damages your immune system and impairs your body's ability to fight infections, preventing infections is extremely important. However, if you do come down with an infection, remember that early recognition and treatment are equally important. Appropriate and timely treatment may prevent your condition from getting worse.

Preventing infection

To help prevent infection, review these guidelines and follow them whenever possible:
- Avoid crowds and people with known infections, such as herpes, influenza, mononucleosis, and cytomegalovirus. Even stay away from people who have minor colds.
- Get adequate sleep at night, and rest often during the day.
- Eat frequent, small meals, even if you've lost your appetite and have to force yourself to eat.
- Practice good hygiene, especially good oral hygiene. Don't use commercial mouthwashes because their high alcohol and sugar content may irritate your mouth and provide a medium for bacterial growth.
- Don't use unprescribed intravenous drugs.
- Don't share needles with anyone.
- Avoid traveling to foreign countries. If you must travel, drink only bottled or boiled water and avoid raw vegetables and fruits to prevent a possible intestinal infection.
- Wear a mask and gloves to clean bird cages, fish tanks, and cat litter boxes.
- Keep rooms clean and well ventilated, and keep air conditioners and humidifiers cleaned and repaired so they don't harbor infectious organisms.

Recognizing signs and symptoms of infection

Contact your doctor immediately if you notice any of these signs or symptoms:
- persistent fever or nighttime sweating not related to a cold or the flu
- swollen lymph nodes in your neck, armpits, or groin that last more than 2 months and aren't related to any other illness
- profound, persistent fatigue unrelieved by rest and not related to increased physical activity, longer work schedules, drug use, or a psychological disorder
- loss of appetite and weight loss
- open sores
- dry, persistent, unproductive cough
- persistent, unexplained diarrhea
- white coating or spots on your tongue or throat, possibly accompanied by soreness, burning, or difficulty swallowing
- blurred vision or persistent, severe headaches
- confusion, depression, uncontrolled excitement, or inappropriate speech
- persistent or spreading rash or skin discoloration
- unexplained bleeding or bruising.

Other care measures
Take the time to educate the patient and his caregivers about other measures that will help them cope with AIDS.

Infection control
Emphasize the importance of prevention or early detection and treatment of infections. Provide a copy of the patient teaching aid *Preventing and recognizing infection in AIDS*.

Preventing AIDS transmission
Besides stressing the importance of prompt treatment, teach the patient how to prevent transmitting AIDS to others. Tell him not to donate blood, blood products, organs, tissue, or sperm. Warn him to inform potential sex partners and health care workers that he's HIV positive. If he uses I.V. drugs, caution him not to share needles and to warn any persons with whom he shared needles in the past that he's infected.

Inform the patient that high-risk sexual practices for AIDS transmission are those that lead to the exchange of body fluids, such as anal or vaginal intercourse without a condom, fellatio without a condom, cunnilingus, insertion of a foreign object into the rectum followed by anal intercourse without a condom, and oral-anal stimulation.

Discuss safer sexual practices with your patient. Tell him that these include hugging, kissing, petting, massaging, mutual masturbation, using sex toys (but not sharing them), and having protected sexual intercourse.

Also teach the patient about precautions in activities of daily living so that friends, roommates, and family members don't contract AIDS.

Dealing with AIDS in children
If your patient is a child, teach his caregivers about the special concerns and precautions involved. Tell them about programs that can help the child cope with a terminal illness.

Coping with AIDS in pregnancy
Caution the pregnant patient that her infant may become infected before birth, during delivery, or during breast-feeding, so caution her not to breast-feed. Advise the female patient of childbearing age to postpone getting pregnant until more is known about the AIDS virus and pregnancy.

Alternative therapy and support services
Tell the patient about alternative therapies if he asks. These treatments include acupuncture, Chinese herbals, megavitamins, coenzyme Q, and diets (such as macrobiotic, immune power, or yeast-control). Suggest that he contact a local or national AIDS organization for information and referrals before starting an alternative therapy. Encourage him to continue with his prescribed regimen even if he uses an alternative therapy and to let the doctor know what other therapies he's trying.

Provide information about local and national AIDS organizations and support groups for patients, their partners, and family members. (See Appendix 2.) Tell the patient about various services, such as one-on-one volunteer counseling and assistance with medical insurance. Urge him to seek support from these organizations, and, if necessary, help him contact them.

Anaphylaxis
A severe allergic reaction, anaphylaxis can be a life-threatening emergency, causing acute respiratory failure and vascular collapse. Even a milder reaction can trigger panic.

Typically, you'll be teaching a patient who has already had anaphylaxis or one who is at risk. To help your patient guard against complications, you'll need to teach him to respond quickly to the earliest signs of anaphylaxis. You'll demonstrate how to use the supplies in an emergency anaphylaxis kit. Above all, you'll discuss how to prevent further reactions by avoiding exposure to known antigens, such as insect stings or certain foods. You'll also encourage him to carry medical identification naming his allergy. This will alert caregivers to his condition should he be unconscious or otherwise unable to speak.

Before teaching a patient about anaphylaxis, make sure you are familiar with the following topics:

• description of anaphylaxis and its signs and symptoms

• common causes of anaphylaxis

• complications, including respiratory failure and cardiovascular collapse

• skin testing and an elimination diet to identify allergens

• importance of immediate treatment after exposure

• how to use an anaphylaxis kit

• how to apply a tourniquet

• avoiding known antigens

• using a medical identification service

• sources of information and support.

ABOUT THE DISORDER

Begin by explaining that anaphylaxis is a severe allergic reaction that occurs after second or subsequent exposures to an antigen. Tell the patient that the first exposure produces no symptoms but causes the body to recognize the antigen and to create antibodies against it. At some subsequent exposure, the body undergoes a major allergic — or anaphylactic — reaction.

Review common antigens and the routes through which they enter the body. Explain, for example, that an antigen may be inhaled, ingested, or injected. Mention that people who react to one antigen are more likely to react to similar or other substances.

Mention that most reactions occur within 30 minutes after exposure. Less typically, they can arise within seconds or up to an hour after exposure. Point out that the greater the sensitivity to the antigen, the more rapid and severe the reaction.

Describe the signs and symptoms that signal an anaphylactic reaction. Usually, initial indications include vague feelings of uneasiness and anxiety, headache, dizziness, numbness, and disorientation. Skin signs and symptoms usually begin with generalized itching followed by redness and, possibly, wheals or hives. Initially, the skin feels clammy, but as redness and swelling develop, the patient is likely to feel warm and uncomfortable. Swelling may affect the eyelids, lips, tongue, palms, and soles. Explain that the patient may feel as if he has a lump in the throat or may have trouble breathing. He also may experience hoarseness, coughing, sneezing, and wheezing.

Complications

Stress that prompt treatment of the earliest symptoms may prevent potentially fatal complications. Warn the patient that an unchecked reaction can lead to respiratory failure or cardiovascular collapse. Total airway obstruction, caused by swollen upper airway structures, is the most common cause of death from anaphylaxis. Severe, prolonged bronchospasm also may cause respiratory failure. Cardiovascular failure may result if chemical mediators released during anaphylaxis cause capillary leakage. Fluids then leave the blood vessels and enter the tissues, and the blood volume drops, causing hypotension, shock, and cardiac arrest.

DIAGNOSTIC WORKUP

Explain that no test can diagnose anaphylaxis, although certain tests can be used to identify antigens. Instead, diagnosis is based on the patient's signs, symptoms, and health history. Advise the patient to give a thorough accounting of previous reactions and potential exposures. Tests that may be done to evaluate the condition during an attack include blood studies, an electrocardiogram, and chest X-rays.

Inform the patient that some sensitivities and antigens may be obvious without testing. For example, if hives and breathing problems occur after he plays with a kitten, he can conclude that cat dander triggers a reaction. In other situations, however, skin testing may be necessary to identify the offending substance.

If appropriate, teach the patient about skin testing and an elimination diet, which may be ordered to screen for sensitivity to various antigens. Reassure him that his reaction to possible antigens is monitored during such testing and that the most common positive reaction is a raised, red, itchy area where the skin was exposed to the antigen. (See *Teaching patients about immune and hematologic tests,* pages 285 and 286.)

Elimination diet
Tell the patient that an elimination diet is used to identify food allergies. First, he keeps a record of everything he eats for at least a week. Next, he removes potentially antigenic foods, such as eggs, milk, and wheat, from the diet. Once his symptoms subside, he reintroduces these foods one at a time to his diet. A reaction after he consumes a certain food — occurring either immediately or over time — identifies the offending substance.

TREATMENTS
Anaphylaxis is always an emergency. Instruct the patient to minimize activity during a reaction. Show him how to use the medications and tourniquet in an anaphylaxis kit. Discuss ways to avoid exposure to the antigens that cause anaphylaxis.

Activity guidelines
Caution the patient not to move around if he's been exposed to an antigen that could cause anaphylaxis. For example, if he's allergic to bee stings, advise him to sit down and minimize all activity if he's stung. Explain that physical activity stimulates blood flow, which can hasten the anaphylactic response.

Dietary modifications
Advise the patient with a food allergy to avoid the offending food in any form. Urge him to read labels to avoid allergens — such as nuts or dyes — that are hidden in food. Remind him to ask about ingredients, especially when eating away from home. Advise children to check with an adult about ingredients of new or unfamiliar foods.

Medications
Demonstrate how to use an emergency kit to treat anaphylaxis. (See *How to use an anaphylaxis kit,* page 254.) Explain that the kit contains alcohol swabs, a tourniquet, a syringe, and two medicines: epinephrine and an antihistamine.

Epinephrine
Tell the patient that this injectable drug, also known as Adrenalin, counteracts anaphylaxis by raising blood pressure and dilating breathing passages. It also inhibits histamine release and offsets the effects of circulating histamine. Alert the patient to possible blurred vision, excitability, eye irritation, headache, hypertension, light-headedness, nausea, restlessness, sweating, or vomiting.

Other care measures
Remind the patient that a prompt response after exposure to the offending antigen can save his life. If the doctor wants him to use an emergency kit, tell him to follow its instructions as soon as he's exposed to the antigen.

 WARNING: Stress that if the patient's condition doesn't improve within 10 minutes after using an emergency anaphylaxis kit, he should call an ambulance for immediate transport to the hospital. If he lives far from an emergency department, tell him to call the ambulance before starting the self-treatment.

If the patient is allergic to insect stings, teach him how to avoid them. If an insect does sting him, instruct him to apply ice packs to the site, if possible. Tell him not to place the ice directly on his skin. Instead, he should wrap the ice in a cloth and then apply it to the affected area. Explain that ice decreases blood flow around the sting and slows the reaction to the antigen.

If the patient is allergic to a medication, remind him to tell his doctor

How to use an anaphylaxis kit

If your patient is susceptible to anaphylactic reactions, teach him how
to use an emergency anaphylaxis kit
if prescribed. Inform him that the kit
contains everything needed to treat
an allergic reaction:
● prefilled syringe containing two
doses of epinephrine
● alcohol swabs
● tourniquet
● antihistamine tablets.

If an insect stings the patient, tell
him to use the kit as follows and to
notify the doctor immediately (or
ask someone else to call).

1. Take the prefilled syringe from the
kit and remove the needle cap. Hold
the syringe with the needle pointing
up. Push in the plunger until it stops,
to expel any air from the syringe.
2. Next, clean about 4" (10 cm) of
the skin on your arm or thigh with
an alcohol swab. (If you're right-
handed, clean your left arm or thigh.
If you're left-handed, clean your right
arm or thigh.)
3. Inject the epinephrine by rotating
the plunger one quarter turn to the
right so it's aligned with the slot.
Insert the entire needle like a dart
into the skin. Push down on the

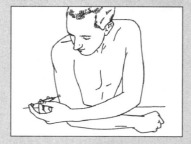

plunger until it stops. It will inject 0.3
ml of the drug for a person age 12 or
over. Withdraw the needle.

Note: The dose and administration
for babies and for children under age
12 must be directed by the doctor.
4. Quickly remove the insect's stinger

if you can see it. Use a dull object,
such as a fingernail or tweezers, to
pull it straight out. Don't pinch,
scrape, or squeeze the stinger. This
may push it farther into the skin and
release more poison. If you can't remove the stinger quickly, stop trying.
Go on to the next step.
5. Chew and swallow the antihistamine tablets. (For children age 12
and under, follow the dosage and
administration directions supplied by
your doctor or provided in the kit.)
6. Next, apply ice to the affected area
(you may use ice cubes in a plastic
bag, ice bags, or any food product
from the freezer such as a poly bag of
vegetables). Wrap the ice product in
a thin layer of cloth or towel to avoid
injury to the skin. Avoid exertion,
keep warm, and see a doctor or go to
a hospital immediately.

Important: If you don't notice an
improvement within 10 minutes,
give a second injection by following
the directions with the kit. If your
syringe has a preset second dose,
don't depress the plunger until
you're ready to give the second injection. Proceed as before, following
the instructions to inject the epinephrine.

Special instructions
● Tell the patient to keep his kit
handy to ensure emergency treatment at all times.
● Instruct him to ask his pharmacist
whether he can store the kit in a
car's glove compartment or must
keep it in a cooler place.
● Tell him to periodically check the
epinephrine in the preloaded syringe. If the solution is pinkish
brown, tell him to replace the syringe.
● Instruct him to make a note of the
kit's expiration date and to renew
the kit just before that date.
● Tell him to dispose of the used needle and syringe safely and properly.

or other caregivers before drugs are prescribed or administered. Point out that if he's allergic to one drug, he's probably sensitive to all drugs in the same family. Tell him to speak up about drug allergies if he's having diagnostic tests that require use of contrast media. Also suggest he wear medical identification, such as a bracelet or necklace, to alert caregivers in emergency situations in which he may be unable to communicate. Finally, tell him how to contact organizations and agencies for further information and support. (See Appendix 2.)

Aplastic anemia

Because aplastic anemia can lead to life-threatening complications, your teaching will emphasize the need for compliance with prescribed treatment. However, the disorder's early clinical features are vague, so your initial teaching will involve preparing the patient for the diagnostic workup, including blood studies and a bone marrow biopsy. After diagnosis, you'll help the patient understand the pathophysiology of this disorder.

Encourage compliance with supportive treatment: restricting activity, maintaining a proper diet, taking prescribed medications, and avoiding infection. As appropriate, teach about a splenectomy or bone marrow transplant. Throughout your teaching, underscore the importance of remaining alert for developing complications, such as infection, bleeding, and worsening anemia.

Before teaching a patient about aplastic anemia, make sure you are familiar with the following topics:
• roles of bone marrow, red and white blood cells, and platelets in aplastic anemia
• complications, such as organ damage, serious infection, and massive bleeding
• diagnostic studies, including blood tests and bone marrow aspiration and biopsy

• activity restrictions and dietary guidelines
• drug therapy
• blood transfusions
• surgery, such as splenectomy and bone marrow transplantation
• preventing infection through isolation, hand washing, and other personal hygiene practices
• preventing injury and reducing stress
• sources of information and support.

ABOUT THE DISORDER

Inform the patient that aplastic anemia results when the bone marrow fails to produce or suppresses all three types of blood cells: red blood cells (RBCs), white blood cells (WBCs), and platelets. (See *Understanding bone marrow's role*, page 256.) Explain that RBCs carry oxygen from the lungs to the rest of the body, WBCs fight infection, and platelets initiate clotting to stanch bleeding.

Inform the patient that signs and symptoms relate directly to blood cell shortages. For example, too few RBCs cause anemia and subsequent weakness, fatigue, and shortness of breath on exertion. A deficiency of WBCs (leukopenia) may result in fever, malaise, and areas of red, swollen, tender skin. Specific shortages of such WBCs as basophils, eosinophils, and especially neutrophils (neutropenia) significantly increase the patient's risk for infection. Thrombocytopenia, a platelet deficiency, commonly results in bruising, superficial bleeding, and petechiae. A deficiency of all of these blood cells (pancytopenia) results in aplastic anemia.

Aplastic anemia usually begins with nonspecific symptoms, such as fatigue, headache, pallor, and shortness of breath. The rate of progression and severity are unpredictable and related to the degree of bone marrow damage.

Explain that aplastic anemia may be congenital or acquired. In about half of all cases, the cause is unknown. In the rest, the cause may be drugs, industrial chemicals, a virus, a congenital abnormality (for instance,

Understanding bone marrow's role

Review bone marrow function with your patient. Explain that marrow is soft connective tissue found mostly in the cavities of long bones, such as the femur, humerus, and sternum. Inform him that marrow, which comes in two types (red and yellow), produces the body's blood cells.

Red marrow — which is found mostly in the cancellous (spongy) tissue at the ends of the long bones (epiphyses) — produces red blood cells, white blood cells, and platelets. *Yellow marrow,* which replaces red marrow as the patient ages, is mostly inactive connective tissue. It lies in the cancellous tissue at the epiphyses and in a canal that runs centrally through the bone.

Fanconi's syndrome), or environmental factors such as radiation.

Complications

Point out that untreated aplastic anemia can result in life-threatening complications, such as myocardial infarction; renal damage; bacterial, viral, or fungal infections; or massive bleeding leading to organ damage or hemorrhagic shock.

DIAGNOSTIC WORKUP

Tell the patient that blood studies will help differentiate aplastic anemia from other blood abnormalities, such as leukemia. A bone marrow biopsy confirms the diagnosis. (See *Teaching patients about immune and hematologic tests*, pages 285 and 286.)

Blood studies

The doctor will order a complete blood count — including an RBC count, total hematocrit and hemoglobin values, RBC indices, WBC count, and WBC differential count — and a platelet count. Inform the patient that repeated blood studies are used to monitor the course of the illness and to measure his response to treatment. The frequency of these tests ranges from daily to monthly, depending on the severity of the illness and the patient's treatment regimen.

TREATMENTS

Inform the patient that the goal of treatment is to prevent complications and make him more comfortable. However, it won't cure the disorder. Explain that even if the cause of aplastic anemia is successfully treated, recovery may take months.

Tell the patient that his treatment regimen will depend on the severity of the disorder and may include drug therapy, blood transfusions, activity restrictions, and a nutritious diet. Occasionally, spontaneous remission occurs with supportive care; more commonly, the disorder progresses, and the doctor recommends bone marrow transplantation or splenectomy.

Activity guidelines

To maintain cardiovascular health, encourage the patient to engage in regular, moderate exercise such as walking. Remind him to avoid contact sports and other traumatic activities. Advise him to pace his daily activities to conserve his energy and avoid shortness of breath.

Dietary modifications

Because bone marrow requires iron and B vitamins to produce blood cells, advise the patient to maintain a diet rich in these nutrients to help boost the number of circulating blood cells. As for food preparation, direct him to cook meats thoroughly, to keep perishable food refrigerated, and to discard food (especially dairy products) still on hand after the expiration date. Following these precautions may help him avoid infections, such as food poisoning from salmonella.

Medications

Tell the patient that aplastic anemia may respond to several medications, such as androgens, corticosteroids, and immunosuppressants. Explain that the doctor may order androgens and corticosteroids to stimulate bone marrow function. The medications may be taken orally (daily) or I.M. (weekly). Emphasize that 2 to 3 months may pass before the patient notices an improvement.

Inform the patient that the doctor may prescribe immunosuppressants (given I.V.) in severe anemia for patients not considered suitable candidates for bone marrow transplantation. Combined with supportive therapy, immunosuppressants may induce partial or complete hematologic remission.

As needed, the patient may receive supportive drug therapy, such as antibiotics to control infection or acetaminophen to control fever.

 WARNING: Caution the patient to avoid taking aspirin, aspirin-containing products, and certain nonsteroidal anti-inflammatory drugs, such as ibuprofen. Explain that these agents may decrease platelet aggregation and cause GI irritation, thereby increasing the risk for bleeding. For safety's sake, urge him to read all nonprescription drug labels carefully.

Androgens

Tell the patient who is receiving androgens — for example, fluoxymesterone (Halo-testin) and oxymetholone (Anadrol) — that these drugs are forms of male hormones. Therefore, a female patient taking androgens may experience a change in voice or menstrual irregularities; a male patient may develop enlarged breasts, frequent or persistent erections, or shrunken testicles. Both sexes may experience headache, nausea and vomiting, swollen arms and legs caused by fluid retention, and weight gain.

Direct the patient to report any of these changes to the doctor, who may adjust the dosage. Advise the patient that he'll need regular blood tests during androgen therapy.

Corticosteroids

Teach the patient about corticosteroids such as prednisone (Deltasone, Meticorten). Warn him that the drug's adverse effects include acne, euphoria, and a puffy face. Advise him to report any of these signs and symptoms, as well as any other adverse reactions to this drug.

Emphasize that he must never abruptly stop taking the medication after he starts therapy; corticosteroids must be discontinued gradually to avoid serious complications. Mention that he'll need regular blood pressure monitoring (to detect hypertension) and blood studies (to detect hyperglycemia) during therapy.

Immunosuppressants

Antilymphocyte globulin and lymphocyte immune globulin (Atgam) are examples of immunosuppressant drugs used in aplastic anemia. The patient is hospitalized for I.V. administration of these medications for up to 10 days. Tell him that adverse reactions to therapy may include serum sickness (chills, fever, flushing, and malaise). Reassure him, however, that simultaneous treatment with a steroid drug — prednisone, for example — minimizes discomfort. He may also receive acetaminophen (Tylenol) — but not aspirin — to control fever. Emphasize that his response to immunosuppressive therapy won't be immediate, so he'll require supportive care during and after treatment.

Experimental drugs

Explain that if standard drug therapy fails, the doctor may suggest medications to stimulate blood cell production. These medications include sargramostim (granulocyte-monocyte colony-stimulating factor) and filgrastim (granulocyte colony-stimulating factor). The patient will probably stay in the hospital during treatment with one of these drugs, and will have frequent blood tests and bone marrow biopsies.

Teaching about blood transfusions

If the doctor orders a blood transfusion, provide information to help your patient understand the procedure.

Purpose

Point out that blood carries food, oxygen, and other important substances for growth and repair of the body's tissues. Therefore, a blood transfusion will help his body maintain its normal functions.

Explain that blood is composed of red blood cells (RBCs), white blood cells (WBCs), and platelets — and that the body needs a certain number of each. Point out that when the number of blood cells (blood count) circulating in his body gets too low, his body can't function properly. For example, too few RBCs impairs the body's ability to carry oxygen, eliminate waste products and poisons, keep warm, and maintain blood pressure. Too few WBCs affects the ability to fight infection. And if the patient doesn't have enough platelets, his blood can't clot properly.

Tell the patient that when his blood count falls below a certain level, the doctor orders a transfusion containing the needed cells. The new blood he receives may contain just one cell type or a mixture.

When to call the doctor

Instruct the patient to call his doctor if he experiences symptoms that may indicate a *low RBC count,* such as short-windedness or constant, rapid breathing, unusually pale skin, difficulty staying warm, or dizziness.

The patient should also contact the doctor if he has symptoms that suggest a *low platelet count,* such as easy bruising, tiny purple or red spots on the skin, bleeding gums, or blood-tinged urine or stools.

Transfusion procedure

Tell the patient that, before the transfusion, a technician collects a sample of his blood to determine his blood type and match it to donor blood. This may be done the day before the transfusion. On the day of the transfusion, a nurse or another trained specialist inserts an I.V. line (tubing connected to a needle) in the patient's arm. Once he's ready for the transfusion, two nurses (or a nurse and a doctor) carefully check and double-check the information on the blood bag to make sure that the blood is specifically for the patient. This may require that they examine his identification bracelet, too.

Explain that during the transfusion, a bag containing the correct blood product is hung above the bed. Then the infusion begins. Tell the patient to expect to have his temperature, pulse rate, blood pressure, and breathing rate taken before and frequently during the infusion.

Inform him that a transfusion of RBCs takes from 2 to 4 hours, and a platelet transfusion takes 15 to 45 minutes.

Possible adverse effects

Assure the patient that his risk for infection is low because of careful blood and donor screening procedures. His chance of getting hepatitis from a blood transfusion is about 1 in 10,000; his chance of getting acquired immunodeficiency syndrome is about 1 in 40,000. (For comparison, point out that his risk of dying in a car accident is 1 in 20,000.)

Occasionally, a transfusion may trigger an *allergic reaction.* Symptoms include fever, chills, and hives during or after the transfusion. If this happens during the procedure,

Teaching about blood transfusions *(continued)*

the nurse will stop the transfusion and return the remaining blood to the blood bank along with a sample of the patient's blood. Then the blood will be examined to determine the cause of his reaction.

Tell the patient that if he has an allergic reaction, he'll receive medications, such as acetaminophen (Tylenol) and diphenhydramine (Benadryl), to ease his symptoms.

When to get immediate help
Rarely, a reaction to a blood transfusion is severe. If the patient experiences any of the following symptoms during or after transfusion, he should notify the doctor or nurse immediately:
- feeling of warmth or flushing
- redness (especially on the face and chest)
- rash or itching
- aching muscles
- pain at the infusion site
- chest pain
- severe headache
- brown urine or pain when urinating.

Procedures
When aplastic anemia causes disability or life-threatening bleeding, the doctor usually orders blood transfusions. Explain that RBC and platelet transfusions may temporarily relieve some symptoms. (See *Teaching about blood transfusions.*)

Surgery
A *splenectomy* may be recommended if the doctor suspects that the spleen is destroying normal RBCs and platelets. Inform the patient that the spleen normally filters old, damaged, and abnormal blood cells from the circulation. Removing the spleen allows older, still-functioning blood cells to survive longer, which increases the number of circulating cells. After a splenectomy, other lymphatic tissue takes on the task of removing dead blood cells but does so at a slower rate.

Bone marrow transplantation is the treatment of choice for severe aplastic anemia. The ideal patient is under age 40 and free from sensitization by excessive blood transfusions. He requires a donor, usually a sibling, who is human leukocyte antigen matched. Explain that tissue typing and matching require a blood sample from both the patient and the potential donor.

Once a match is found, the doctor collects healthy bone marrow from the donor's iliac crest in the operating room. The marrow cells then are purified and diluted with heparin. Next, the new bone marrow is infused into the patient through a Hickman catheter, which is placed under the collarbone.

Advise the patient that he'll be hospitalized for 2 to 3 months. Clarify the risk of graft rejection, graft-versus-host disease (GVHD), and serious infection. Point out that he'll undergo long-term follow-up and treatment with oral immunosuppressants to control GVHD and ensure long-term survival.

Other care measures
Inform the patient with a low WBC count that he may require isolation to prevent infection. If he's in the hospital, this may include special airflow rooms, protective isolation techniques, or simply hand washing. Recommendations vary because of controversy over the mechanism of infection acquisition. If the patient requires only protective isolation, he should expect visitors to wear masks in addition to washing their hands thoroughly.

If the patient is caring for himself at home, stress the importance of following strict personal hygiene practices and minimizing exposure to infection. Teach him to take his temperature two to three times daily. Instruct him to report signs of infection, including chills, fever, and red, swollen, tender areas on his skin. Also advise him to report any severe anemia symptoms, such as headache, ringing in the ears, and light-headedness. Urge him to report any chest pain at once or to go to the nearest emergency department.

WARNING: Because of the blood's decreased ability to clot, caution the patient to avoid injury — for example, by using an electric razor and by avoiding sharp instruments or tools. Urge him to be especially careful when trimming his nails. Remind him to inspect his surroundings for safety. Suggest that he clear hallways of clutter, install lights on stairways, discard slippery throw rugs or doormats, and install grab bars in the bathroom.

Because of the intensity of aplastic anemia treatments, offer emotional support to the patient and his family, and, as necessary, refer them to other sources of support and information. (See Appendix 2.) Encourage him to practice stress-reduction and relaxation techniques, such as deep breathing, guided imagery, and biofeedback.

Hemophilia

A rare, inherited bleeding disorder, hemophilia affects about 1 in 4,000 males. Fortunately, early recognition and treatment of bleeding episodes can prevent the many complications that were common before clotting factor concentrates and home I.V. infusion programs were developed. Most likely, you'll emphasize this point as you explain the patient's condition and discuss measures he can take to manage bleeding episodes.

Before teaching the patient with hemophilia, make sure you are familiar with the following topics:
• normal and abnormal clotting processes
• hemophilic inheritance patterns

• type and severity of the patient's hemophilia
• importance of recognizing bleeding episodes and seeking prompt treatment
• diagnostic tests such as blood studies
• activity restrictions to avoid injury
• medications
• administration of I.V. clotting factors
• prevention of hepatitis and acquired immunodeficiency syndrome (AIDS)
• importance of avoiding aspirin and other drugs that affect platelets
• first-aid measures
• preventive dental care
• sources of information and support.

ABOUT THE DISORDER

Explain how the body normally responds to bleeding: First, the injured blood vessels constrict to impede blood flow. Platelets then rush to the injury site to plug leaking capillaries. Next, clotting factors (special plasma proteins) activate to form a firm fibrin clot. This clot continually breaks down and re-forms until the injury heals.

Tell the patient that, in a person who has hemophilia, an injured vessel constricts and platelets plug the capillaries as usual. But because one of the blood's 10 clotting factors is missing or abnormal, the clotting process goes awry. Compare the hemophilic clotting process to the domino effect, with the 10 clotting factors as the dominoes. Explain that the removal or misalignment of one falling domino in the chain breaks the chain reaction. Interrupted in this way, the clotting process produces a mushy, ineffective clot.

Make it clear that the patient doesn't bleed faster than anyone else. However, because of the missing or defective clotting factor, he may have prolonged or delayed oozing. Explain that bleeding typically occurs with injuries to the kidneys, joints, muscles, and subcutaneous tissue, where the missing factor plays the most important role in coagulation. Identify which of the patient's clotting factors is defective or missing.

Tell him that hemophilia is inherited and almost always affects males because the causative genetic abnormality occurs on the X chromosome. Women have two X chromosomes, so they have two chances to inherit an X chromosome with the normal gene. Men have an X and a Y chromosome, so they have only one chance to inherit the normal gene. If a woman has an X chromosome with a hemophilia gene on it, she's considered a carrier.

Review the patient's type of hemophilia and classify it as mild, moderate, or severe. Tell him that the severity depends on the degree of his clotting factor deficiency.

If the patient has *mild hemophilia,* explain that prolonged bleeding follows major trauma, surgery, or tooth extractions. Postoperative bleeding continues as a slow ooze or stops and starts again, up to 8 days after surgery.

If the patient has *moderate hemophilia*, tell him that he may bleed abnormally after relatively mild injuries, such as a hard bump or a sprain. Bleeding episodes may occur as often as once a month or as seldom as once every several years. The patient may experience occasional spontaneous bleeding.

With *severe hemophilia*, the first symptom typically is excessive bleeding after circumcision. Later, spontaneous bleeding or severe bleeding after minor injuries may cause hematomas (large swellings of blood) beneath the skin and within muscles. Bleeding into joints and muscles causes pain, swelling, extreme tenderness and, possibly, permanent deformity.

Even in people who don't have hemophilia, small blood vessels in the tissue surrounding joints rupture from time to time. Normally, the bleeding stops almost immediately. But in severe hemophilia, the vessel keeps oozing until pressure in the joint becomes great enough to stop the bleeding. This usually takes several days. The only other way to stop the bleeding is to administer the missing clotting factor. People with severe hemophilia may have bleeding episodes as often as once a week.

Complications
Urge the patient and his family to comply with treatment measures. Point out that most hemophiliacs can now expect a normal life span, although damage from abnormal bleeding still poses a serious threat. For instance, bleeding near nerves may cause nerve inflammation and degeneration, pain, abnormal sensations (such as numbness, tingling, and prickling), and muscle shrinkage.

If bleeding impairs blood flow through a major vessel, decreased blood supply and gangrene may result. Of greater concern is bleeding within the brain, skull, heart, throat, or tongue, which can cause shock and death. To prevent serious blood loss and chronic joint disease, the hemophiliac must learn how to recognize the symptoms of internal bleeding and respond to them promptly. (See *Recognizing and managing bleeding*, page 262.)

DIAGNOSTIC WORKUP
Explain that a family or personal history of bleeding after trauma or surgery (including tooth extractions) or of spontaneous bleeding into muscles or joints usually indicates a defect in the hemostatic mechanism. However, the patient will need specific clotting factor assays to confirm and identify the type and severity of hemophilia.

Inform the patient that blood studies are the key diagnostic tool for assessing hemophilia. Additional tests may be done periodically to evaluate complications caused by bleeding. For example, computed tomography scans are used to evaluate suspected bleeding within the skull, arthroscopy or arthrography for certain joint problems, and endoscopy for GI bleeding.

Inform the patient that the usual blood tests for any suspected bleed-

Recognizing and managing bleeding

Bleeding in hemophilia may occur spontaneously or because of an injury. Inform your patient and his family about possible types of bleeding and their signs and symptoms. Accordingly, advise them when to call for medical help.

BLEEDING SITE	SIGNS AND SYMPTOMS	TEACHING POINTS
Intracranial	Change in personality or wakefulness (level of consciousness), headache, nausea	Instruct the patient or his family to notify the doctor immediately and to treat symptoms as an emergency.
Joints (affects the knees, followed by elbows, ankles, shoulders, hips, and wrists)	(Joint pain and swelling, joint tingling and warmth (at onset of hemorrhage)	Tell the patient to begin antihemophilic factor (AHF) infusions and then to notify the doctor.
Muscles	Pain and reduced function of affected muscle; tingling, numbness, or pain in a large area away from the affected site (referred pain)	Urge the patient to notify the doctor. An AHF infusion might be started if the patient is reasonably certain that bleeding results from recent injury.
Subcutaneous tissue or skin	Pain, bruising, and swelling at the site (delayed oozing also may occur after an injury)	Show the patient how to apply appropriate topical agents, such as ice packs or absorbable gelatin sponges (Gelfoam), to stop bleeding.
Kidney	Pain in the lower back near the waist, decreased urine output	Notify the doctor. An AHF infusion might be started if bleeding results from a known recent injury.
Heart (cardiac tamponade)	Chest tightness, shortness of breath, swelling (usually occurs in hemophiliacs who are very young or who have severe disease)	Instruct the patient to contact the doctor or go to the nearest emergency department at once.

ing disorder are bleeding time, platelet count, coagulation screenings, and clotting factor assays. Once test findings confirm the diagnosis, regularly required tests include specific clotting factor assays and an occasional inhibitor screen, all of which can be done with one blood sample. Describe the bleeding time test. (See *Teaching patients about immune and hematologic tests*, pages 285 and 286.)

TREATMENTS

Inform the patient that he may go

for years without requiring treatment, depending on the severity of the disorder. Emphasize, however, that he must always act cautiously to prevent injury and, when necessary, receive I.V. clotting factors promptly.

Activity guidelines
Tell your patient to get regular, moderate exercise. Explain that strong muscles protect the joints. These, in turn, can guard against bleeding into the joints. Add that isometric exercises that strengthen surrounding muscles can help prevent muscle weakness and recurrent joint bleeding. For example, quadriceps (thigh) exercises may be done after bleeding into the knee joint.

Urge the patient, though, to avoid sports such as football, lacrosse, and boxing, which obviously increase the risk of serious bleeding. Stress that all hemophiliacs — even those with mild hemophilia — must avoid rough contact sports or activities that increase the risk of bleeding within the skull. Tell patients with chronic joint disease to avoid such sports as soccer, basketball, skiing, aerobic exercises, and ice hockey because they stress the joints and carry a high risk for joint injury.

Besides avoiding certain sports, caution the patient to refrain from activities that increase his risk for injury and prolonged bleeding. These include heavy lifting and carrying and using potentially harmful equipment such as power tools.

Alternatively, encourage the patient to take up swimming, hiking, or bicycling. If the patient is a child, review appropriate safety precautions with his parents. For example, the child may require supervision and protective apparel, such as a helmet, elbow and knee pads, and leg guards, to prevent injury.

Medications
Inform your patient or his family that the primary treatment for hemophilia is I.V. administration of the missing clotting factor. Which replacement factor or other preparation

Clotting factor replacement products

Some of the products available for clotting factor replacement include:
● cryoprecipitate, a frozen human plasma product containing mostly factor VII
● prothrombin complex concentrate, which contains factors II, VII, IX, and X
● purified factor VIII
● fresh frozen human plasma, which contains factors VIII and IX
● anti-inhibitor coagulant complex, derived from the plasma of people with factor VIII inhibitor
● factor IX.

These products are purified to minimize the risk of passing on communicable diseases, such as hepatitis and human immunodeficiency virus. Some are heated under high pressure; others are treated with substances called *monoclonal antibodies*. Consequently, the risk of disease transmission is minimal.

the patient receives depends on the type and severity of his hemophilia. He may need repeated infusions because clotting factors have a short half-life. (See *Clotting factor replacement products.*)

Patients with mild hemophilia and those undergoing minor surgical procedures such as tooth extraction may receive desmopressin (DDAVP). This drug stimulates the release of stored factor VIII in the body and can temporarily raise factor VIII levels high enough to control minor bleeding.

Procedures
Teach the patient or his parents how to give a clotting factor infusion, how to care for veins, how to mix the infusion and calculate the dosage, and how to keep accurate records.

Explain possible complications, such as blood-borne infection and factor inhibitor development related to replacement factor procedures.

Administering home infusions

Most parents learn to administer clotting factors to their hemophilic child by the time he enters school. To qualify for home infusion, the child must have reasonably accessible veins and must be able to remain still.

Hemophilic children usually learn to perform self-infusion between ages 8 and 12. Reinforce the doctor's or nurse's instructions on performing the technique.

Protecting veins

Because of the need for lifelong therapy, emphasize that the patient must take steps to preserve his veins. Instruct him not to apply pressure to the puncture site until after he removes the needle. Warn him that putting pressure on the needle as it's withdrawn will damage the vein. After removing the needle, though, he must apply firm pressure with one finger for 3 to 5 minutes. Tell him to keep his arm straight, not bent.

Also instruct him to remind health care professionals to use stainless steel butterfly needles whenever possible and to remove them after each infusion. The reason: Plastic inside-the-needle catheters may inflame and scar the vein, especially if they're left in place for several days. Also, a new venipuncture should be performed for each infusion, except when continuous I.V. fluids or antibiotics are needed, or in patients for whom venipuncture is especially difficult, such as young children.

Keeping infusion records

Advise the patient and his family to keep accurate treatment records. For example, tell them to write down the problem that required an infusion treatment, the nature of the treatment, and the treatment outcome. Tell them to send or take this information to the hemophilia treatment center at least once a month.

For minor bleeding episodes, explain that most hemophiliacs are taught to first infuse the clotting factor concentrate and then record the treatment. For major bleeding episodes, tell the patient to first infuse the clotting factor concentrate, then call the doctor or hemophilia treatment center for further instructions. Also instruct him to record the facts about the bleeding episode.

Reviewing possible complications

Emphasize that self-infusion may be complicated by infection. Hepatitis, for example, may be transmitted through blood products. Urge the patient to be immunized against hepatitis B. (No vaccines exist for hepatitis C or D.)

 WARNING: To prevent spreading blood-borne communicable diseases (such as hepatitis) to family members and others, tell the patient to dispose of all needles, syringes, and blood-contaminated waste in a hard plastic or cardboard container and return the container to the hospital or hemophilia treatment center for disposal. Advise him to place larger wastes contaminated with blood in an impermeable plastic bag and return this package as well.

The patient may be concerned about the risk of contracting AIDS through blood products. Explain that all donated blood and plasma is screened for antibodies to human immunodeficiency virus (HIV), the virus that causes AIDS. Also, all freeze-dried blood products are now routinely heat-treated to kill HIV. Because of these precautions, it's highly unlikely that he'll contract AIDS through blood products.

Of course, a hemophiliac who received clotting factor concentrate before these products were heat-treated may already be infected with HIV. This is also true of a patient who received cryoprecipitate and plasma before blood donors were screened carefully. This patient needs your reassurance. If appropriate, consult a hemophilia treatment center for follow-up information and counseling.

Between 10% and 20% of people with severe hemophilia will develop inhibitors. This means that their body produces an abnormal factor VIII or IX that recognizes the normal (infused) factors as foreign proteins. In response, the body produces antibodies, called *inhibitors,* against normal factors VIII and IX. The antibodies destroy the normal clotting factor as quickly as it's infused.

Because of this risk, advise the patient to call his doctor if home infusions don't seem to be controlling bleeding episodes. Factor inhibitor levels can be measured to diagnose this condition. If it's confirmed, the patient may be treated with anti-inhibitor coagulant complex.

Additional occasional treatment with DDAVP or aminocaproic acid (Amicar) may help. Explain that the severity of this condition commonly depends on the severity of hemophilia.

Other care measures

Taking measures to avoid bleeding, learning first-aid techniques, and observing general precautions can help your patient cope with hemophilia.

For the child with hemophilia, keep in mind that emotional problems can be as disabling as physical ones. Remind parents that being overprotective and permissive — even withdrawing from the child — are typical parental responses to hemophilia. Unfortunately, these responses may cause serious social or emotional problems in the child.

Observing general precautions

Tell the patient to wear medical identification, such as a necklace or bracelet, to ensure that he receives clotting factor infusions as soon as possible after a major accident or loss of consciousness.

Preventive dental care is especially important for someone with hemophilia. Make sure he understands that he can have cavities filled and teeth extracted, but he'll need clotting factor infusions before some of these procedures. Emphasize that poor

dental hygiene can lead to bleeding from inflamed gums.

Because of the patient's extensive home care needs, the doctor or nurse usually refers the patient to the nearest comprehensive hemophilia center for evaluation and follow-up teaching. Encourage interested family members to go, too. Explain that these centers typically offer carrier testing, prenatal diagnosis, and other genetic counseling services.

Finally, provide the names of organizations that can offer the patient and his family further information and support. (See Appendix 2.)

Iron deficiency anemia

For patients with iron deficiency anemia, you'll need to focus on promoting compliance with therapy. Affecting 10% to 30% of adults in North America, iron deficiency anemia is most common in premenopausal women, premature and low-birth-weight infants, children, and adolescent girls. Because the disorder is so common, many patients consider it trivial and fail to comply with treatment. As a result, you'll need to convince patients that iron deficiency can lead to severe problems.

Begin by explaining the disorder and its characteristic signs and symptoms. Point out the complications if anemia goes untreated, and explain laboratory tests to diagnose the disorder. Finally, discuss the treatment regimen, including an iron-rich diet, iron supplements, and adequate rest and follow-up care.

Before teaching the patient with iron deficiency anemia, make sure you are familiar with the following topics:
• explanation of iron deficiency anemia, including the role of red blood cells (RBCs) and iron
• signs and symptoms of iron deficiency anemia
• causes and age-related risk factors
• diagnostic blood studies
• role of diet in treatment, including

ways to stimulate the appetite and how to choose iron-rich foods
• iron supplements
• importance of continuing care, obtaining adequate rest, and treating infections promptly
• sources of information and support.

ABOUT THE DISORDER

Inform the patient that the body's iron reserves can be rapidly depleted when its demand for iron isn't met. Discuss the role of RBCs. Explain how body tissues become starved for oxygen (hypoxia) when iron deficiency impairs the body's oxygen-transporting capacity.

Point out that signs and symptoms of iron deficiency anemia usually don't develop until the problem is severe, so the patient may postpone seeking medical attention. Classic advanced signs and symptoms include dyspnea with exertion, fatigue, listlessness, pallor, inability to concentrate, irritability, headache, frequent infections, and tachycardia. A cardinal sign is pica, the desire to eat nonfood substances such as dirt or ice. Other key signs of long-standing iron deficiency include brittle, spoon-shaped nails, cracks in the corners of the mouth, smooth tongue, dysphagia, vasomotor disturbances, numbness and tingling of the hands and feet, and neuralgic pain.

Tailor your teaching about iron deficiency anemia to the patient's age. If the patient is an infant, tell the parents that natural iron stores are depleted by age 4 to 6 months, so an infant given prolonged, unsupplemented breast-feedings or bottle feedings (especially of cow's milk) typically has iron deficiency anemia.

Tell the teenager and her parents that a rapid growth period such as adolescence increases the body's need for iron. If the body must draw on unreplenished iron stores, anemia results. If your patient is a woman, explain that she may have iron deficiency from blood loss during menstruation, especially if her iron stores are already low. Tell a pregnant patient that much of her body's iron supply is diverted to the fetus for RBC formation.

Mention that iron deficiency anemia also may result from chronic diarrhea, gastrectomy, celiac disease and other iron malabsorption disorders, erythrocyte trauma caused by heart valve replacement, and blood loss from traumatic injury, GI bleeding, cancer, or varices.

Complications

Stress that failure to comply with therapy can lead to a chronic lack of oxygen, possibly producing persistent fatigue and dyspnea, increased susceptibility to infection, and other advanced symptoms of iron deficiency. The body tries to compensate for oxygen deprivation by increasing both heart rate and cardiac output, resulting in tachycardia.

DIAGNOSTIC WORKUP

Explain that the doctor will order blood tests to diagnose iron deficiency anemia and to determine its severity. Routine tests to measure iron levels include serum iron, total iron-binding capacity, and ferritin analyses. A complete blood count may be ordered to evaluate hemoglobin levels and detect morphologic changes in RBCs. Add that blood tests may be repeated to monitor the patient's progress through treatment.

TREATMENTS

Inform the patient that iron deficiency anemia typically improves with iron supplementation and an iron-rich diet. Instruct the patient to get adequate rest, treat infections promptly, and keep all follow-up medical appointments. If her disorder is particularly severe, she may need blood transfusions.

Dietary modifications

Inform the patient that diet alone can't cure iron deficiency anemia but that it does play a leading role in therapy. Discuss which foods contain the most iron, and encourage her to include them in her daily diet. (See *Choosing iron-rich foods*.) Explore the

Choosing iron-rich foods

To help your patient choose iron-rich foods, tell her that although many everyday foods contain large amounts of iron, the body typically absorbs only a small portion of it. For this reason, she needs to choose foods that contain lots of iron.

Which foods should she choose? First of all, advise her to pick foods from all of the four major groups — milk and dairy, meat, bread and cereal, and fruit and vegetable. Then tell her to modify the amount from each group by considering her other dietary needs. For instance, if she needs to cut back on cholesterol, she shouldn't choose liver.

Selecting wisely

Explain that the iron in grains and vegetables isn't absorbed as readily as the iron in meat, fish, and poultry.

On the other hand, eating meat, fish, or poultry *along with* grains and vegetables increases iron absorption. So does eating a food that contains vitamin C, such as an orange, a tomato, or a potato. In fact, eating a tomato with a hamburger quadruples iron absorption. (On the other hand, drinking tea with the same meal lowers iron absorption.)

Iron requirements

Tell your patient that the recommended amounts of dietary iron are 18 mg/day for women age 50 and under and 10 mg/day for men and women over age 50. The doctor will tell her exactly how much iron she should consume.

Advise the patient to consult the following table to find the foods highest in iron.

FOOD	QUANTITY	IRON (MG)
Oysters	3 ounces	13.2
Beef liver	3 ounces	7.5
Prune juice	½ cup	5.2
Clams	2 ounces	4.2
Walnuts	½ cup	3.7
Ground beef	3 ounces	3.0
Chickpeas	½ cup	3.0
Bran flakes	½ cup	2.8
Pork roast	3 ounces	2.7
Cashews	½ cup	2.6
Shrimp	3 ounces	2.6
Raisins	½ cup	2.5
Navy beans	½ cup	2.5

(continued)

Choosing iron-rich foods *(continued)*

FOOD	QUANTITY	IRON (MG)
Sardines	3 ounces	2.5
Spinach	½ cup	2.4
Lima beans	½ cup	2.3
Kidney beans	½ cup	2.2
Turkey, dark meat	3 ounces	2.0
Prunes	½ cup	1.9
Roast beef	3 ounces	1.8
Green peas	½ cup	1.5
Peanuts	½ cup	1.5
Potato	1	1.1
Sweet potato	½ cup	1.0
Green beans	½ cup	1.0
Egg	1	1.0
Turkey, light meat	3 ounces	1.0

patient's eating habits. Does she have a poor appetite? This may contribute to the disorder.

Medications

Explain that the doctor may prescribe iron supplements to replenish the patient's iron supply. These supplements are usually taken orally and are the safest, most effective, and least expensive treatment. However, they may be given parenterally if the patient doesn't take oral supplements as prescribed or if they trigger an adverse reaction, such as nausea or constipation.

 TIPS AND TIMESAVERS: Inform the patient that although she'll need a prescription for

some supplements, she can obtain others over the counter. Teach her how to take the iron supplement her doctor prescribes, and point out possible adverse effects.

Other care measures

Encourage the patient to keep follow-up appointments with the doctor and to continue the prescribed therapy even after her condition improves. Explain that once her hemoglobin levels return to normal, she'll probably need to continue therapy for at least 2 more months to replenish the body's depleted iron reserves. Caution her also that iron deficiency may recur.

Advise the patient to pace her activities to include frequent rest periods. If shortness of breath, weakness, light-headedness, or palpitations develop during the day, suggest changing positions or moving about slowly to minimize dizziness and other symptoms.

If the patient is a child, promote health maintenance through immunizations and prompt treatment of infections.

Explain to the patient with severe iron deficiency anemia that she may need transfusions of packed RBCs. This treatment increases circulating hemoglobin levels and improves tissue oxygenation. Supplied by I.V. infusion, a packed RBC transfusion may take up to 2 hours to complete.

Rheumatoid arthritis

Afflicted with an insidious, chronic, and painful inflammatory disorder, the patient with rheumatoid arthritis (RA) can easily become discouraged. However, you can help him overcome this feeling by pointing out that effective treatments for inflammation and joint pain do exist. Discovering what best meets his individual needs may take time, though. Consequently, you'll need to motivate the patient to experiment with self-care measures and assistive devices.

Your teaching should include an explanation of how the disease occurs. You'll also want to teach the patient about blood and synovial fluid tests and X-rays. What's more, you'll need to point out the significance of medication, diet, and a balanced program of exercise and rest. In severe RA, you may need to discuss surgery.

Before teaching the patient with RA, make sure you are familiar with the following topics:
• description of RA
• explanation of its suspected cause
• importance of complying with treatment to prevent complications
• blood tests and, if ordered, synovial fluid analysis
• use of salicylates or other medication such as nonsteroidal anti-inflammatory drugs (NSAIDs)
• balanced program of rest and activity, with tips for improving quality of sleep
• exercise program
• dietary considerations, including devices to ease meal preparation
• surgical options, when appropriate
• use of good body mechanics and assistive devices
• application of heat or cold
• discussion of sexual activity and alternative treatments
• sources of information and support.

ABOUT THE DISORDER

Early on, the patient with RA may experience pain, tenderness, swelling, or stiffness in the synovial joints (the shoulder, elbow, wrist, hand, hip, knee, and foot). Explain that he has a chronic, systemic inflammatory disorder. The course of the disorder is difficult to predict; it may progress slowly or rapidly, with exacerbations and remissions.

Tell the patient that the cause of RA is unknown, but that researchers suspect that it involves an autoimmune response within the joint. (See *What happens in rheumatoid arthritis*, page 270.)

Tell the patient that these autoimmune responses lead to inflammation and pannus — thickening of the synovial membranes. Inflammation may spread to the cartilage, tendons, ligaments and, eventually, bone. The patient may suffer joint deformities, subluxations, contractures, pain, and loss of function.

Complications

Warn the patient that improperly treated RA can lead to excruciating joint pain. If he fails to follow his drug regimen, irreversible joint damage and severe deformities may occur. If he doesn't follow his prescribed exercise program, muscle strength and joint mobility may be reduced. Weakness in hip flexor and quadriceps muscles can also lead to gait problems, demanding extra energy

INSIGHT INTO ILLNESSES

What happens in rheumatoid arthritis

To help your patient understand what causes the pain and swelling of rheumatoid arthritis (RA), begin by describing the structure of a normal joint. Show him the location of the synovium on this illustration. Explain that synovium is the inner layer of an articular capsule that surrounds a freely movable joint and secretes the thick fluid that normally lubricates the joint.

Next, describe how RA is characterized by an autoimmune response. Synovial lymphocytes (B cells) produce immunoglobulin G (IgG), which acts as an antigen. This stimulates an immune response within the joint, with the production of anti-IgG antibodies (rheumatoid factors), leading to the formation of immune complexes.

Explain that the immune complexes activate the classic and alternative complement systems. This activation initiates the inflammatory response, which results in progressive enlargement and thickening of the synovium and damage to cartilage and bone.

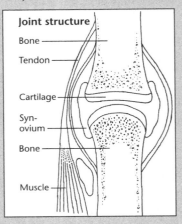

Joint structure

Bone

Tendon

Cartilage

Synovium

Bone

Muscle

and placing further stress on other joints.

DIAGNOSTIC WORKUP

Teach the patient about three blood tests: rheumatoid factor (RF), erythrocyte sedimentation rate (ESR), and complete blood count (CBC). Tell him that each requires a small blood sample.

The RF test, which detects anti–immunoglobulin G antibodies, is positive in about 80% of RA patients. The ESR may detect inflammation. The CBC can be used to detect anemia, a frequent finding in RA. No single blood test provides a conclusive diagnosis.

Also teach the patient about synovial fluid analysis, which can help determine the cause of joint inflammation and swelling. (See *Teaching patients about immune and hematologic tests,* pages 285 and 286.)

Because X-rays of affected joints are used to help assess damage, tell the patient that he may undergo repeat X-rays at varying intervals to monitor bone erosion and joint deformity.

TREATMENTS

Your goal is to impart the knowledge and skills needed to effectively manage a chronic illness. Emphasize that the patient's well-being depends on his willingness to comply with the treatment regimen and thereby prevent worsening pain and deformity.

Activity guidelines

Highlight the importance of balancing activity with rest. Recommend sleeping 8 to 10 hours a night and lying down for ½ hour twice each day. If the patient experiences a flare-up, advise him to simplify his schedule. Tell him that it's appropriate to ask for help with daily tasks.

Counsel the patient who can't sleep well because of pain. Tell him to maintain correct body position during rest, with joints extended rather than flexed. Advise using a firm mattress (supported by a bed board) and a small, flat pillow. If splints are prescribed, tell the patient to wear them in bed and whenever possible during the day. Caution against placing a pillow under his knees, which fosters joint deformity. Impress on the patient the importance of using good body mechanics at all times.

Encourage the patient to pace himself and to set realistic goals for activities. How can he know when it's time to slow down? He may experience increased pain or fatigue and progressive loss of dexterity in involved joints. If pain lasts for 2 hours or more after completing a task, the patient should do a little less the next time or find ways to simplify his effort. Provide appropriate suggestions to help the patient conserve his energy. (See *Energy-saving tips*.)

Exercise

Explain that exercise can make flexing and extending joints easier, reduce pain and stiffness, and help prevent loss of joint function. It may even help the patient regain joint function.

Recommend an exercise program as part of the patient's daily routine. Remind him to consult with his doctor or therapist before beginning. Underscore the importance of staying within reasonable limits; an exercise program shouldn't be too difficult in light of his condition.

 WARNING: Caution the patient against performing strenuous exercise during acute inflammatory episodes.

If the patient experiences muscle cramping or pain while exercising, advise him to stop exercising and gently massage the cramped muscle. When symptoms diminish, he can resume activity. Encourage him to take advan-

> # Energy-saving tips
>
> The patient with rheumatoid arthritis needs to conserve his energy. Suggest that he:
> - use dressing aids, including a long-handled shoehorn, a reacher, elastic shoelaces, a zipper pull, and a buttonhook
> - wear mittens if he has trouble putting his fingers into gloves
> - use helpful household items, such as a handheld shower nozzle, hand rails, grab bars, and easy-to-open drawers
> - keep needed materials, utensils, and tools organized and handy
> - when possible, sit down while performing activities that may tire him, such as dressing or cooking, to prevent stress on weight-bearing joints.

tage of moments when he has the least pain and stiffness and the most energy and when his medication achieves its peak.

Discuss the significance of therapeutic and recreational exercise. Therapeutic exercises are prescribed by a doctor or physical or occupational therapist to meet the patient's individual needs with maximum efficiency. A therapeutic program may include range-of-motion exercises to improve joint mobility and flexibility and strengthening exercises.

Recreational exercises, such as group exercises, sports, games, crafts, and hobbies, can help maintain or improve strength, joint mobility, and endurance. However, they cannot substitute for a therapeutic exercise program. A local Arthritis Foundation chapter may be able to recommend a group exercise program adapted for people with arthritis.

Dietary modifications

Explain the importance of a balanced diet. Foods high in vitamins, proteins, and iron promote tissue building and repair. Make sure the patient knows how to select foods from the four basic food groups to meet daily requirements. Advise frequent, small meals if his appetite is poor.

 TIPS AND TIMESAVERS: Teach techniques for making meal preparation easier. Tell the patient to plan breaks between cooking chores. When symptoms become severe, suggest eating convenience foods. Also promote the use of assistive devices and appliances for meal preparation and eating.

Medications

Help the patient understand that the goal of drug therapy is to control inflammation and pain and arrest the progress of RA. Achieving this may require several types of drugs:
• *Anti-inflammatory drugs* reduce inflammation, thereby diminishing pain. NSAIDs work by blocking prostaglandin synthesis. (Prostaglandins precipitate the inflammatory response, which includes edema, pain, warmth, and redness at the site of tissue injury.)
• *Corticosteroids* inhibit the immune response by suppressing or preventing cell-mediated immune reactions.
• *Disease-modifying agents,* such as gold compounds and antimalarials, slow the disease process.
• *Immunosuppressants,* such as azathioprine, methotrexate, and cyclophosphamide, inhibit the autoimmune response seen in RA. Because immunosuppressant therapy heightens the risk of severe infection, teach the patient infection control measures.

To help the patient remember his medication schedule, assist him in devising a medication calendar. Urge him to notify the doctor if symptoms worsen during therapy. If he has weak or deformed hands or if moving them hurts, suggest that he ask his pharmacist not to use childproof caps.

Surgery

Joint surgery may relieve pain, increase mobility, and improve appearance. Describe relevant surgical procedures, which may include:

• synovectomy — removal of the synovium to reduce pain and swelling
• osteotomy — cutting and resetting a bone to correct a deformity
• resection — removal of a bone or part of a bone, commonly performed on the feet to increase comfort when walking
• arthrodesis — bone fusion to diminish pain
• arthroplasty — repairing or replacing joints to reduce pain and increase flexibility and mobility.

Urge the patient to comply with his prescribed postsurgical regimen. Physical therapy constitutes a key part of this regimen. Tell him that he'll experience muscle — not joint — pain early on during therapy. Assure him that this will decrease with time. Depending on the type of surgery, he may require several months of therapy.

Other care measures
Coping with RA can be made easier by learning about proper clothing and heat and cold therapy.

Appropriate clothing
Because cold drafts can cause muscle tension, advise the patient to wear warm clothing. Foot pain may be relieved by inserting special pads or metatarsal bars in his shoes. A severe foot deformity may call for custom-made shoes.

Heat and cold therapy
Advise the patient that applying heat and cold locally may relieve pain and inflammation. Applying heat before exercising will also relieve stiffness. Encourage him to experiment to determine what works best for him.

Tell the patient that he doesn't need to purchase costly devices for applying heat or cold; home methods usually prove effective. For moist heat, suggest that he stand in a warm shower, soak in a tub, or apply warm wet towels to stiff or painful joints. Explain that mild heat will produce results; it should feel soothing, not hot. For dry heat, recommend wrapping a heating pad in a towel before placing it against the skin.

If the patient has diminished sensation, tell him never to set the heating pad on the highest setting, and tell him to check often for burns. Advise him to use heat for about 20 minutes to achieve full benefit.

For cold application, suggest using moist towels or ice packs for 10 to 15 minutes. To make an ice pack, the patient can fill a plastic bag with crushed ice.

The patient may also benefit from using a combination of heat and cold. Instruct him to first soak his hands or feet in warm water (110° F [43.3° C]) for about 3 minutes and then soak them in cold water (65° F [18.3° C]) for about a minute. He should repeat this process three times, ending with warm water.

Special patient concerns
Because arthritis changes the way the patient looks and moves, he may need reassurance that he can still enjoy a satisfying sexual relationship.

Advise the woman of childbearing age with RA to let her doctor know if she plans to become pregnant. He may adjust her medication dosage.

To help the patient cope with RA, refer him to an organization that can offer further information and support. (See Appendix 2.)

Alternative treatments
Make it clear that RA has no miracle cures, despite claims to the contrary. Encourage the patient to notify you, his doctor, or the local chapter of the Arthritis Foundation *before* trying any alternative treatment.

Sickle cell syndrome
Sickle cell syndrome includes sickle cell anemia (SCA) and sickle cell trait, among other disorders. SCA is a chronic and incurable inherited blood disease, which occurs mostly in blacks and sometimes in persons from Mediterranean cultures. Shrouded by myth and misinformation, this painful disease calls for sensitive teaching. Because patients and families typically experience fear and anxiety, your

teaching will focus on relieving apprehension and discomfort, preventing sickle cell crises, avoiding complications, and understanding hereditary transmission.

Because the patient with SCA usually has periodic crises, he may be discouraged and depressed, which can delay learning. You may need to help him express his feelings before implementing your teaching plan. Also, because SCA is a chronic disease, you'll need to determine how much the patient already knows before you start teaching. If he's been hospitalized before, point out that there's always more to learn about his conditions. And the more he learns, the better prepared he'll be to guard against complications.

Before teaching your patient with sickle cell syndrome, make sure you are familiar with the following topics:
• explanation of SCA, sickle cell trait, and inheritance patterns
• complications of SCA — especially those requiring immediate medical attention such as vaso-occlusive crisis
• precipitating factors for vaso-occlusive crisis
• blood tests and other diagnostic procedures
• principles of good nutrition, especially adequate intake of fluids and foods containing folic acid
• infection prevention measures, including immunizations and prophylaxis
• home care for vaso-occlusive crisis
• special care measures, including genetic counseling and precautions related to surgery and pregnancy
• sources of information and support.

ABOUT THE DISORDER
Explain that SCA results from an inherited mutation in hemoglobin, the blood component that carries oxygen to body tissues. Red blood cells (RBCs) containing this substance (hemoglobin S) have normal oxygen capacity but become abnormally rigid, rough, and elongated (sickle-shaped) when they lose oxygen. In contrast, normal RBCs, which carry normal hemoglobin A, are disklike and pliable.

INSIGHT INTO ILLNESSES

The sickle cell cycle: A closer look

Use these illustrations to show the patient the difference between normal and sickled red blood cells (RBCs) and to illustrate how sickle cell anemia (SCA) threatens his health.

Normal RBCs
Point out that normal RBCs look like disks with an indented center. Their round shape and pliability ease their circulation through the blood vessels.

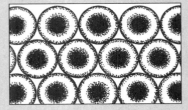

Sickle-shaped RBCs
RBCs that contain hemoglobin S, the genetic defect responsible for SCA, can become sickle- or crescent-shaped when they deliver oxygen. As these cells circulate, their shape causes them to tangle, trapping one another and jamming the blood vessels.

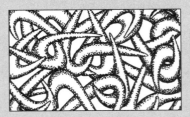

Consequently, oxygen isn't delivered to body tissues and ischemia results. This sets up a risky situation: Clogged vessels lead to capillary blood backups. Then hypoxia increases, and more RBCs are needed to meet increased oxygen needs. As more RBCs lose oxygen, more sickling occurs, and a dangerous cycle begins. Without interruption, the "sickle cycle" can be life-threatening.

Inform the patient that sickling typically occurs with activities or conditions that increase the body's need for oxygen, such as running at high altitudes. Inform him, too, that as sickle cells increase, they tend to clump together, obstructing circulation and depriving tissues of oxygen. (See *The sickle cell cycle: A closer look.*) Warn him that without intervention, tiny obstructions can become large infarctions. Explain that heavy concentrations of sickled cells can thicken the blood and slow circulation. Dehydration — from vomiting, diarrhea, excessive sweating, or diuretic use — causes the blood to thicken and makes the condition worse.

Reassure the patient that reoxy-genation usually returns most sickled cells to a normal, round shape, but some cells may remain permanently deformed. That's when chronic anemia occurs, because deformed RBCs survive for only 15 to 20 days. (Normally formed RBCs survive and function for about 120 days.)

Include an explanation of inheritance patterns and the sickle cell trait as you discuss SCA and the risk of passing on the disorder to children. Explain that persons with sickle cell trait can pass on the gene that causes SCA, but they don't have the disease itself.

Complications
Urge the patient to comply with pre-

scribed therapy. Emphasize that he's susceptible to serious infection, especially meningitis, pneumonia, and sepsis. One reason for this is the spleen's inability to function properly, which limits the body's defenses. Inform the patient that serious infection can start suddenly and quickly worsen. Although young children are at greater risk, SCA patients of any age can incur serious infection.

Besides risking infection, the patient also risks vaso-occlusive crisis. The most common complication of SCA, this painful condition can result from infection, dehydration, and excessive fatigue.

DIAGNOSTIC WORKUP
Tell the patient and his family that blood tests — notably hemoglobin electrophoresis — can confirm the SCA diagnosis. If SCA is confirmed, all family members should be tested.

Describe other tests as needed, such as routine blood counts, blood chemistry profiles, and urinalysis to detect early organ damage. Complications may call for additional blood tests and possibly X-rays. Tell the patient that the doctor may order a lateral chest X-ray to detect the "Lincoln log deformity." This spinal abnormality develops in many adults and some adolescents with SCA, leaving the vertebrae resembling logs that form the corner of a cabin.

Explain that another simple diagnostic tool is an ophthalmoscopic examination to detect corkscrew- or comma-shaped vessels in the conjunctivae, another possible sign of SCA.

TREATMENTS
Although SCA can't be cured, treatments can alleviate symptoms and prevent painful crises. Urge the patient to modify his activities and to adopt eating habits that ensure adequate dietary folic acid. Discuss such infection prevention measures as routine immunizations. Highlight the signs and symptoms of vaso-occlusive crisis and home care measures.

Activity guidelines
Inform the patient that he can participate in physical activities that promote health and fitness, such as gym classes, as long as he rests frequently, increases his fluid intake, and doesn't overdo it. Emphasize that fatigue can contribute to vaso-occlusive crisis.

 WARNING: Caution the patient with splenomegaly to avoid contact sports to minimize the risk of a ruptured spleen.

Dietary modifications
Adequate nutrition is essential for patients with SCA. Because folic acid deficiency exacerbates anemia and may lead to bone marrow depression from increased demands to replace RBCs, urge the patient to add folic acid–rich foods (leafy, green vegetables) to his diet. Also, remind him to avoid consuming alcohol and smoking cigarettes.

To maintain adequate hydration and minimize RBC sickling, suggest that parents offer a child with SCA more fluids, such as eggnog, ice pops, and milk shakes.

Medications
Although drugs can't cure SCA, certain vaccines, anti-infectives, and chelating agents can minimize complications resulting from SCA or from possible transfusion therapy. Other medications such as analgesics may help relieve the pain of vaso-occlusive crisis.

Emphasize infection prevention measures, especially for a child with SCA. Tell parents that immunization against childhood diseases is a must, as is strict adherence to a prescribed medication regimen when an infection develops.

Vaccines
Discuss the advantages of polyvalent pneumococcal vaccine, which the child may receive at age 6 months and again at age 2 years, with booster vaccines every 4 years. Mention the *Haemophilus influenzae* B vaccine as another immunization to consider.

Explain that the child usually receives this vaccine at age 15 months.

Anti-infective drugs
Review prophylactic anti-infective therapy. Low-dose oral penicillin given twice daily until age 6 may reduce the child's risk for pneumococcal infections. After age 6, this preventive measure may not be needed. Although parents must understand the importance of complying with these measures, they should also realize that prophylaxis isn't foolproof. They'll still have to watch for early signs and symptoms of infection. Typically, appropriate antibiotic therapy is prescribed to treat infections. Warn parents that the child may need to be hospitalized for antibiotic therapy.

Chelating agent
If a patient with SCA receives regular transfusions, he may require deferoxamine (Desferal), a chelating agent. This medication helps to remove dangerous iron deposits caused by repeated transfusions. The patient can take the drug at home, but he or his parents will need detailed instructions on how to mix and administer it.

Instruct the patient or his parents to contact the doctor as soon as possible if the following adverse reactions occur: dyspnea, hearing or visual impairment, pain at the injection site, or skin rash. Explain that the drug may color urine orange red.

Analgesics
The patient with SCA may need medication to relieve pain, especially that related to vaso-occlusive crisis. Recommend acetaminophen. Or, if the doctor prescribes a narcotic analgesic, tell the patient to follow his instructions and to report persistent pain.

Other care measures
Because sickle cell disorders affect not only the patient, but also those closest to him, make sure to provide guidelines for giving crisis care, maintaining emotional and physical support, and obtaining genetic and psychological counseling as needed.

Crisis care
Review the signs and symptoms of vaso-occlusive crisis so that the patient or his parents will recognize and treat it early. As appropriate, explain how to care for this condition at home.

Inform parents that an infant's first vaso-occlusive crisis may be called the "hand-foot crisis" because the infant's hands or feet, or both, swell and become painful. Advise them to begin home treatment measures but to call the doctor if symptoms persist or worsen.

If the patient must be hospitalized for a vaso-occlusive crisis, explain that I.V. fluids and parenteral analgesics may be given. Sometimes the patient also may receive oxygen and blood transfusions.

Review signs and symptoms that warrant immediate medical attention. For example, instruct parents of young children (ages 8 to 24 months) to report signs of acute sequestration crisis. Without treatment, this sudden massive entrapment of RBCs in the spleen and liver can lead to hypovolemic shock and death. Stress that this crisis, though rare, is a medical emergency.

Other symptoms requiring urgent care include a temperature over 101° F (38.3° C), stiff neck, difficulty speaking or walking, numbness, weakness or in infants, priapism.

Emotional support
Because delayed growth and late puberty are common among SCA patients, reassure adolescent patients that they will grow and mature. Tell them they should catch up with their friends by age 17 or 18.

General health promotion
Forewarn parents that urinary frequency may prevail and that bedwetting may begin around age 6. Explain that this results not from disobedience or behavior problems but from the SCA patient's inability to concentrate urine.

Encourage parents to schedule their child for a yearly eye examination to detect and treat retinal damage resulting from SCA. Stress meticulous leg and foot care because leg ulcers commonly develop during the late teens.

Promote normal intellectual and social development by cautioning parents against overprotectiveness. Although the SCA patient must avoid strenuous exercise, he can safely enjoy most everyday activities.

Counseling

Refer parents of children with SCA for genetic counseling to answer their questions about SCA in future children. Recommend screening for other family members to determine whether they're SCA carriers.

Besides genetic counseling, parents may benefit from psychological counseling to help them cope with possible feelings of guilt. Recommend an appropriate support group.

Special situations

Discuss how special conditions, such as surgery or pregnancy, may affect SCA patients. Urge the patient to make sure all health care providers know that he has SCA before he undergoes any treatment, especially major surgery. That's because during any procedure that requires general anesthesia, the patient with SCA will need adequate ventilation to prevent hypoxic crisis. Also urge the patient to wear medical identification stating that he has SCA.

Inform women that SCA makes pregnancy hazardous. Also hazardous is use of oral contraceptives. If appropriate, refer female patients to a gynecologist for counseling. However, if the patient *does* become pregnant, offer guidelines for maintaining a balanced diet and advise her to ask her doctor about taking a folic acid supplement.

Recognize that, in men with SCA, sudden, painful bouts of priapism may develop. Reassure the patient that these common episodes have no permanent, harmful effects.

Finally, because SCA affects all body systems and many aspects of a patient's lifestyle, it requires multidisciplinary care involving hematologists, nurses, social workers, and other therapists. Encourage the patient to take full advantage of these and other available resources. (See Appendix 2.)

Systemic lupus erythematosus

A chronic inflammatory disorder, systemic lupus erythematosus (SLE) poses difficult but not insurmountable teaching problems. The disorder's chronic nature, its periodic flare-ups, and its unpredictable remissions can interfere with learning and hinder compliance. When the patient experiences a long remission, for instance, she may lose her motivation to comply with therapy. Alternatively, she may meticulously comply with it but become discouraged when flare-ups persist. Before your teaching can succeed, you'll have to help her accept the reality of lifelong treatment and periodic flare-ups.

During the early stages of SLE, you'll need to prepare the patient for a lengthy diagnostic workup. After diagnosis, your focus turns to helping her understand the disorder and the importance of adhering to prescribed treatment. You'll also encourage her to perform gentle exercises, maintain a proper diet, and take other steps to preserve health. And you'll reinforce the need to minimize exposure to sunlight and possibly prepare her for apheresis. What's more, you may need to advise her about pregnancy and family planning.

Before teaching your patient with SLE, make sure you are familiar with the following topics:
• explanation of the disorder, especially its unpredictable exacerbations and remissions
• complications of SLE
• need for repeated diagnostic tests
• importance of gentle exercise and ample rest

- drug therapy
- apheresis to treat acute flare-ups or life-threatening complications
- preventing infection and skin breakdown
- minimizing exposure to sunlight
- coping with Raynaud's phenomenon
- pregnancy and family planning, if needed
- sources of information and support.

ABOUT THE DISORDER

Explain that SLE is a chronic disorder that leads to structural changes in the connective tissue, the fibers that support many other body tissues. Its unpredictable course includes exacerbations interspersed with long periods of complete or near-complete remission.

Tell the patient that SLE may produce only mild effects. However, its effects on the heart, blood vessels, kidneys, lungs, and central nervous system (CNS) may be life-threatening. It strikes women eight times as often as men and has a higher incidence among nonwhites, especially among blacks. Most patients are between ages 20 and 50.

Inform the patient that SLE causes various signs and symptoms. The most common are a butterfly-shaped rash on the face (facial erythema), hair loss, stiff and aching joints, musculoskeletal deformity, and photosensitivity. The patient may also experience fatigue, weight loss, chills, fever, sensitivity to heat and cold, and musculoskeletal pain.

Explain the pathophysiology of SLE. Point out that, although the cause of the disorder remains uncertain, researchers believe antibodies develop against the body's own tissues — mostly deoxyribonucleic acid (DNA) but sometimes ribonucleic acid, clotting factors, and blood cells. This autoimmune response generates immune complexes, which damage connective tissue and cause inflammation. Explain that because immune complexes may reside anywhere in the body, different symp-

toms appear at different times, with varying severity. (See *Immunity gone awry*.)

Point out that heredity may predispose some patients to SLE; the disorder has been found in certain families for several generations. Explain that certain factors may trigger the onset of symptoms; these include physiologic or emotional stress, streptococcal or viral infection, inadequate rest, or exposure to direct or indirect sunlight, ultraviolet light, vaccines, or X-rays. Throughout the course of illness, these same factors may trigger periodic flare-ups. Certain drugs, including sulfonamides, hydralazine, procainamide, penicillin and other antibiotics, and some oral contraceptives, also may cause acute exacerbations.

Complications

Explain that failure to comply with treatment will intensify the risk of exacerbations, but that even full compliance can't guarantee protection against a flare-up. Communicating this reality early in treatment may help the patient avoid needless self-recrimination later.

Because SLE is a systemic disease, complications depend largely on the organs affected. The patient may develop vasculitis, possibly leading to infarctive ulcers, necrotic leg ulcers, or digital gangrene; Raynaud's phenomenon; cardiopulmonary abnormalities such as myocarditis, endocarditis, tachycardia, parenchymal infiltrates, and pneumonitis; renal abnormalities such as hematuria, urinary tract infections, and kidney failure; and such CNS complications as emotional instability, organic brain syndrome, and headache.

DIAGNOSTIC WORKUP

Advise the patient that definitive diagnosis of SLE may require months of observation, many laboratory tests, renal biopsy and, possibly, measurement of the patient's response to different medications. Ask her to pro-

INSIGHT INTO ILLNESSES

Immunity gone awry

Inform the patient with systemic lupus erythematosus (SLE) that she has an *autoimmune disease* in which her immune system malfunctions. Normally, antibodies fight off harmful bacteria. In SLE, they attack her body's own healthy tissues. Tell her that no one knows for sure why this happens.

Overproduction of antibodies by plasma cells (perhaps the first stage in SLE development)

↓

Immune complex formation, consisting of antibodies and antigens

↓

Circulation of immune complexes to various sites, including the kidneys, joints, brain, skin, and heart, with deposition of immune complexes at these sites

vide a precise history of her symptoms to aid diagnosis.

Inform the patient that blood tests will help evaluate her immune system and detect certain antibodies. The antinuclear antibody test yields positive results in about 95% of SLE patients. A positive lupus erythematosus factor test strongly suggests SLE, especially in the presence of clinical symptoms. However, the anti-DNA antibody test remains the most specific test for SLE; it rarely gives positive results in other disorders. Tests may be repeated periodically to monitor the effectiveness of therapy.

Tell the patient that she may have a complete blood count, an erythrocyte sedimentation rate, urinalysis, a chest X-ray, an electrocardiogram, and renal function tests to evaluate

the effects of SLE. A renal biopsy may also be ordered.

TREATMENTS

Point out that treatment for SLE combines drug therapy and measures to prevent complications. These measures may include gentle exercise, ample rest, dietary changes, precautions against infection and photosensitivity reactions, coping with Raynaud's phenomenon, preparing for apheresis, and family planning for women in their childbearing years.

Activity guidelines

If the patient suffers from joint stiffness and inflammation, inform her about the benefits of moderate exercise, such as range-of-motion exercises, to promote optimal health and maintain joint mobility. Recommend using moist or dry heat before exercising to decrease discomfort. Warn her not to exercise to the point of fatigue, to stop during a flare-up, and to resume exercise slowly thereafter.

Because fatigue commonly occurs in SLE, recommend 10 to 12 hours of sleep each night and periodic rests during the day. Make sure the patient understands the need to curtail activities before she tires. Encourage her to maintain a calm, stable environment, if possible, and to practice relaxation exercises and other stress-reduction techniques.

Dietary modifications
Although no diet will cure or even improve SLE, recommend foods high in protein, vitamins, and iron to help the patient maintain optimum nutrition and prevent anemia.

 TIPS AND TIMESAVERS: If the patient has lost weight, suggest increasing caloric intake with between-meal snacks or commercially available high-protein, high-calorie supplements.

Medications
Explain that the doctor will tailor drug therapy to the patient's symptoms and severity of illness.

If the patient takes aspirin or other nonsteroidal anti-inflammatory drugs (NSAIDs), explain that these drugs not only relieve pain and fever, but also fight inflammation. Warn her that common adverse effects include gastric upset and ulcers. Advise her to report unintended weight gain and GI symptoms, including loss of appetite, nausea, vomiting, diarrhea, and abdominal cramps. Tell her to call her doctor immediately if she has black, tarry stools or if her vomit contains blood or resembles coffee grounds.

For severe SLE or acute exacerbations, systemic corticosteroids are the treatment of choice. Initial high dosages often bring noticeable improvement within 48 hours. When symptoms come under control, dosage is tapered slowly. Although corticosteroids may provide dramatic symptomatic relief, their long-term use can cause severe adverse reactions. Consequently, advise the patient to report mood disturbances, GI upset, acne, fever, easy bruising, weight gain, menstrual irregularities, and unusual tiredness.

 WARNING: Caution the patient never to stop a corticosteroid or alter the dosage without consulting her doctor. Also instruct her to inform the dentist or doctor of corticosteroid therapy before undergoing any dental work or surgery.

Topical corticosteroids may also be used to treat skin or mucosal lesions. Demonstrate proper application of cream to the patient and warn her not to use nonprescription preparations without her doctor's approval. Local adverse effects may include burning, itching, irritation, dryness, acne, hypopigmentation, hypertrichosis, allergic contact dermatitis, secondary infection, and atrophy.

Antimalarial drugs may be used to treat skin and mucosal lesions. Tell the patient taking these drugs to report mild nausea, vomiting, diarrhea, ringing in her ears or loss of hearing, mood changes, sore throat, fever, and unusual bleeding or bruising. Because antimalarials can cause retinopathy, recommend that an ophthalmologist examine her eyes every 3 to 4 months to detect early signs of retinal damage. If she notices any changes in her vision, such as blurring or blind spots, tell her to contact her doctor immediately. Inform her that she must take the antimalarial regularly and that she may not achieve full benefits for up to 6 months.

If the patient fails to respond to NSAIDs, corticosteroids, or antimalarials, the doctor may prescribe an immunosuppressive drug. (See *Precautions during immunosuppressive therapy.*)

Procedures
If the patient has life-threatening complications or an acute flare-up that resists corticosteroids, she may undergo therapeutic apheresis. Explain that a needle will be inserted

in each arm and that her blood will be pumped through a machine to remove the circulating immune complexes that exacerbate her disorder. Tell her that her pulse and blood pressure will be monitored and that she should report any tingling sensations around her mouth or in her hands or feet.

Other care measures
Underscore the importance of minimizing exposure to infection, especially if the patient takes corticosteroids, which suppress the immune response. Advise her to avoid crowds and people with known infections and to consult her doctor about influenza and pneumococcal vaccines. Caution against excessive bathing because it can dry or break down the skin, leaving it vulnerable to infection. However, each day she should clean and pat dry areas where two skin surfaces touch, such as the underarm or genital area. Tell her to regularly inspect these areas for signs of infection or skin breakdown.

Mouth care
Emphasize meticulous mouth care for preventing and treating oral lesions. Advise the patient to use a soft toothbrush and to avoid commercial mouthwashes because of their high sugar content and the irritating and drying effect of the alcohol base. Instruct her to have regular dental checkups and to call her doctor upon noticing white plaques in her mouth; these are possible signs of fungal infection. Suggest soft, bland foods if she has open sores.

Sunlight exposure
Inform the patient that sunlight exposure may cause severe urticaria and bullous lesions. Even brief exposure (20 minutes or less) may produce a rash. Caution the patient to avoid sunlight, even when reflected from sand or snow.

Coping with Raynaud's phenomenon
If the patient has Raynaud's phenom-

Precautions during immunosuppressive therapy

If your patient is receiving an immunosuppressive drug, explain that these drugs hinder the inflammatory responses that lead to symptoms of systemic lupus erythematosus but can cause serious adverse reactions. Tell her to watch for and immediately report unusual bleeding or bruising, chills, fever, and sore throat. Forewarn her that she may experience some hair loss; hair will grow back when she stops taking the drug.

Be sure to encourage the patient to comply with regular blood tests, which can be used to determine if the drug interferes with blood cell production.

enon (a common occurrence in SLE), tell her to protect her hands and feet from cold temperatures to prevent vasospasm. Instruct her to avoid cold water and to wear gloves when handling cold items such as frozen foods.

Family planning
If the patient is in her childbearing years, provide counseling about pregnancy and family planning, as needed. Explain that she may experience menstrual irregularities during flareups but her normal cycle will resume during remissions. If she wishes to become pregnant, tell her that keeping her disorder under control and obtaining good prenatal care increase her chances of having a healthy baby. Advise choosing an obstetrician who specializes in high-risk pregnancies, ideally one with experience in caring for pregnant SLE patients.

If the patient wishes to avoid pregnancy, discuss birth control options. Explain that oral contraceptives may aggravate the disorder and that many doctors recommend a diaphragm. If your patient is unfamiliar with the diaphragm, explain how to obtain and use one. Warn her against becoming pregnant and possibly exposing a fetus to potentially teratogenic medications.

Other advice
Tell the patient to call the doctor if fever, cough, or skin rash occurs or if chest, abdominal, muscle, or joint pain worsens.

Finally, provide the names of organizations that can offer further information and support. (See Appendix 2.)

Thrombocytopenia

In teaching your patient about thrombocytopenia, you'll need to emphasize the importance of taking precautions against accidental bleeding — without unduly frightening the patient. You must also explain what platelets are and how they function before you discuss implications and treatment options. Understanding this disorder will help the patient and his family cope with its limitations, take realistic but not excessive precautions, and respond to treatment recommendations.

Before teaching your patient with thrombocytopenia, make sure you are familiar with the following topics:
• description of platelets and their role in clotting
• possible causes of thrombocytopenia
• severity of the patient's thrombocytopenia
• signs and symptoms of bleeding that should be reported
• identifying purpuric lesions
• bleeding complications
• platelet counts and other diagnostic tests
• activity restrictions
• platelet infusions and possible reactions
• immunosuppressive agents
• treatment of local bleeding
• explanation of splenectomy, if performed

• importance of taking precautions against accidental bleeding
• sources of information and support.

ABOUT THE DISORDER
Explain that thrombocytopenia is a congenital or acquired bleeding disorder marked by a shortage of platelets (thrombocytes) — blood cells needed for normal blood clotting. Point out that the disorder may have several causes. These include decreased or defective platelet production in the bone marrow, abnormal platelet sequestration (collection) in the spleen, increased platelet destruction in the bloodstream, or conditions related to infection, the use of some drugs, a primary immune disorder or other disease, or a vitamin deficiency. Identify the cause of the patient's disorder, if known.

Reassure the patient that in many instances thrombocytopenia resolves spontaneously. Then discuss the role of platelets. Explain that these blood cells are essential for normal blood clotting.

Describe the normal clotting process. Tell the patient that, when a cut occurs, the blood vessels constrict in an attempt to stop the bleeding. Platelets rush to the injured area, stick to the edges of the torn vessels, and clump together, forming a plug that temporarily stops the bleeding until a clot can form. A clot then builds within the platelet plug; without the platelet plug, a clot cannot form. Even when the patient isn't injured, platelets help maintain vascular integrity by filling small gaps in blood vessel walls. This prevents blood from leaking out of the vessels.

In thrombocytopenia, decreased platelet function impairs blood clotting after a vascular injury and allows red blood cells to escape from the circulatory system through small gaps in undamaged vessels. This produces the petechiae, ecchymoses, and mucous membrane bleeding that commonly accompany this disorder. The severity of these signs varies with the

Identifying purpuric lesions

Clarify the terms that the patient's doctor may use to describe a rash or a bruise. Tell the patient that the purpuric lesions (purplish discoloration from blood seeping into the skin) associated with spontaneous bleeding in thrombocytopenia include petechiae, ecchymoses, and hematomas.

Petechiae
Painless, round, and as tiny as pinpoints (1 to 3 mm in diameter), these red or brown lesions result from leakage of red blood cells into cutaneous tissue. Inform the patient that petechiae usually occur on dependent portions of the body, appearing and fading in crops and sometimes grouping to form ecchymoses.

Ecchymoses
Another form of blood leakage and larger than petechiae, these purple, blue, or yellow-green bruises vary in size and shape. Tell the patient that these bruises can occur anywhere on the body as a result of traumatic

injury. In patients with bleeding disorders, ecchymoses usually appear on the arms and legs.

Hematomas
If your patient has a palpable ecchymosis that's painful and swollen, he has a hematoma. Usually the result of traumatic injury, superficial hematomas are red, whereas deep hematomas are blue. Although their size varies widely, hematomas typically exceed 1 cm in diameter.

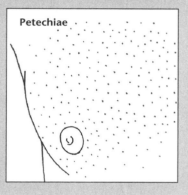

degree of thrombocytopenia. (See *Identifying purpuric lesions*.)

Inform the patient that a normal platelet count ranges from 150,000 to 400,000 platelets/µl of blood. Usually, abnormal bleeding doesn't occur, even with surgery, unless the platelet count drops below 100,000/µl.

Review the severity of the patient's disorder and describe the symptoms of abnormal bleeding. If, for example, his platelet count decreases to between 30,000 and 50,000/µl, tell him to expect bruising with minor trauma.

If his platelet count decreases further — to between 15,000 and 30,000/µl — warn him to expect spontaneous bruising and petechiae, most prominently on his arms and

legs; a woman with a platelet count in this range may have menorrhagia.

If the patient's platelet count falls to less than 15,000/µl, tell him that he may experience spontaneous bruising or (after minor trauma) mucosal bleeding, generalized purpura, epistaxis, hematuria, and GI or intracranial bleeding.

Without alarming the patient, emphasize the symptoms of intracranial bleeding, including persistent headache, mood changes, nausea, vomiting, and drowsiness. Instruct him to report any of these symptoms immediately, even if he hasn't suffered a head injury.

Additionally, capillary or mucosal bleeding may lead to GI bleeding, epistaxis, menorrhagia, or gingival or urinary tract bleeding. Explain the significance of black, tarry stools or "coffee-ground" emesis. Tell the patient that by reporting bleeding signs promptly, he may prevent serious blood loss from a tiny ulcer or other internal lesion.

Complications

Urge the patient to comply with treatment recommendations and activity restrictions to avoid the dangers of abnormal bleeding. Warn him that severe thrombocytopenia can cause acute hemorrhage, which may be fatal without immediate therapy. The most common sites of severe bleeding include the brain and the GI tract, although intrapulmonary bleeding or cardiac tamponade also can occur.

DIAGNOSTIC WORKUP

Advise the patient that he may need to provide frequent blood samples. For example, he may have his platelet count evaluated often. This relatively simple test requires only a small venous blood sample.

The patient may need to provide a blood sample for a blood count after a platelet infusion, especially if he's received repeated infusions. Test results will reveal whether his condition is responding to infusion therapy or whether the platelets are being destroyed.

Platelet antibody studies require a larger blood sample. Tell the patient that these studies can determine why his platelet count is low and help direct treatment.

Occasionally, a patient will need platelet survival studies. These tests help the doctor differentiate between ineffective platelet production and inappropriate platelet destruction. (Platelet production disorders may occur after radiation exposure, medication ingestion, or an infectious disease. They also may occur idiopathically. Inappropriate platelet destruction may occur with splenic disease and platelet antibody disorders.)

Bone marrow study and biopsy

Patients with severe thrombocytopenia usually require a bone marrow study to determine the number, size, and cytoplasmic maturity of the megakaryocytes (the bone marrow cells that release mature platelets). This information may identify ineffective platelet production as the cause of thrombocytopenia and rule out a malignant disease. The patient may also have a bone marrow biopsy. (See *Teaching patients about immune and hematologic tests,* pages 285 and 286.)

TREATMENTS

Explain that typical treatment for thrombocytopenia includes activity restrictions to prevent injury and medications to depress the immune response. Additional therapy may involve platelet transfusions or surgery such as splenectomy. Emphasize self-care measures to prevent bleeding episodes. These include performing meticulous oral hygiene and informing all health care providers that he has thrombocytopenia.

Activity guidelines

Advise the patient that the lower his platelet count falls, the more cautious he must be in his activities. If he has severe thrombocytopenia, instruct him to avoid sports and other strenuous physical activities in which he might twist a joint, strain a muscle, sustain hard blows or kicks, or traumatize vital organs. Explain that even minor bumps or scrapes can cause bleeding. In extreme situations, spontaneous hemorrhage may occur.

If this is the case for your patient, suggest that a family member or other caregiver provide supervision and assistance to prevent injury and to monitor for bleeding. (See *How to avoid excessive bleeding*, page 287.)

Medications

Inform the patient that corticosteroids may be prescribed to suppress his immune response if the dis-

Teaching patients about immune and hematologic tests

TEST AND PURPOSE	TEACHING POINTS
Bleeding time • To assess hemostasis • To detect bleeding disorders, such as hemophilia	• Explain that this test measures the time it takes to form a clot and stop bleeding. Tell the patient that it usually takes 10 to 20 minutes. • Tell him that the site (the forearm) is cleaned with antiseptic. A blood pressure cuff is applied to the upper arm and two tiny cuts are made on the forearm. Then filter paper is used to blot drops of blood until a platelet plug forms and oozing stops.
Bone marrow aspiration and biopsy • To assess the number, size, and cytoplasmic maturation of megakaryocytes, red cell precursors, and white cell precursors • To determine if thrombocytopenia, leukopenia, or anemia results from decreased or abnormal production and to determine possible cause	• Explain that this test evaluates blood cells made in bone marrow and takes 5 to 10 minutes. • Discuss what happens during the test: The skin over the iliac crest (the bony protrusion just above the buttock) is cleaned with antiseptic solution and anesthetized. A hollow needle with a stylet is introduced into the bone marrow cavity. The stylet is removed, a syringe attached, and a small volume (0.5 ml) of blood and marrow is aspirated. For biopsy, a small skin incision (3 to 4 mm) is made so a larger hollow needle can be introduced and a tiny core of bone marrow is removed through the needle. Warn the patient that he may experience brief discomfort when the marrow is aspirated. • Explain that pressure will be applied for 10 to 15 minutes after this procedure. Tell the patient that he can expect slight soreness over the puncture site but should report bleeding or severe pain.
Skin testing • To confirm allergic sensitization and help identify its cause	• Tell the patient that skin tests evaluate the immune system after application or injection of small doses of antigens. Inform him that he needn't restrict food or fluids before the test. • Explain what happens during *intradermal skin testing:* The doctor injects antigens into the patient's skin at spaced intervals on the forearm or interscapular area. At the same time, he injects a control substance (which should cause no reaction). After 15 to 30 minutes, the doctor inspects the injection sites for wheals and surrounding erythema, which indicate a positive reaction. This test can detect allergies to pollen, feathers, animal dander, and dust. • Tell the patient scheduled for *scratch testing* that in this alternative to intradermal testing, the doctor cleans areas of the patient's skin with alcohol. When the skin dries, the doctor uses an instrument to make a superficial scratch (about 1 to 4 mm long) on the patient's skin, then applies an extract con-

(continued)

Teaching patients about immune and hematologic tests *(continued)*

TEST AND PURPOSE	TEACHING POINTS
Skin testing *(continued)*	taining the test antigen. After waiting 30 minutes, the site is checked for erythema. ● If the doctor suspects allergies to fibers, detergents, perfumes, or cosmetics, he may order *patch testing*. Inform the patient that a gauze pad is saturated with the suspected antigen and taped to the patient's skin. After 48 hours, the doctor removes the patch, inspects the skin, and grades the response. A plus sign (+) signifies erythema only; ++ indicates erythema and papules; +++ indicates erythema, papules, and vesicles; ++++ signifies erythema, papules, vesicles, and bullae or ulceration.
Synovial fluid analysis ● To help diagnose rheumatoid arthritis	● Tell the patient that this test helps determine the cause of joint inflammation and swelling and helps to identify which type of arthritis he has. If glucose testing of synovial fluid is ordered, instruct him to fast for 6 to 12 hours before the test; otherwise, inform him he needn't restrict food or fluids. ● Describe the aspiration process: A needle is inserted, usually in the knee joint, to obtain a fluid sample. Warn the patient that although he will be given a local anesthetic, he may feel temporary discomfort when the needle penetrates the joint. ● Tell the patient to report increased pain or fever (indications of joint infection) after the test.

order doesn't resolve spontaneously. Mention whether therapy will be brief or long-term. Also describe possible adverse effects. Tell the female patient to inform her doctor if she's pregnant, suspects she's pregnant, plans to become pregnant, or is breast-feeding.

WARNING: Tell the patient *never* to stop taking corticosteroids without consulting the doctor because abrupt withdrawal may cause serious adverse effects. The doctor will instruct the patient how to taper the dosage gradually.

For safety's sake, recommend that the patient on corticosteroids wear medical identification describing his condition and treatment. Also advise

him to keep his medicine away from children and to dispose of unused medication properly.

Remind the patient to inform health care providers that he's taking a corticosteroid before receiving any vaccinations, skin tests, surgery, or treatment for serious injuries or infections. Also inform the patient that he's at increased risk for infection.

If the patient is receiving high doses of corticosteroids, forewarn him about possible cushingoid effects. Reassure him that these effects typically subside after therapy ends. Suggest that he calculate his caloric intake to prevent weight gain. Encourage him to take the drug with meals to prevent GI upset.

How to avoid excessive bleeding

Because your patient has a tendency to bleed easily and for a longer time than normal, he may need to change his daily activities and modify his living habits. Provide the following list of general do's and don'ts to help him function safely and avoid excessive bleeding.

Do's
● Use an electric razor.
● Wear gloves when washing dishes, raking, or gardening.
● Take your temperature only by mouth.
● Wear socks and shoes that fit properly. Footwear that's too large can cause abrasions. Footwear that's too small can pinch the blood vessels in your feet.
● Regularly check your urine, stools, and sputum for blood.
● Use a thimble while hand sewing.
● Wear a medical identification necklace or bracelet that states your bleeding disorder.
● Inform all health care workers of your condition before undergoing any procedure, including routine dental care.
● Use a nasal spray containing normal saline solution or run a vaporizer to moisturize your breathing passages and prevent nosebleeds.
● Use a soft toothbrush and floss gently unless your doctor advises otherwise.
● Take stool softeners as needed. Eat sensibly to avoid constipation and subsequent straining and bleeding.
● Keep your head elevated when lying down.

Don'ts
● Avoid shaving, cutting paper, or removing paint with a straight-edged razor blade.
● Never go barefoot. Always protect your feet with shoes.
● Avoid leaving knives, scissors, thumbtacks or other sharp objects on countertops or tables where they could accidentally cut you. Store them in protective containers instead.
● Refrain from contact sports and general roughhousing.
● If possible, avoid intramuscular or subcutaneous injections.
● Avoid plucking your eyebrows.
● Reject substances that increase your risk for bleeding — for example, alcohol, nicotine, caffeine, or products containing aspirin or ibuprofen.

If corticosteroid therapy fails to increase the platelet count, tell the patient that other immunosuppressive agents may be tried.

Procedures
Tell the patient that he may need an I.V. infusion of platelets to stop episodic abnormal bleeding caused by a low platelet count. If platelet destruction results from an immune disorder, however, platelet infusions may have only minimal effect and may be reserved for life-threatening bleeding.

If appropriate, discuss immune globulin treatment. Mention that it achieves moderate success in some patients who have immune thrombocytopenia.

Tell the patient who is receiving repeated platelet infusions that he may produce antibodies to the white blood cells contained in the platelets. If this reaction produces fever and chills, reassure him that these symptoms aren't serious, just uncomfortable. Advise him that acetaminophen (Tylenol) may be used to decrease or prevent discomfort.

The patient also may develop antibodies to plasma proteins, which typically causes hives. Explain that he may be given an antihistamine before a platelet infusion to prevent this reaction.

Surgery

Splenectomy may be necessary to correct thrombocytopenia caused by platelet destruction. Because the spleen acts as the primary site of platelet removal and antibody production, a splenectomy usually significantly reduces platelet destruction. Indications that thrombocytopenia may result from hypersplenism include abdominal pain, nausea, vomiting, and an enlarged, tender spleen.

Other care measures

Encourage good dental hygiene to avoid bleeding and to prevent the need for tooth extractions or restorations. Advise the patient to use a soft toothbrush.

 TIPS AND TIMESAVERS: Demonstrate proper tooth flossing technique. Tell the patient to avoid using a sawing motion that cuts the gums. (If his platelet count drops below 30,000/µl, he may have to stop flossing altogether.) Also instruct him to avoid using toothpicks.

If the patient experiences frequent nosebleeds, advise him to use a humidifier at night. Suggest also that he moisten his inner nostrils twice a day with an anti-infective ointment, such as Neosporin Ointment.

Self-monitoring

Teach the patient to monitor his condition by examining his skin for ecchymoses and petechiae. Ideally, he should have someone else check skin areas that he has difficulty seeing. Tell him to report any bleeding from the mucous membranes or GI tract as well as any new petechiae or ecchymoses.

Show the patient how to test his stools for occult blood. Instruct a female patient to report increased menstrual flow to her doctor. Advise the patient to carry medical identification to alert others that he has thrombocytopenia.

10

Urinary conditions

Acute renal failure

When teaching about acute renal failure (ARF), you may be dealing with a patient who is troubled by the initial sign of the disorder — a sudden decrease in urination (oliguria) or, rarely, total absence of urination (anuria). The patient may also be frightened by the prospect of losing kidney function or becoming dependent on dialysis. To address his fears, your teaching must emphasize that early detection and aggressive therapy can usually reverse ARF and prevent its progression to chronic renal failure.

As always, effective treatment hinges on the patient's compliance. To involve him in his care, you'll need to teach him to monitor his fluid balance daily by taking his blood pressure, weighing himself, and recording his fluid intake and output. Active self-care also requires teaching him to recognize the signs and symptoms of ARF and related complications and helping him to accept activity limits and a prescribed diet. If the patient is scheduled for dialysis, you'll review the process, including preparations and aftercare.

Before teaching a patient about ARF, make sure you are familiar with the following topics:
• description of ARF and its causes
• signs and symptoms of kidney dysfunction
• importance of treatment in preventing complications
• preparation for diagnostic tests, such as blood and urine studies and kidney-ureter-bladder (KUB) radiography, renal ultrasonography, or other imaging studies
• activity limitations
• diet and fluid restrictions, as indicated and ordered
• self-care measures, including how to monitor fluid balance, weight, and blood pressure
• medication precautions
• treatments, such as hemodialysis or peritoneal dialysis, if ordered
• preparation for surgery, if appropriate
• sources of information and support.

ABOUT THE DISORDER
Inform your patient that ARF is the sudden inability of the kidneys to remove waste materials from the blood and to maintain proper fluid and electrolyte balance. This means that the body retains metabolic wastes and its fluid, electrolyte, and acid-base balances are dramatically altered. Then tell him whether his disorder is classified as prerenal, intrarenal, or postrenal.

Explain that *prerenal failure* results from conditions outside the kidneys that impair renal perfusion. These conditions include heart failure and other cardiovascular disorders, hypovolemia, and renovascular obstruction. *Intrarenal failure* results from disorders that damage the kidneys themselves, such as acute tubular necrosis. *Postrenal failure* results from bilateral obstruction of urinary outflow caused, for example, by renal calculi or ureteral constriction.

Assure the patient that ARF is usually reversible with early and appropriate intervention. Roughly 50% to 60% of patients regain most or all of their kidney function.

Complications

Emphasize that compliance with therapy may help prevent serious complications, including uremia, hypervolemia, hypovolemia, and hyperkalemia. What's more, it may prevent or delay chronic renal failure.

Define *uremia* as an accumulation of protein waste products in the blood. Explain that when these waste products reach toxic levels, such complications as uremic pericarditis and uremic pneumonitis may result. Instruct the patient to watch for and report signs and symptoms of uremia, including nausea, vomiting, headache, decreased level of consciousness, dizziness, decreased visual acuity, urinous breath odor, and elevated blood pressure.

Tell the patient that *hypervolemia* is an abnormal increase in the volume of fluid circulating in the body. This excess fluid may accumulate in the vessels or tissues. Unchecked, hypervolemia can result in such serious complications as hypertension, heart failure, and pulmonary edema. Teach the patient to watch for and report signs of hypervolemia, such as sudden weight gain, swollen hands and feet, and increased blood pressure.

Explain that *hypovolemia,* an abnormal decrease in the volume of fluid circulating in the body, can progress to shock if it's untreated. Teach the patient to watch for and report indications of hypovolemia, such as weight loss, dry skin and mucous membranes, decreased urine output, muscle cramps, fatigue, dizziness, and decreased blood pressure.

Point out that *hyperkalemia* occurs when too much potassium accumulates in the blood. Mention that hyperkalemia can cause an irregular heart rhythm, possibly leading to cardiac arrest and death. Instruct the patient to notify the doctor if he experiences weakness, malaise, nausea, diarrhea, or abdominal cramps — all warning signs and symptoms of hyperkalemia.

DIAGNOSTIC WORKUP

Tell the patient that he will be carefully screened for preexisting conditions, especially exposure to nephrotoxic substances, that may predispose him to decreased kidney function. Instruct him about the routine blood and urine tests used to evaluate renal function.

Blood tests may include a complete blood count, arterial blood gas (ABG) studies, serum electrolyte levels, and tests to determine serum protein, creatinine, uric acid, and blood urea nitrogen (BUN) levels. *Note:* If the patient has an arteriovenous access device for dialysis, instruct him to tell the phlebotomist not to use the affected arm when drawing blood for ABG analysis.

Inform the patient that he will undergo follow-up blood tests regularly during treatment to ensure that ARF is being properly managed.

Urine tests

Teach the patient that urine studies will be done to evaluate his kidneys' ability to dilute and concentrate urine, to determine the extent of kidney failure, and to check for infection. If he will undergo tests for urine osmolality, sodium levels, and creatinine clearance, teach him how to collect the urine specimen properly.

Other studies

Teach the patient about such diagnostic studies as computed tomography scan, KUB radiography, magnetic resonance imaging, renal angiography, renal ultrasonography, and retrograde ureteropyelography, if ordered. (See *Teaching patients about renal and urologic tests,* pages 302 to 309.) Explain that these tests can detect abnormal kidney size or shape, fluid accumulation, and obstruction of urinary outflow. Point out that if diagnostic results are inconclusive, the doctor may order renal biopsy to help diagnose ARF.

TREATMENTS

Tell the patient that treatment aims at eliminating the precipitating causes of ARF, preventing progression to chronic renal failure, and maintaining or improving the patient's quality of life. Inform him that treatment usually involves activity restrictions, dietary changes, medications and, possibly, dialysis and surgery. Point out the importance of diligent monitoring of fluid, electrolyte, and acid-base balance; taking measures to prevent infection; and recognizing signs and symptoms of kidney failure.

Activity guidelines

Instruct the patient with severe ARF to limit his activity to conserve energy. However, tell him that the doctor may want to monitor him for improved endurance to physical activity when his condition warrants an increased activity level.

If the doctor wants the patient to monitor his heart rate, blood pressure, and respiratory rate during exercise, advise him that his heart rate should not rise more than 20 beats per minute over his resting heart rate, his blood pressure should not increase more than 20 mm Hg over his resting blood pressure, and his respirations should not rise above 20 breaths per minute, with normal depth and pattern. If the doctor orders bed rest, teach the patient early, progressive ambulation techniques, as appropriate.

Dietary modifications

Although diet alone can't treat ARF, it does play an important role in therapy. Collaborate with the doctor and the dietitian to teach the patient how to adjust his diet.

Explain that a diet high in carbohydrates and low in protein, sodium, potassium, and phosphorus can prevent further kidney damage while maintaining nutritional balance. Inform the patient that his diet is based on his renal function, so he must follow the diet prescribed by the doctor or dietitian. Be sure to include family members in your dietary teaching, especially those who prepare the patient's meals. (See *Restricting potassium and sodium intake*.)

Depending on the cause and stage of ARF, the patient may be instructed

---

Restricting potassium and sodium intake

If the doctor prescribes a diet low in potassium and sodium, review which foods the patient should avoid.

Foods high in potassium

Apricots
Artichokes
Avocado
Bananas
Cantaloupe
Carrots
Cauliflower
Chocolate
Dried beans, peas
Dried fruit
Liver
Nuts
Oranges
Peanuts
Potatoes
Prune juice
Pumpkin
Spinach
Sweet potatoes
Tomatoes
Watermelon

Foods high in sodium

Bouillon
Canned foods
Celery
Cheeses
Chinese food
Dried fruit
Frozen foods
Monosodium glutamate
Mustard
Olives
Pickles
Preserved meat
Salad dressing and prepared
  sauces
Sauerkraut
Snack foods (crackers, chips,
  pretzels)
Soy sauce

to either restrict or increase his fluid intake.

 TIPS AND TIMESAVERS: If the patient must restrict fluids, suggest that he suck on ice chips if he gets thirsty. Remind him to include the ice chips as part of his daily fluid intake.

Advise him to divide his fluid amounts over the day. To avoid overload, show him how to measure his fluid intake and urine output precisely.

Medications

Inform the patient that the doctor may recommend discontinuing the medications he normally takes, especially if they're concentrated in the kidneys and excreted in the urine. Explain that because ARF delays urine excretion, the patient is at increased risk for toxic drug reactions.

 WARNING: Instruct the patient not to discontinue or adjust the dosages of any medications without the doctor's approval.

Procedures

If ARF does not respond promptly to other treatment measures, the patient will probably need to undergo dialysis. Explain the purpose and type of dialysis the patient will receive — hemodialysis, peritoneal dialysis, or continuous arteriovenous hemofiltration (CAVH). Make sure he understands what to expect during and after the procedure.

Hemodialysis

If the patient will undergo hemodialysis, explain that a surgeon will catheterize the subclavian or femoral veins. (Rarely, a fistula may be created to access the patient's blood.) Point out that the blood will leave his body through the catheter or fistula, circulate through a dialyzer that removes waste products, and return to his body. Tell the patient that the process takes 3 to 5 hours and is repeated approximately three to four times a week until the patient's own

kidney function improves. Advise him that after hemodialysis, he may feel tired for several hours as his body adjusts to the treatment.

Peritoneal dialysis

Tell the patient that this procedure may be performed manually, by an automatic or semiautomatic cycler machine, or as continuous ambulatory peritoneal dialysis. With all methods, a catheter will be inserted into the peritoneal cavity through a small incision in his abdomen. Explain that a dialysate solution will be instilled through the catheter into the peritoneal cavity, where it remains long enough to allow excess fluid, electrolytes, and accumulated wastes to move through the peritoneal membrane into the dialysate. After the prescribed dwelling time, the dialysate will be drained from the patient's peritoneal cavity, taking toxins with it.

Continuous arteriovenous hemofiltration

Tell the patient who will undergo CAVH (also called continuous renal replacement therapy [CRRT]) that this relatively new dialysis procedure filters fluid, solutes, and electrolytes from the blood and infuses a replacement solution. If appropriate, mention that CAVH is much less likely than conventional hemodialysis to cause hypotension, cramps, nausea, vomiting, and headache because it withdraws fluid more slowly.

Inform him that catheters will be inserted into his thigh, or an internal arteriovenous fistula or external arteriovenous shunt may be used. A hemofilter then removes water and toxic solutes from his blood, and replacement fluid is infused. Assure the patient that he will be monitored closely during the procedure. Tell him to report any pain at the catheter insertion sites.

Surgery

If the patient has postrenal ARF, treatment usually includes catheteri-

How to measure fluid intake and output

The doctor will probably want your patient to keep a daily record of his fluid intake and output. Explain to the patient that this record can help the doctor judge his progress and response to treatment.

What are intake and output?

Inform the patient that fluid *intake* includes everything he drinks, such as water, fruit juice, and soda. It also includes foods that become liquid at room temperature, such as gelatin, custard, and ice cream. Intake even includes fluids, liquid medicines, and solutions delivered through tubing into one of the veins (intravenously) or into his stomach.

Explain that *output* includes everything that leaves his body as a fluid, such as urine, drainage from a wound, diarrhea, and vomitus.

Because the patient's intake should balance his output, urge him to keep very accurate records. Tell him to measure fluids whenever possible instead of guessing the amount.

Measuring intake

Instruct the patient to measure and record the amount of fluid he has with each meal, with medicine, and between meals. Tell him to pour any liquid into a measuring cup or other graduated container before putting it in a glass or cup. Inform him that labels on cans and bottles indicate exact amounts.

Tell the patient not to forget to subtract any amount he doesn't drink. The difference, of course, is his intake amount.

If the patient is receiving medicine or nutrition intravenously or through a stomach tube, instruct him to record the amounts of fluid he uses.

Measuring output

Before throwing away any urine from a bedpan, urinal, or portable toilet, the patient (or his caregiver) should measure and record the amount. Advise him to keep a measuring container handy just for this purpose.

If the patient has a drainage bag in place, instruct him or his caregiver to measure and record the amount of fluid in the bag before discarding it. Finally, advise the patient to measure and record any vomitus or liquid bowel movements as output.

Converting to metric measurements

The doctor may want the patient to measure his fluid intake and output metrically. To convert fluid ounces (oz) to the metric equivalent of milliliters (ml), instruct the patient to multiply by 30. To convert ml to oz, tell him to divide by 30.

APPROXIMATE EQUIVALENTS

Household	Metric
1 quart (32 oz)	1,000 ml
1 pint (16 oz)	500 ml
1 measuring cup (8 oz)	240 ml
2 tablespoons (1 oz)	30 ml

zation to drain urine from the bladder and a surgical or nonsurgical procedure to free the obstruction. If the patient requires surgery, explain the procedure to him, including who will perform it and where, and how long it will take. For example, you may need to teach him about removal of calculi from a ureter.

Other care measures

Prepare the patient for home care by teaching him how to monitor his fluid balance. Show him how to measure and record his daily weight, blood pressure, and fluid intake and output. (See *How to measure fluid intake and output*, page 293.)

Instruct the patient to weigh himself at the same time each day, using the same scale and wearing the same type of clothing. Tell him to notify the doctor if his weight increases or decreases by more than 5% from one day to the next.

Show the patient the proper technique for taking accurate blood pressure readings, and instruct him to compare each blood pressure reading with his baseline reading. Tell him to notify the doctor if his blood pressure exceeds the desired reading the doctor has specified for him.

Also encourage the patient to monitor his temperature and to stay alert for signs and symptoms of possible urinary infection, such as a change in the odor, color, or consistency of his urine.

Be sure to acknowledge the patient's fear of losing kidney function or becoming dependent on dialysis. To allay his fears, stress that early detection and aggressive therapy can usually reverse ARF and prevent its progression to chronic renal failure.

Finally, refer both the patient and his family to a local group or national organization for information and support. (See Appendix 2.)

Chronic renal failure

Chronic renal failure is the irreversible failure of normal kidney function. Thanks to dialysis and kidney transplantation, patients with this condition are surviving longer than ever before. As a result, you'll have more opportunities to teach the patient how to manage this life-threatening disorder. Above all, you'll be challenged to convince him that

complying with prescribed treatment really can improve his quality of life despite the disorder's irreversible and progressive course.

To promote compliance, you'll need to provide thorough teaching about regular exercise, dietary changes, medications, and such therapies as hemodialysis, peritoneal dialysis, and kidney transplantation. You'll also need to offer emotional support to help him cope with life-style changes, frequent hospitalizations, long-term complications, and the prospect of a shortened life.

Before teaching a patient about chronic renal failure, make sure you are familiar with the following topics:
• explanation of the disorder and the extent of nephron damage
• importance of treatment to delay onset of end-stage renal disease and prevent complications
• preparation for blood and urine tests and for other scheduled diagnostic studies, such as radiography and renal ultrasonography, biopsy, and bone X-rays
• prescribed exercise, diet, and fluid restrictions
• drugs and their administration
• explanation of hemodialysis or peritoneal dialysis (if ordered)
• preparation for kidney transplantation or nephrectomy, if indicated
• symptom management, depression, and sexual concerns
• sources of information and support.

ABOUT THE DISORDER

Tell the patient that chronic renal failure results from progressive, irreversible damage to the nephrons — the kidneys' structural and functional units. Explain that in the earliest stage of renal disease, about 50% of renal tissue has already been damaged but that no signs or symptoms occur. During this stage, too, the effects of other conditions (such as hypertension), dehydration, or nephrotoxic drugs may cause rapid, sometimes irreversible, renal failure.

In the second stage, called *renal insufficiency,* up to 80% of renal tissue is destroyed. With the kidneys unable to concentrate urine, the patient may experience dehydration and anemia. In the third stage, *chronic renal failure,* more than 80% of renal tissue is damaged. The patient experiences increasing fatigue, anorexia, weakness, decreased attention span, weight loss, and behavioral changes. In *end-stage renal disease,* more than 90% of renal tissue is damaged, and dialysis or transplantation becomes necessary. Signs and symptoms worsen and may include nausea, vomiting, dyspnea, drowsiness, and increased edema.

Complications
Stress that failure to comply with prescribed therapy can hasten the progression of renal disease, increase the risk and severity of complications, and shorten the patient's life. Discuss potential complications, such as anemia, hyperkalemia, hypertension, pericarditis, fluid overload, coronary artery disease, and bone disease.

DIAGNOSTIC WORKUP
Describe the routine blood and urine tests the patient will undergo to evaluate renal function, detect complications, and monitor treatment. Tell the patient about radiologic tests to visualize abnormalities and renal biopsy to permit histologic examination of tissue.

Blood and urine studies
Blood studies include a complete blood count, coagulation studies (such as activated partial thromboplastin time and prothrombin time), serum electrolyte levels, serum creatinine, blood urea nitrogen and, periodically, serum calcium and phosphorus analyses.

Urine studies include urinalysis with microscopic study, creatinine clearance and protein loss determinations, and cultures (if infection is suspected). If a clean-catch midstream specimen is needed, teach the patient how to collect this specimen. (See *How to collect a urine specimen,* page 296.) For a 24-hour urine specimen, instruct the patient to save all urine during the collection period. (See *Collecting a 24-hour urine specimen,* page 297.)

Radiologic studies
Teach the patient about radiologic studies, such as kidney-ureter-bladder radiography and renal ultrasonography, to determine kidney size and to detect cystic disease. (See *Teaching patients about renal and urologic tests,* pages 302 to 309.) If appropriate, tell him that he will undergo a chest X-ray to assess heart size and identify pulmonary edema. Explain that he may have bone and skeletal X-rays annually to detect the presence or progression of bone disease. Stress the importance of returning to the doctor for follow-up studies.

TREATMENTS
Describe treatments for chronic renal failure, such as dietary modifications and drug therapy. If the patient has end-stage renal disease, describe treatment options, such as hemodialysis and peritoneal dialysis. If appropriate, teach him about kidney transplantation or nephrectomy. Tell him how to manage symptoms of renal failure, such as dry skin, bad breath, and muscle cramps. Also discuss sexual difficulties.

Activity guidelines
Emphasize the need for regular exercise to maintain muscle strength and mobility and to prevent bone demineralization. Advise the patient to avoid excessive fatigue, and urge him to conserve energy by alternating activity periods with rest periods.

 WARNING: Advise the patient to protect his dialysis access site during exercise.

Dietary modifications
In collaboration with the doctor and dietitian, teach the patient about dietary restrictions. Inform him that a diet high in calories but low in protein, sodium, potassium, and phosphorus helps avoid taxing the kidneys and may even slow progression of renal disease. To ensure adequate

How to collect a urine specimen

If the doctor wants your patient to provide a urine specimen, explain that the specimen should not contain germs from the patient's hands or genitals. To ensure that the patient collects an appropriate specimen, caution against drinking a lot of water before the test because this could affect the accuracy of test results. Then provide the following instructions.

For a man

1. Wash your hands thoroughly. Open the package of disposable wipes that you were given, and place it on a clean, dry, nearby surface.

2. Remove the lid from the specimen cup and place it flat side down. *Don't touch the inside of the cup or lid.*

3. Prepare to urinate (if you're uncircumcised, first pull back your foreskin). Using a disposable wipe, clean the head of your penis from the urethral opening toward you, as shown at the top of the next column. Then discard the used wipe.

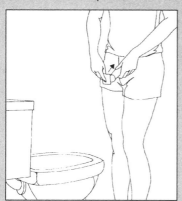

4. Urinate a small amount into the toilet. After 1 or 2 seconds, catch about 1 oz (30 ml) of urine in the specimen cup.

A health care professional will tell you how far to fill the cup. As a rule, you'll fill it about one-fourth or more. *Don't* allow the cup to touch your penis at any time. When you're done, place the lid on the cup and return it to the health care professional.

For a woman

1. Wash your hands thoroughly. Open the package of disposable wipes that you received, and place it on a clean, dry, nearby surface.

2. Remove the lid from the specimen cup and place it flat side down. *Don't touch the inside of the cup or lid.*

3. Sit as far back on the toilet as possible. Spread your labia apart with one hand, keeping the folds separated for the rest of the procedure.

4. Using the disposable wipes, clean the area between the labia and around the urethra thoroughly from front to back. Use a new wipe for each stroke.

5. Urinate a small amount into the toilet. After 1 or 2 seconds, hold the specimen cup below your urine stream and catch about 1 oz (30 ml) of urine in the cup. Don't allow the cup to touch your skin at any time.

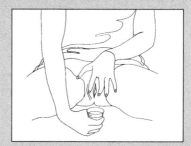

6. Place the lid back on the cup and then return it to the health care professional.

vitamin intake, encourage him to take prescribed vitamin supplements.

Explain to the patient that his dietary needs will change as his disease progresses. Emphasize that he will have to carefully regulate his fluid intake based on his urine output.

Medications

Tell the patient that the doctor may prescribe drugs to help control the systemic effects of renal failure and to relieve symptoms. Instruct the patient to inform other health practitioners (such as his dentist and pharmacist) that he has chronic kidney disease so that any prescribed medications will be appropriate. Also advise him to have all prescriptions filled by the same pharmacy to ensure an accurate record of medications. Caution the patient not to take over-the-counter drugs unless his doctor approves their use.

Dialysis

If the patient requires dialysis, explain its purpose, and discuss the two types: hemodialysis and peritoneal dialysis. Point out that dialysis does not cure or reverse renal disease and will not compensate for loss of the kidney's endocrine or metabolic functions.

Hemodialysis

If hemodialysis is selected, tell the patient that he'll undergo surgery to create a vascular access called a native arteriovenous fistula — a connection between an artery and a vein — or a graft arteriovenous fistula — a synthetic bridge between an artery and a vein. This connection ensures adequate blood flow for hemodialysis. The graft takes 4 to 6 weeks to "mature" before it's ready for use.

Explain that for hemodialysis, two needles are placed in the fistula or graft. Blood leaves the body through one needle, circulates through the dialyzer (which removes wastes and excess fluid and electrolytes), and then returns to the patient through the other needle.

Collecting a 24-hour urine specimen

For a 24-hour urine specimen, the patient must save all urine voided during the collection period. Provide the following instructions.

Discard the first voided urine

When the patient is ready to start the collection period, tell him to void. Then tell him to discard this urine so he starts the collection time with an empty bladder. Instruct him to record the time.

Add preservative

Tell the patient to collect urine from subsequent voidings. After pouring the first urine specimen into the collection bottle, he should add the required preservative and then refrigerate the bottle or keep it on ice until the next voiding. The hospitalized patient should notify the nurse or other caregiver after each voiding to avoid contaminating the urine with stool or toilet tissue.

Important reminders

- Tell the patient to collect all urine voided during the 24-hour period.
- Instruct him to void just before the collection period ends and then add this last specimen to the container.
- If the patient accidentally discards a specimen during the collection period, he must start over, or discuss a possible shortened collection time with the doctor.

Tell the patient that the procedure is repeated three times a week and takes up to 4 hours each time. He is awake during treatment and has minimal discomfort from the needle insertion. However, he is likely to feel tired for several hours after dialysis. Instruct the patient to notify the nurse if he experiences any symptoms, especially dizziness, hot or cold flashes, and headache or nausea, during hemodialysis. These symptoms may reflect hypotension, a common complication.

Emphasize that the patient will need to continue hemodialysis for life unless he receives a successful transplant or changes to peritoneal dialysis.

Peritoneal dialysis

Peritoneal dialysis is often the treatment of choice for patients who don't want to undergo hemodialysis or transplantation. This type of dialysis may be performed using an automatic cycler machine (continuous cyclical peritoneal dialysis, or CCPD) or using four to six fluid exchanges daily (continuous ambulatory peritoneal dialysis, or CAPD).

If the patient chooses CCPD or CAPD, inform him that a catheter will be inserted into the peritoneal cavity through a small incision in his abdomen. Explain that after the catheter site heals, dialysate solution will be instilled through the catheter into the peritoneal cavity, where it will remain for a specified time to allow excess fluid and electrolytes and accumulated wastes to pass through the peritoneal membrane into the dialysate. At the end of the prescribed time, the dialysate is drained and new solution instilled.

Surgery

If appropriate, teach the patient about nephrectomy or kidney transplantation.

Nephrectomy

Nephrectomy — the removal of part or all of a kidney — is indicated if the kidneys are severely infected, greatly enlarged from cystic disease, or causing renin-induced hypertension. Show the patient the incision site — in the flank over the affected kidney.

Tell him that the surgery takes 2 to 3 hours and that afterward he may have a catheter in his bladder to monitor urine volume, depending on his renal disease stage. In early renal failure, urine is manufactured, so he may have a catheter. In later renal failure, decreased urine volume makes measurement less important than avoiding the infection associated with catheter use, so a catheter may not be used. A drain may be placed to remove fluid from the surgical site and help prevent infection.

Inform the patient that, to manage pain, he may undergo epidural anesthesia during the initial postoperative period. Tell him that full recovery takes 6 to 8 weeks, but further interventions will be needed if kidney function is inadequate.

Kidney transplantation

Kidney transplantation is the treatment of choice for patients with end-stage renal disease, especially for patients who want to avoid dialysis or improve their quality of life. Also, the cost of maintaining a successful kidney transplant is one-third that of dialysis.

Tell the transplant candidate that the treatment, if successful, will restore renal function. Stress that he'll need medical follow-up for the rest of his life. Inform him that the donor kidney can come from a healthy family member or from a cadaver. Tell him that before transplantation, he'll have a comprehensive examination and tests to identify and treat any disorders that might complicate recovery.

Review what to expect before surgery. If a cadaver kidney will be used, the patient will be notified when a kidney is available; then surgery will be performed immediately. Stress the importance of staying healthy during the waiting period so the surgery can be performed safely on short notice.

The surgery usually takes 3 to 4 hours. Afterward, the patient will be monitored closely in an intensive care or transplant unit. He'll have a catheter in his bladder to monitor urine output and will receive immunosuppressive drugs to prevent rejection. Explain that immunosuppressive therapy will continue as long as the transplanted kidney remains in place.

Other care measures
Teach the patient how to manage signs and symptoms of renal failure. Pruritus, which results from dry skin, calcium and phosphorus imbalances, and uremic toxins, can be relieved by antipruritic drugs, by avoiding daily bathing and deodorant soaps, and by using moisturizing soaps and lotions. Tell the patient to promptly report muscle cramps to the doctor so that he can treat their cause.

 TIPS AND TIMESAVERS: To minimize uremic mouth odor, encourage good oral hygiene and regular dental visits.

Managing psychological problems
Recognize that lifelong kidney disease disrupts the patient's normal activities, lifestyle, and relationships and may trigger serious depression. Also, sexual dysfunction can occur. Both physiologic and psychological problems, which may hamper sexual activity, are more common in hemodialysis patients than in peritoneal dialysis patients. However, in any patient with chronic renal failure, anemia may cause fatigue and weakness. Medications, especially antihypertensives, can cause impotence. Altered body image, resulting from pallor, discolored skin, uremic mouth odor, or the presence of a vascular access or peritoneal catheter, may contribute to sexual difficulties.

To help the patient deal with his sexual concerns, encourage him to follow his treatment regimen closely; this should improve his feelings of well-being. And although dialysis doesn't completely restore health, it may minimize complications, thus improving the patient's outlook. If antihypertensive drugs cause impotence, the patient should discuss with the doctor the option of changing drugs.

Give the patient an opportunity to talk openly about psychological obstacles. Ask for a sexual history and encourage him to share his feelings. Advise him to pursue sexual activity when he's most energetic — perhaps in the morning or after a rest. Explain that time pressures and stress inhibit sexual pleasure. Because role reversal may affect his relationship with his partner, be sure to include his spouse in your discussion. Reassure them that sexual activity won't damage the patient's health.

If intercourse isn't possible, discuss other forms of sexual expression, such as touching, stroking, and caressing. Advise the patient that a close, supportive relationship with his partner is crucial in managing his disorder.

Finally, refer the patient and his family to a local or national organization that can help him cope with chronic renal failure. (See Appendix 2.)

Hydronephrosis
A urinary tract obstruction, hydronephrosis begins insidiously, without signs or symptoms. However, eventually it may cause pain severe enough to necessitate hospitalization.

In fact, the patient who experiences acute pain from this disorder may be hunched over, clutching his abdomen in distress. Or he may pace the floor or begin to vomit. Whatever his symptoms, you'll need to explain — to the extent his condition permits — that his pain results from a urinary tract blockage and will cease when the obstruction is relieved.

Review the tests the patient will undergo to locate the obstruction, assess kidney damage, and determine its cause. Inform him about medications to relieve discomfort and, if necessary, about catheterization or nephrostomy tube insertion to promote urine drainage. Finally, teach him how to recognize signs and symptoms of another obstruction.

Before teaching a patient about hydronephrosis, make sure you are familiar with the following topics:
• normal renal structures and functions
• how hydronephrosis affects the kidneys
• signs and symptoms of hydronephrosis
• complications, especially infection
• diagnostic studies, including antegrade pyelography, cystoscopy, retrograde cystography, renal ultrasonography, and excretory urography

• medications to minimize pain, control nausea and vomiting, and combat infection
• urinary bladder catheterization to promote urine flow
• nephrostomy tube care
• surgery to remove a urinary tract obstruction
• other care measures, such as increasing fluid intake to counterbalance postobstructive diuresis and recognizing signs and symptoms of infection and additional obstruction.

ABOUT THE DISORDER
Inform the patient that hydronephrosis is characterized by dilation of the renal pelvis and calyces with urine. Dilation is more common in one kidney, although it can affect both if the obstruction is in the bladder or urethra. (See *Teaching about renal structures and functions*.)

Point out that dilation results from an obstruction in the urinary tract, which may be caused by a calculus, a tumor, a kink in the ureter, an infection or inflammation, or scar tissue. In older men, obstruction may result from prostatic hyperplasia. Although the muscles in the affected area contract to force urine around the obstruction, urine eventually backs up into the kidney, filling the organ beyond its capacity and exerting pressure on the renal wall. This results in renal dilation and loss of function.

Emphasize that the damaging effects of hydronephrosis depend on the obstruction's duration, extent, and location. As hydronephrosis progresses, tissue expansion and muscle spasms around the obstructed area produce pain. Usually localized, pain may occur during activity or urination. Dull flank pain suggests slowly developing hydronephrosis. Pain that radiates to the genitalia and the flank occurs when ureteral smooth muscle increases peristaltic motion to dislodge the obstruction or force urine around it.

Complications
Explain that pooled urine in the dilated renal pelvis produces a culture

medium for bacteria, increasing the patient's risk for infection. Furthermore, such an infection exacerbates renal damage and, left untreated, can lead to life-threatening illness.

What's more, calculi may form in the dilated renal pelvis, adding to renal damage. Over time, pressure from backed-up urine in the kidney may cause irreversible nephron destruction and renal failure.

DIAGNOSTIC WORKUP
Prepare the patient for an in-depth examination of the urinary tract, including such diagnostic tests as antegrade pyelography, computed tomography, cystoscopy, retrograde cystography, renal ultrasonography, and excretory urography. Tell him that these tests can confirm the diagnosis, locate the obstruction, and assess the damage. (See *Teaching patients about renal and urologic tests,* pages 302 to 309.)

The patient will also undergo blood and urine studies (blood urea nitrogen, serum creatinine, and urinalysis) to determine the adequacy of renal function.

TREATMENTS
Clarify treatment goals, such as pain relief, infection control, and removal of urinary tract obstruction. Then discuss drug therapy options and surgery, if appropriate.

Medications
Advise the patient with severe, colicky pain that he may receive narcotic pain relievers (such as morphine or meperidine [Demerol]), antispasmodics (such as propantheline bromide [Pro-Banthine]), and antiemetics (such as prochlorperazine [Compazine]). Antibiotics may be prescribed to control infection.

 WARNING: Instruct the patient taking narcotic analgesics to take these drugs only as directed. Advise him to seek medical attention if he experiences an abnormally slow heartbeat (bradycardia), abnormally slow breathing (bradypnea), shortness of breath (dys-

pnea), light-headedness or fainting (hypotension), confusion, severe dizziness, restlessness, or weakness. He should also watch for dry mouth, nausea, and vomiting. Emphasize that drug tolerance may develop with long-term use.

Inform the patient who is taking antispasmodics that adverse effects of these drugs include constipation, decreased sweating, dizziness, drowsiness, and dry mucous membranes.

If the patient receives antiemetics to control nausea and vomiting, inform him about possible adverse effects, such as dizziness, dry mouth, and sedation.

Advise the patient taking any of these drugs not to participate in activities requiring mental or physical alertness, such as driving a car or operating heavy machinery, until he knows the full effects of the medication. Suggest that he use ice chips or sugarless hard candy or gum to relieve dry mouth.

The doctor may prescribe antibiotics to prevent or treat infection. Instruct the patient to complete the full course of medication. Advise him to watch for and report adverse effects, such as hematuria, difficulty breathing or swallowing, hives, itching, numbness and tingling, sore throat, fever, unusual fatigue and weakness, and other reactions associated with the specific drug.

Procedures
If urine retention and bladder distention accompany hydronephrosis, the patient may need to catheterize himself intermittently or have an indwelling catheter to promote continuous urine flow and prevent recurrent obstruction. Demonstrate how to care for the catheter and drainage bag, and show him how to care for surrounding skin to prevent breakdown and infection.

Surgery
Explain that the doctor may recommend using a nephrostomy tube to drain urine from the renal pelvis, or

(Text continues on page 309.)

Teaching patients about renal and urologic tests

TEST AND PURPOSE	TEACHING POINTS
Antegrade pyelography • To evaluate obstruction of the upper collecting system by stricture, stone, clot, or tumor • To evaluate hydronephrosis revealed during excretory urography or ultrasonography and to enable placement of a percutaneous nephrostomy tube • To evaluate the function of the upper collecting system after ureteral surgery or urinary diversion • To assess renal functional reserve before surgery	• Explain to the patient that this test allows radiographic examination of the kidney. Tell him that it takes about 1 hour. • Discuss what happens during the test: The patient will be positioned prone on an X-ray table and given a sedative to help him relax. Next, the skin over the kidney will be cleaned with an antiseptic solution and numbed with a local anesthetic. Then a needle will be inserted into the kidney to inject contrast medium. Explain that urine may also be collected from the kidney for testing and that a tube will be left in the kidney for drainage, if necessary. Warn him that he may feel mild discomfort as the local anesthetic is injected and transient burning and flushing from the contrast medium. Mention that the X-ray machine will make loud, clacking sounds as it exposes films of the kidney. • Describe what happens after the test: The patient's blood pressure, heart rate, and respirations will be monitored every 15 minutes for the first hour, every 30 minutes for the second hour, and every 2 hours for the next 24 hours. Also, his dressing will be checked for blood or urine leakage, and his fluid intake and urine output will be monitored for 24 hours. If a nephrostomy tube was inserted, note that it will be checked to be sure that it's patent and draining well. • Instruct the patient to report posttest chills, fever, and rapid pulse or respirations to the doctor immediately. Also tell him to report pain in the abdomen or flank or sudden onset of chest pain or dyspnea.
Cystometry • To evaluate detrusor muscle function and tonicity • To help determine the cause of bladder dysfunction	• Explain to the patient that this test evaluates bladder function, especially as it relates to the urgency to void and the ability to suppress voiding. Tell him that the test takes about 40 minutes. Ask him to urinate just before the test. • Explain what happens during the test: The patient will be placed in a supine position on an examining table, and a catheter will be passed into the bladder. As fluid is instilled into the bladder, he'll be asked to report his sensations, such as a strong urge to void, nausea, flushing, or a feeling of warmth. • Warn the patient that he may experience transient urinary burning or frequency after the test.

Teaching patients about renal and urologic tests *(continued)*

TEST AND PURPOSE	TEACHING POINTS
Cystoscopy • To visualize internal bladder structures • To help confirm hydronephrosis • To locate an obstruction associated with hydronephrosis	• Explain to the patient that this 20-minute test usually is performed in the doctor's office. Tell him that he may receive a general anesthetic; if so, he should not eat for 8 hours before the test. If he'll have a local anesthetic, he may receive a sedative to help him relax before the test. (If the patient is a woman, she will not receive any anesthetic.) If the doctor plans to take bladder X-rays, describe the preparation he may receive to clean his bowels to ensure sharper, clearer X-ray images. • Describe what happens during the test: The patient lies supine (with hips and knees flexed) on an X-ray table. The genitalia are cleaned with an antiseptic solution, and he's covered with a sterile drape. Next, the doctor administers a local anesthetic, if appropriate, and introduces the cystoscope through the urethra and into the bladder. Explain that the bladder is filled with irrigating solution and the cystoscope is rotated to inspect the bladder wall surface. If a local anesthetic is used, warn the patient that he may feel a burning sensation as the cystoscope advances through the urethra. He may also feel an urgent need to void as the bladder fills with irrigating solution.
Cystourethroscopy • To directly visualize the bladder wall, ureteral orifices, and urethra • To provide a channel for invasive procedures, such as biopsy, lesion resection, removal of calculi, or passage of a ureteral catheter to the renal pelvis	• Explain to the patient that this test permits visualization of the bladder and urethra. Tell him that it takes about 20 minutes. • If a general anesthetic has been ordered, inform the patient that he must fast for 8 hours before the test. If a local anesthetic has been ordered, tell the patient that he may receive a sedative before the test to help him relax. • Describe what happens during the test: The patient will be positioned supine on an X-ray table, with his hips and knees flexed. His genitalia will be cleaned with an antiseptic solution, and he'll be draped. Then the doctor will administer a local anesthetic, if appropriate, and introduce the cystourethroscope through the urethra into the bladder. Next, he'll fill the bladder with irrigating solution and rotate the scope to inspect the entire surface of the bladder wall. If a local anesthetic was used, warn the patient that he may feel a burning sensation when the cystourethroscope is passed through the urethra. He may also feel an urgent need to urinate as the bladder is filled with irrigating solution.

(continued)

Teaching patients about renal and urologic tests *(continued)*

TEST AND PURPOSE	TEACHING POINTS
Cystourethroscopy *(continued)*	• Describe what happens after the test: The patient's blood pressure, heart rate, and respirations will be monitored every 15 minutes for the first hour after the test, then every hour until stable. Instruct him to drink plenty of fluids and to take the prescribed analgesics. However, he should avoid alcohol for 48 hours after the test. Reassure him that urinary burning and frequency will soon subside. Instruct him to take antibiotics, as ordered, to prevent bacterial infection. • Tell the patient to report flank or abdominal pain, chills, fever, or decreased urine output to the doctor immediately. In addition, tell him to notify the doctor if he doesn't void within 8 hours after the test or if bright red blood continues to appear after three voidings.
Excretory urography (intravenous pyelography) • To determine the size, shape, and position of the kidneys, their internal structures, and perirenal tissues • To evaluate and localize urinary obstruction and abnormal accumulation of fluid • To assess and diagnose complications following kidney transplantation	• Explain to the patient that this test evaluates the kidneys and urinary tract. Tell him that it takes about 1 hour. • Discuss pretest preparation: The patient should drink plenty of fluids and then fast for 8 hours before the test. Inform him that he may receive a laxative or other bowel preparation before the test. • Explain what happens during the test: The patient will be placed in a supine position on an X-ray table. After injection of a contrast medium, X-rays will be taken at specific intervals. Mention that a belt may be placed around his hips to keep the contrast medium at a certain level. Warn the patient that the X-ray machine will make loud, clacking sounds as it exposes films. Also warn him that he may experience a transient burning sensation and metallic taste when the contrast medium is injected; tell him to report these and any other sensations to the doctor. • Instruct the patient to report symptoms of delayed reaction to the contrast medium.
External sphincter electromyography • To assess neuromuscular function of the external urinary sphincter • To assess the coordination of bladder and sphincter muscle activity	• Explain to the patient that this test evaluates how well his bladder and urinary sphincter muscles work together. Tell him who will perform the test and where, and that it takes about 30 minutes to 1 hour. • Describe what happens during the test: If skin electrodes will be used, show the patient where they'll be placed. Tell him that a technician will first clean and possibly shave the areas before applying the electrodes. If needle electrodes will be used,

Teaching patients about renal and urologic tests (continued)

TEST AND PURPOSE	TEACHING POINTS
External sphincter electromyography *(continued)*	also show the patient where they'll be placed. Tell him that he'll feel slight discomfort when the electrodes are inserted. Explain that the needles will be connected to wires leading to the recorder; assure the patient that there's no danger of electric shock. If an anal plug will be used, inform him that only the tip will be inserted into the rectum and that he may feel fullness or an urge to defecate. Reassure him that a bowel movement rarely occurs. • After the test, tell the patient to drink 2 to 3 qt (2 to 3 L) of fluids daily and to take warm sitz baths to ease posttest discomfort.
Kidney-ureter-bladder radiography • To evaluate the size, structure, and position of the kidneys • To screen for abnormalities (such as calcifications) in the region of the kidneys, ureters, and bladder	• Explain that this test shows the position of the urinary system organs and helps detect abnormalities in them. Tell the patient that the test takes only a few minutes. Inform him that he needn't restrict food or fluids. • Describe what happens during the test: The patient is placed in the supine position in correct body alignment on a radiographic table. His arms are extended overhead, and the iliac crests are checked for symmetrical positioning. If the patient can't extend his arms or stand, he may lie on his left side with his right arm up. Assure the male patient that his gonads will be shielded to prevent irradiation of the testes. (The female patient's ovaries can't be shielded because they're too close to the kidneys, ureters, and bladder.) Then a single X-ray is taken.
Nephrotomography and renal computed tomography • To differentiate between a renal cyst and a solid tumor • To detect and evaluate pathologic renal conditions, such as tumor, obstruction, calculi, polycystic kidney disease, congenital anomalies, and abnormal fluid accumulation around the kidneys	• Explain to the patient that this test helps detect renal abnormalities by providing cross-sectional images of the kidney. In renal computed tomography, a computer translates these images for display on an oscilloscope screen. Tell him that the test takes about 1 hour. • Instruct the patient to fast for 8 hours before the test if he's scheduled to receive a contrast medium. If he has a history of hypersensitivity to iodine or iodine-containing foods, inform him that the doctor may forgo administration of the contrast medium or may prescribe antiallergenic prophylaxis. • Describe what happens during the test: The patient will be positioned on an X-ray table and will hear loud, clacking sounds as the scanner rotates around the body. Explain that he'll be asked to lie still to avoid distorting the X-ray films. After a se-

(continued)

Teaching patients about renal and urologic tests (continued)

TEST AND PURPOSE	TEACHING POINTS
Nephrotomography and renal computed tomography (continued)	ries of films is taken, the patient may receive an injection of contrast medium. Warn him that he may experience transient flushing, headache, and metallic taste as well as a burning or stinging sensation at the injection site. • If the patient received a contrast medium, tell him to report any posttest flushing, nausea, itching, or sneezing to the doctor.
Radionuclide renal imaging • To detect and assess functional and structural renal abnormalities (such as lesions), renovascular hypertension, and acute and chronic renal disease (such as glomerulonephritis) • To assess renal transplantation • To assess renal injury due to trauma or obstruction of the urinary tract	• Explain to the patient that this test permits evaluation of kidney structure, blood flow, and function. Tell him that it takes about 1½ hours. • Describe pretest preparations: Pregnant women and young children may receive a super-saturated solution of potassium iodide 1 to 3 hours before the test to block thyroid uptake of iodine. • Explain what happens during the test: After the patient receives an injection of a radionuclide, several series of X-ray films will be taken of his bladder. Mention that he may experience transient flushing and nausea as the radionuclide is injected. However, emphasize that he'll receive only a small amount of radionuclide and that it's usually excreted within 24 hours. • Instruct the patient to flush the toilet immediately after each voiding for 24 hours after the test, as a radiation precaution.
Renal biopsy • To aid diagnosis of renal parenchymal disease • To monitor progressive renal disease and to assess effectiveness of treatment	• Explain to the patient that this test helps diagnose kidney disorders. Tell him that it takes about 15 minutes. Mention that the biopsy needle is in the kidney for only a few seconds. • Instruct him to restrict food and fluids for 8 hours before the test. Inform him that he'll receive a mild sedative before the test to help him relax. • Explain what happens during the biopsy: The patient will be placed in a prone position with a sandbag under his abdomen. After the biopsy site is numbed with a local anesthetic, he'll be asked to hold his breath as the biopsy needle is inserted through his back into the kidney. Warn him that he may experience a pinching pain as the needle is inserted. • Describe what happens after the test: Pressure will be applied to the biopsy site to stop superficial bleeding; then a pressure dressing will be applied. Instruct the patient to lie flat on his back without moving for at least 12 hours to prevent bleeding.

Teaching patients about renal and urologic tests *(continued)*

TEST AND PURPOSE	TEACHING POINTS
Renal or penile arteriography • To demonstrate the configuration of renal or penile vasculature • To determine the cause of renovascular hypertension, such as stenosis, thrombotic occlusion, emboli, or aneurysms • To evaluate chronic renal disease or renal failure • To investigate renal masses and renal trauma • To detect complications following renal transplantation, such as a nonfunctioning shunt or rejection of the donor organ • To help differentiate between organic and psychogenic impotence	• Explain to the patient that this test permits visualization of vessels in the kidneys or penis. Tell him that it takes about 1 hour. • Describe pretest preparation: The patient must fast for 8 hours before the test. Tell him that he may receive a narcotic analgesic and a sedative before the test to help him relax. Instruct him to remove all metallic objects and to void just before the test. • Explain what happens during the test: The patient will be placed in a supine position on an X-ray table, and a peripheral I.V. infusion will be started. The skin over the arterial puncture site will be cleaned with antiseptic solution, and a local anesthetic will be injected. Then the femoral artery will be punctured and cannulated for instillation of a contrast medium. Warn the patient that he may experience transient discomfort (flushing, burning sensation, and nausea) as the contrast medium is injected. After this injection, a series of rapid-sequence X-ray films will be taken. Then the catheter will be removed and pressure applied to the puncture site for 15 minutes to stop bleeding. • Discuss what happens after the test: The patient will be kept flat in bed for 8 to 12 hours and nonambulatory for 24 hours after the test. His blood pressure, heart rate, and respirations will be monitored every 15 minutes for 1 hour, then every 30 minutes for 2 hours, then once every hour until they're stable. His popliteal and dorsalis pedis pulses will be monitored every 4 hours.
Renal ultrasonography • To determine the size, shape, and position of the kidneys, their internal structures, and perirenal tissues • To evaluate and localize urinary obstruction and abnormal accumulation of fluid • To assess and diagnose complications following kidney transplantation	• Explain to the patient that this test helps detect abnormalities in the kidneys. Tell him that it takes about 30 minutes. Reassure him that the test is safe and painless; in fact, it may feel like a back rub. • Describe what happens during the test: The patient will be placed in a prone position and the area to be scanned will be exposed. The technician will then apply ultrasound jelly and guide a transducer over this area. During the test, the patient may be asked to breathe deeply to assess kidney movement during respiration. *(continued)*

Teaching patients about renal and urologic tests *(continued)*

TEST AND PURPOSE	TEACHING POINTS
Retrograde cystography, ureteropyelography, or urethrography • To diagnose bladder rupture without urethral involvement, neurogenic bladder, recurrent urinary tract infections, reflux, diverticula, and tumors • To diagnose urethral strictures, laceration, diverticula, and congenital abnormalities • To examine the renal collecting system when excretory urography is contraindicated or inconclusive	• Explain to the patient that this test evaluates the structure and integrity of the bladder, renal collecting system, or urethra. Tell him that it takes about 30 minutes to 1 hour. • Describe pretest preparation: If a general anesthetic is ordered, tell the patient to fast for 8 hours before the test. However, before retrograde ureteropyelography, he must drink plenty of fluids to ensure adequate urine flow. • Explain what happens during the test: *For retrograde urethrography and retrograde cystography,* tell the patient that he'll be placed in a supine position on an X-ray table. A catheter will be inserted into the urethra (for urethrography) or the bladder (for cystography); then a contrast medium will be instilled through the catheter. He'll be asked to assume various positions while X-ray films are taken. *For retrograde ureteropyelography,* tell the patient that he'll be positioned on an X-ray table with his legs in stirrups and that a contrast medium will be injected through a urethral catheter. X-ray films will be taken while the catheter is in place and again after it's withdrawn. Warn the patient that he may experience some discomfort when the catheter is inserted and when the contrast medium is instilled through the catheter. Also mention that the X-ray machine will make loud, clacking sounds as it exposes the films. • Describe what happens after the test: *After retrograde urethrography,* instruct the patient to report flushing, nausea, itching, or sneezing to the doctor immediately. *After retrograde cystography or ureteropyelography,* tell him that his blood pressure, heart rate, and respirations will be monitored frequently until stable. His urine volume and color will also be monitored. Have the patient notify the doctor if blood continues to appear in his urine after the third voiding or if he develops chills, fever, or increased pulse or respiration rate.
Uroflometry • To evaluate lower urinary tract function • To demonstrate bladder outlet obstruction	• Explain to the patient that this test evaluates his pattern of urination. Tell him that it takes about 10 to 15 minutes. • Advise the patient not to urinate for several hours before the test and to increase his fluid intake so that he'll have a full bladder and a strong urge to void. • Explain what happens during the test: The male patient will be asked to void while standing; the

Teaching patients about renal and urologic tests *(continued)*

TEST AND PURPOSE	TEACHING POINTS
Uroflometry *(continued)*	female patient, while sitting. Tell the patient that he'll void into a special commode chair with a funnel that measures his urine flow rate and the amount of time he takes to void. Assure him that he'll have complete privacy during the test. To help ensure accurate results, instruct him to remain as still as possible while voiding.
Voiding cystourethrography ● To detect abnormalities of the bladder and urethra, such as vesicoureteral reflux, neurogenic bladder, prostatic hyperplasia, urethral strictures, or diverticula	● Explain to the patient that this test permits assessment of the bladder and the urethra. Tell him that it takes about 30 to 45 minutes. ● Explain what happens during the test: The patient will be placed in a supine position, and a catheter will be inserted into his bladder. Then a contrast medium will be instilled through the catheter. Tell him that he may experience a feeling of fullness and an urge to void when the contrast medium is instilled. Explain that he'll be asked to assume various positions for X-ray films of his bladder and urethra. ● Describe what happens after the test: The time, color, and amount of each voiding will be observed and recorded. The patient should drink plenty of fluids to reduce burning on urination and to flush out any residual contrast medium. Tell him to report chills or fever, because these may indicate urinary infection.

he may suggest surgery (depending on the obstruction) to relieve the blockage that causes hydronephrosis.

Nephrostomy tube
Inserted through the patient's flank and into the kidney, a nephrostomy tube allows urine to drain from the kidney, preventing renal damage from the increased pressure associated with continuous urine formation without adequate urine flow. If appropriate, teach the patient how to care for the nephrostomy tube. Demonstrate the technique for cleaning and changing the tubing and drainage bag. Tell him to change the dressing daily.

Urinary tract surgery
To relieve a urinary tract obstruction, the surgeon may perform ureterolithotomy (removal of a calculus from the ureter), cystoscopy with prostatic resection, or removal of a bladder tumor. Explain that nephrectomy may be done to remove an irreparably damaged kidney.

Before surgery, reinforce and clarify the doctor's explanations. Answer the patient's questions and listen to his concerns. Tell him which type of anesthetic he'll receive, and advise him of any preoperative food or fluid restrictions or bowel preparation. Outline what he can expect after surgery by discussing pain relief, breathing and coughing techniques, and ambulation.

Other care measures

Emphasize that removal of a urinary tract obstruction relieves pressure on the renal parenchyma, and untrapped urine begins to flow freely. Warn the patient, however, that diuresis after removal of a urinary tract obstruction can lead to fluid depletion. Advise him to drink at least 2 qt (2 L) of fluid daily. Reassure him that postobstructive diuresis normally ceases as the kidneys readjust.

Finally, tell the patient to contact the doctor if chills, fever, pain, anorexia, or general malaise occur. These are signs and symptoms of infection, which suggest another obstruction and further hydronephrosis.

Neurogenic bladder

One of your primary goals when caring for a patient with this disorder is to guide him through a lengthy diagnostic workup to identify his bladder dysfunction. Affecting more than 1 million Americans of all ages, neurogenic bladder results from altered bladder innervation and may lead to urinary tract infections (UTIs), hydronephrosis, and calculi formation.

Fortunately, you can help the patient minimize or prevent these complications by encouraging strict compliance with treatment. However, you'll be challenged to help him overcome anxiety and squeamishness about performing many treatments himself, such as bladder training and intermittent self-catheterization.

Other areas to cover in your teaching include conservative treatment, such as drug and diet therapy. If necessary, explain the use of indwelling urethral catheters, an artificial urinary sphincter implant, or a bladder pacemaker. Discuss major surgery, such as cutaneous ureterostomy and ileal conduit, if appropriate. Of course, in addition to tests and treatments, your teaching should address background information about the causes, sign and symptoms, types of neurogenic bladder, and possible complications.

Before teaching your patient about neurogenic bladder, make sure you are familiar with the following topics:
• comparison of normal and neurogenic bladder function
• causes of neurogenic bladder
• types of neurogenic bladder — spastic and flaccid — and the signs and symptoms
• diagnostic procedures, including excretory urography, cystourethroscopy, cystometry, external sphincter electromyography, uroflometry, retrograde cystography, and voiding cystourethrography
• importance of adequate fluid intake
• prescribed medications and adverse reactions
• role of bladder training and intermittent self-catheterization
• caring for an indwelling catheter
• use of an artificial urinary sphincter implant and a bladder pacemaker
• cutaneous ureterostomy and ileal conduit
• sources of information and support.

ABOUT THE DISORDER

Inform the patient that neurogenic bladder (also known as neuromuscular bladder dysfunction, neurogenic bladder dysfunction, or neuropathic bladder disorder) involves an interruption or delay in normal nerve impulse transmission from the spinal cord to the bladder. This leads to inadequate bladder storage capacity and voiding problems, such as incontinence and incomplete emptying. Underlying causes are myriad and include such conditions as multiple sclerosis, stroke, dementia, tumors, and lesions.

Point out that signs and symptoms of neurogenic bladder vary with the cause and its effect on the bladder. The condition is classified as spastic or flaccid.

Spastic neurogenic bladder

Tell the patient that spastic neurogenic bladder, which affects the upper motor neurons, results from spinal cord damage above the S2, S3, or S4 sacral segments. Signs and symptoms include loss of conscious sensation in the bladder, decreased bladder capacity, hypertrophy of the bladder wall, spontaneous detrusor muscle contractions, urinary sphincter spasms, urinary frequency and retention, recurrent UTIs, and lack of urinary control, including stress incontinence.

Flaccid neurogenic bladder
Explain that flaccid neurogenic bladder, which affects the lower motor neurons, results from spinal cord damage — usually traumatic injury at or below the S2, S3, or S4 sacral segments. The bladder becomes flaccid, resulting in overfilling and overdistention, less efficient bladder and detrusor muscle contractions, and lack of bladder sensation, so the patient doesn't realize when his bladder is full. Other effects include urine retention, UTIs, and overflow incontinence.

Complications
Warn the patient that untreated neurogenic bladder can lead to recurrent UTIs, calculi formation, hydronephrosis, and renal failure (a life-threatening complication).

DIAGNOSTIC WORKUP
Inform the patient that the doctor will first take a thorough medical history, emphasizing neurologic and urologic problems. Then he'll order routine laboratory tests, including a urinalysis and urine culture, to screen for renal or urinary tract disease and UTI. Mention that he may also order several other diagnostic tests, including excretory urography, cystourethroscopy, urodynamic tests (cystometry, external sphincter electromyography, and uroflometry), retrograde cystography, and voiding cystourethrography. (See *Teaching patients about renal and urologic tests,* pages 302 to 309.)

TREATMENTS
Inform the patient that treatment for neurogenic bladder aims to maintain bladder function, control infection, and prevent incontinence. Discuss conservative measures first, such as bladder training techniques, increased fluid intake, medication, and intermittent self-catheterization. If these measures are unsuccessful, the doctor may insert an indwelling catheter temporarily or implant an artificial urinary sphincter or a bladder pacemaker. If all else fails, urinary diversion surgery may be needed.

Dietary modifications
Advise the patient to drink 8 to 10 glasses (at least 2 qt [2 L]) of fluids a day to flush his urinary system and to reduce the risk of UTIs. He should drink 8 oz (240 ml) every 2 hours and try to void 30 minutes later.

 TIPS AND TIMESAVERS: Remind the patient to count as fluids any foods that are liquids at room temperature, such as gelatin, pudding, or ice cream.

Recommend drinking cranberry juice daily to help keep the urine acidic, thereby decreasing the risk of UTIs. Instruct the patient to avoid foods rich in calcium and phosphorus to reduce the risk of developing kidney stones. In addition, the doctor may suggest taking ascorbic acid (vitamin C) to help maintain urine acidity.

Medications
Explain that drug therapy is usually the first-line treatment for neurogenic bladder. Medications can correct incontinence by helping the bladder empty more efficiently and improving coordination between the detrusor muscle and urethral sphincter. Drugs used to treat neurogenic bladder may include anticholinergics such as propantheline bromide (Pro-Banthine), antispasmodics such as flavoxate hydrochloride (Urispas), cholinergics such as bethanechol (Urecholine), and external sphincter relaxants such as dantrolene sodium (Dantrium).

Procedures
Explain to the patient that certain

self-care measures can help him empty his bladder and avoid UTIs. These measures include bladder-training techniques — manual stimulation, Credé's method, and Valsalva's maneuver — intermittent self-catheterization, and the use of an indwelling catheter. If he will practice any of these methods, instruct him to record what time he voids, the length of time between voidings, his fluid intake, and his urine output. Teach him the signs and symptoms of a full bladder — discomfort and distention around the bladder, restlessness, and sweating.

Manual stimulation
If the patient has a spastic neurogenic bladder, teach him to activate urination and relax the urethral sphincter by stimulating "trigger areas." Tell him to sit on the toilet and stroke his abdomen or genitalia, then pull gently on his pubic hair. Or he can digitally stimulate the anal sphincter.

Credé's method
If the patient has a flaccid neurogenic bladder, teach him to manually empty the bladder. Instruct him to sit on the toilet and apply pressure to his abdomen over the bladder, moving his fingers downward in a "milking" motion.

Valsalva's maneuver
This method is also effective for the patient with a flaccid neurogenic bladder. Instruct him to sit on the toilet, then forcibly exhale while keeping his mouth closed. This helps the bladder release urine and promotes complete emptying.

Intermittent self-catheterization
In conjunction with a bladder training program, intermittent self-catheterization is especially useful for a patient with a flaccid neurogenic bladder.

Indwelling catheterization
Usually, indwelling catheterization is reserved for patients who lack the

manual dexterity to perform a bladder training program, such as those with multiple sclerosis or other neuromuscular problems. If your patient has an indwelling catheter, teach him and his family how to care for it at home and how to cope with any problems. Discuss what to do if the catheter becomes blocked and how to recognize signs and symptoms of infection. Urge the patient to contact the doctor or nurse if these problems arise. (See *Preventing bladder infection from an indwelling catheter.*)

Surgery
Inform the patient that the doctor may implant an artificial urinary sphincter or a bladder pacemaker if diet, drug therapy, and bladder training fail to improve his bladder function. If necessary, an alternate route for urine excretion may be surgically created. Two such procedures are cutaneous ureterostomy and ileal conduit.

Tell the patient that a *cutaneous ureterostomy* is the simplest type of urinary diversion surgery. In this procedure, one or both ureters are dissected from the bladder and brought through the abdominal skin surface to form one or two stomas. The exact stoma site is often chosen during surgery, based on the length of ureter available.

Explain that an *ileal conduit* involves connecting the ureters to a small portion of the ileum excised especially for the procedure, followed by creation of a stoma from one end of the ileal segment. The stoma will be located somewhere in the lower abdomen, probably below the waistline.

Preoperative and postoperative considerations
Tell the patient who is scheduled for one of these procedures that, because he will receive a general anesthetic, he'll have to fast for 8 hours before surgery. Point out that after surgery, his vital signs will be monitored until he's stable, and his dressings will be checked periodically and changed at

Preventing bladder infection from an indwelling catheter

If your patient has an indwelling catheter, teach him ways to prevent or at least control bladder infection.

Fluid and medication guidelines

Instruct the patient to drink at least eight 8-oz (240 ml) glasses of fluid a day, including cranberry juice (which keeps the urine acidic). Advise him to take any medications prescribed by the doctor.

Catheter care

Tell the patient to wash the catheter area with soap and water twice a day to keep it from becoming irritated or infected. Also instruct him to wash the rectal area whenever he has a bowel movement. He should dry the skin gently but thoroughly.

Instruct the patient to wash the drainage tubing and bag with soap and water once a day, followed by a rinse with a solution made from about 1 part white vinegar to 7 parts water. Tell him to empty his leg drainage bag every 2 or 4 hours and to empty his bedside drainage bag at least every 8 hours.

Stress the need to always keep the drainage bag below bladder level. Warn the patient never to pull on the catheter. Tell him to disconnect it from the drainage tubing only to clean the bag. Caution him never to remove the catheter himself unless the doctor or nurse has given him instructions.

Other instructions

Advise a woman to always wipe from front to back after bowel movements and to do the same when washing and drying the genital area. Explain that this prevents contamination of the catheter and urinary tract with germs from the rectum.

Signs and symptoms to report

Advise the patient to call the doctor right away if he has:
- urine leakage or discharge around the catheter
- pain in the bladder area
- abdominal pain and fullness
- scanty urine flow
- blood or particles in his urine
- temperature above 100° F (37.7° C)
- cloudy urine
- discharge around the catheter.

least once every shift. Also, he will have a nasogastric tube in place after surgery.

Review the doctor's explanation of the urine collection device that will be used after surgery. Encourage the patient to handle the device to help ease his acceptance of it. Reassure him that he'll receive complete training on how to use it after he returns from surgery.

If possible, arrange for a visit by a well-adjusted ostomy patient who can provide a firsthand account of the operation and offer some insight into the realities of ongoing stoma

and collection-device care. As appropriate, include the patient's family in your preoperative teaching — especially if they'll be providing much of the routine care after discharge.

Home care
If the patient will be discharged with an indwelling urethral catheter, explain how to care for it and how to handle problems. Make sure that the patient and any caregivers know how to care for the stoma and change the ostomy pouch. Stress the importance of keeping scheduled follow-up appointments with the doctor and en-

terostomal therapist to evaluate stoma care and make any necessary changes in equipment. For instance, stoma shrinkage, which normally occurs within 8 weeks after surgery, may require a change in pouch size to ensure a tight fit.

Reassure the patient that he should be able to return to work soon after discharge. However, if his job requires heavy lifting, he should talk to his doctor before resuming work. Explain that he can safely participate in most sports, even strenuous ones, but suggest that he avoid contact sports such as wrestling.

If the patient expresses doubts or insecurity about his sexuality related to the stoma and collection device, recommend sexual counseling. Reassure the female patient that pregnancy should pose no special problems. But urge her to consult with her doctor before she becomes pregnant.

Finally, refer the patient and his family to a support group (See Appendix 2.)

Renal calculi

Because the overwhelming majority of renal calculi, or kidney stones, don't exceed 5 mm in diameter, most of your patient teaching will involve explaining measures to promote their natural passage, such as vigorous hydration and use of diuretics.

However, for patients with larger stones, your approach will differ significantly. These sometimes excruciatingly painful stones require removal or disintegration to avoid urinary tract obstruction. Depending on the size and location of the calculi, you'll need to teach the patient about such procedures as extracorporeal shock wave lithotripsy (ESWL) or surgery. To prevent calculi from recurring, your teaching must then stress compliance with prescribed dietary restrictions and drug therapy, if appropriate.

Before teaching your patient about renal calculi, make sure you are familiar with the following topics:
• explanation of how calculi form

and precipitate in the urine, including factors that influence their formation
• types of calculi and where they form in the urinary tract
• diagnostic tests, such as blood and urine tests to determine the cause and composition of calculi, and radiography or ultrasonography to pinpoint their location
• importance of treatment to prevent urinary tract obstruction
• drugs to prevent recurrent calculi
• importance of following prescribed dietary restrictions and fluid recommendations to prevent calculi recurrence
• preparation for procedures such as ESWL to remove calculi
• preparation for surgery, if indicated
• home care of a nephrostomy tube, if appropriate
• signs and symptoms of infection
• sources of information and support.

ABOUT THE DISORDER
Tell the patient that the kidneys excrete several substances that are insoluble and that are normally excreted with minimal crystal formation. However, diet, medications, metabolic abnormalities, systemic disease, or infection can increase the tendency for crystals to form and stones to develop. Explain that calculi usually begin when tiny specks of undissolved material precipitate and remain in the urinary tract. As more material clings to these specks, they gradually develop into calculi.

Inform the patient that calculi typically form in the kidneys but can develop anywhere in the urinary tract, including the ureters and bladder. Point out that although the cause of calculi is unknown, many factors have been linked to their formation. (See *Risk factors for renal calculi*.)

Stress that calculi can vary in size from minute granular deposits — called sand or gravel — to bladder stones the size of an orange. Small calculi seldom cause problems because they're easily carried through the ureter and passed in the urine. A

Risk factors for renal calculi

Discuss with your patient the following predisposing factors for renal calculi:
- metabolic disorders, including cystinuria, renal tubular acidosis, hypercalcemia, hyperoxaluria, hyperuricuria, and hypomagnesemia
- family history of calculi
- geography — the U.S. northwest, southeast, and southwest are known "calculi belts"
- climate — exposure to sunlight increases vitamin D production (and calcium absorption).
- diet — eating too much animal protein can raise calcium oxalate and uric acid levels by 50% in calculus-forming patients.
- dehydration — diminished water intake and reduced urine production concentrate calculus-forming substances.
- obesity
- urinary tract abnormalities
- sedentary jobs (linked to upper urinary tract calculi)
- obstruction — urinary stasis (as in spinal cord injury) allows calculus constituents to accumulate.
- drug therapy — certain medications, vitamins C and D, and calcium supplements can promote calculi development; for instance, adrenocorticosteroids elevate urine calcium levels, as do phosphate-binding nonabsorbable antacids, which also increase urine pH.

Chemotherapeutic agents and external radiation may cause cellular breakdown and acute hyperuricemia. Furosemide may cause hyperuricemia, too, whereas aspirin and probenecid raise urine uric acid levels in hyperuricemia.

larger calculus, however, may cause excruciating pain if it enters the ureter. It may also become lodged there. (See *Where calculi form,* page 316.)

Complications
Explain that calculi too large for natural passage cause obstruction in the urinary tract. Unless calculi are removed, urine trapped above the obstruction may set the stage for renal infection. Eventually, the kidney's collection system may also become abnormally dilated — holding up to several liters of urine. Called hydronephrosis, this condition may lead to renal insufficiency if untreated. (See "Hydronephrosis," page 299.)

DIAGNOSTIC WORKUP
Inform the patient that the doctor will take a thorough medical history, focusing on the type, location, and duration of pain and the presence of any fever. Then he'll order blood, urine, and imaging tests to diagnose and evaluate renal calculi. Blood will

be drawn for a complete blood count and to determine calcium, phosphorus, blood urea nitrogen, creatinine, glucose, uric acid, and electrolyte levels. Explain that tests to measure serum calcium and phosphorus may be repeated on three different days to determine average levels; instruct the patient to fast for 8 hours before each test.

Teach the patient how to collect a clean-catch urine specimen and 24-hour urine collection for routine urinalysis and urine cultures and to check for infections. Then describe the imaging tests the patient may undergo. (See *Teaching patients about renal and urologic tests,* pages 302 to 309.)

TREATMENTS
Explain that the goals of treatment are to identify the type of calculus and eradicate it, control pain, prevent nephron destruction and infection, relieve the obstruction, and prevent calculus recurrence. Inform the patient that treatments may involve

INSIGHT INTO ILLNESSES

Where calculi form

Point out to the patient that calculi may form at various sites in the urinary tract, including the kidneys, ureters, and bladder. This illustration shows common sites of calculi formation.

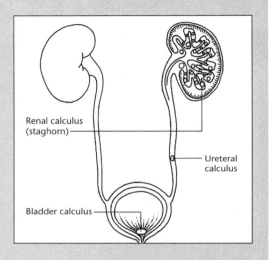

Renal calculus (staghorn)

Ureteral calculus

Bladder calculus

dietary and fluid changes, medications, calculi removal techniques and, possibly, surgery.

Dietary modifications
Explain that, because most renal calculi contain calcium combined with phosphate and some other substances, the patient should reduce his intake of calcium and phosphorus. Emphasize that nutritional therapy also plays an important role in the prevention of calculi recurrence. In collaboration with a dietitian, teach the patient which foods to eliminate from the diet.

TIPS AND TIMESAVERS: Inform the patient that he may need to reduce or eliminate his intake of cheese (for its calcium); beets, spinach, chocolate, and tea (for their oxalate); and carbonated soft drinks (for their phosphorus).

Advise the patient to restrict protein, limiting meat consumption to once a day or less. If he is on a nonrestricted fluid diet, instruct him to drink at least 12 glasses of fluid a day, to keep urine volume at about 2 quarts daily.

Medications
Explain that drug therapy depends on the composition of the patient's calculi and will continue indefinitely to prevent calculi from recurring. The doctor may also prescribe ammonium chloride or acetohydroxamic acid (Lithostat) to acidify the urine, which will help to prevent further stone formation.

Procedures
As appropriate, teach the patient about invasive and noninvasive procedures to remove his calculi. Such procedures include ESWL, percutaneous nephrolithotomy, endoscopic stone manipulation, ultrasonic endoscopy, percutaneous ultrasonic lithotripsy, and laser lithotripsy.

Chemolysis may be used alone or in combination with these treatments.

Extracorporeal shock wave lithotripsy

Explain that ESWL successfully removes calculi in 75% of patients with ureteral calculi. Tell the patient scheduled for this procedure that he will sit in a large water tank or tub; the water transmits high-pressure shock waves into the body. Or he will lie on a stretcher over a water-filled cushion; the cushion, containing a shock electrode and reflector, is coupled to the stretcher by a layer of ultrasonic gel and placed against the patient's lower back. Explain that the procedure using the water-filled cushion can be performed with a sedative-analgesic rather than a general anesthetic because improved shock generators keep shock-wave intensity high but below the patient's pain threshold.

Endoscopic stone manipulation

Tell the patient that this procedure is used to remove small calculi (less than 0.4" [1 cm] in diameter) in the lower third of the ureter. Using a cystoscope, the doctor inserts special loops or basket catheters into the ureter to capture and remove the calculus.

Inform the patient that a ureteroscope may allow visualization and calculi removal in the middle third of the ureter. Ureteral probes or electrohydraulic shock waves are used to fragment and remove a large calculus. If the doctor is unable to remove the calculus, he may leave a loop or ureteral catheter in place to dilate the ureter for later manipulation. He may also leave a ureteral catheter in place after the procedure to prevent obstruction from edema.

Ultrasonic endoscopy

Inform the patient scheduled for ultrasonic endoscopy that, in this procedure, the trapped calculus is fragmented with an ultrasonic probe and then removed by suction. A J-stent — a catheter that helps to pass the calculus and drain urine — is usually left in place until after discharge.

Percutaneous ultrasonic lithotripsy

Tell the patient that this procedure (also called percutaneous nephrolithotripsy) removes kidney or upper ureteral calculi. Explain that the doctor uses an electrohydraulic or ultrasonic probe to fragment large calculi with electrical or ultrasonic energy. He removes larger fragments with a basket catheter and smaller pieces with continuous suction through a nephroscope. Afterward, he places a catheter in the tract to drain the kidney and control bleeding (a possible major complication). The external lumen of the large nephrostomy catheter and its inflated balloon (if the doctor uses a balloon catheter) is used to apply direct pressure to bleeding areas.

Laser lithotripsy

Explain that this procedure directs laser light through a ureteroscope to the calculus, where strobe-light pulsations create tiny shock waves. These pulsations fragment calculi without damaging the ureteral wall.

Chemolysis

Describe how this procedure uses drugs to break up calculi. Tell the patient that the drugs are delivered through a nephrostomy tube to renal calculi or through a catheter to bladder and ureteral calculi. Hemiacidrin is used for struvite dissolution; sodium bicarbonate for uric acid dissolution.

Surgery

Before the advent of lithotripsy, surgical removal of kidney stones was the major mode of therapy. Today, however, surgery is performed on only about 1% to 2% of patients.

If the patient requires surgery to remove calculi, reinforce the doctor's explanations and answer any questions. Depending on the type and location of the calculi, surgery may involve pyelolithotomy, ureterolithotomy, nephrolithotomy, percutaneous nephrostomy, or nephrectomy. Tell the patient what type of anesthetic he'll receive — local, spinal, or general — and advise him of any preoperative food and fluid restrictions or bowel preparation.

Other care measures

After most calculi removals, instruct the patient to strain his urine after voiding and to save any solid material for analysis. Explain that knowing the composition of calculi will help the doctor pinpoint what's causing them to form.

Advise the patient to watch for and report continuing passage of bloody urine and signs or symptoms of infection — increased pain, inability to void, change in the color or odor of his urine, or temperature exceeding 101° F (38.3° C).

Urinary tract infection

Among the most common urologic disorders, urinary tract infections (UTIs) affect people of all ages. They are about 10 times more common in females than in males. UTIs don't always cause signs or symptoms, so your teaching must emphasize prevention as well as treatment.

Establishing a good rapport with your patient is especially important because you'll need to discuss preventive measures that may require her to adopt new dietary and personal hygiene habits and new voiding patterns. Your teaching will also include the pathophysiology and risks of UTIs, test procedures, and drug therapy.

Before teaching your patient about UTIs, make sure you are familiar with the following topics:
• types of UTIs, including their signs and symptoms
• risk factors for UTIs
• complications such as renal disease
• diagnostic tests, such as urinalysis and radiography
• activity and diet guidelines

• prescribed medications such as antibiotics
• explanation of surgery, if necessary
• preventive measures, including healthful hygiene practices and urination patterns.

ABOUT THE DISORDER

Inform the patient that the naturally sterile urinary tract can harbor infection when bacteria enter the nonsterile area near the urethra. Explain that lower UTIs, such as urethritis and cystitis, involve the urethra, bladder, or both, whereas upper UTIs (called pyelonephritis) affect the kidneys. (See *Sites of urinary tract infection*.)

Tell the patient that symptoms may develop rapidly (if at all) over a few hours or a few days. Although symptoms may resolve without treatment, residual infection is common, and symptoms are likely to recur.

Explain that lower UTIs usually produce urinary urgency and frequency, dysuria, bladder cramps or spasms, itching, a feeling of warmth during urination, and nocturia. Males may complain of urethral discharge. If the bladder wall is inflamed, the patient may also have fever and hematuria. Other common symptoms include abdominal pain or tenderness over the bladder, chills, flank pain, low back pain, malaise, nausea, and vomiting.

Explain that upper UTIs cause similar symptoms, including urinary urgency and frequency, burning during urination, dysuria, nocturia, and hematuria. The urine may appear cloudy and have an ammonia or fish-like odor. Other typical signs and symptoms include a temperature of 102° F (38.9° C) or higher, chills, flank pain, anorexia, and fatigue.

To help your patient understand why prevention ranks high in self-care, identify common UTI risk factors. (See *Reviewing risk factors for urinary tract infection*, page 320.)

Complications

Warn the patient that complications, such as chronic pyelonephritis — a leading cause of end-stage renal dis-

INSIGHT INTO ILLNESSES

Sites of urinary tract infection

Use a simple illustration like this one to enhance your teaching on urinary tract infections (UTIs). Then identify the patient's specific infection and the affected area. If appropriate, name the organism causing the patient's UTI.

Lower UTI

If your patient has urethritis (an infection of the urethra) or cystitis (an infection of the urethra and the bladder), point out the urethra and the bladder. Explain that lower UTIs result from infection by bacteria, such as *Escherichia coli* or *Klebsiella*,

Proteus, Enterobacter, Pseudomonas, or *Serratia* species.

Upper UTI

If your patient has pyelonephritis (an infection of the kidneys and renal pelvis), show her where the kidneys lie. Explain that infectious bacteria usually are normal intestinal and fecal flora that grow readily in urine. Mention that the most common causative organism is *E. coli.* Other disease-causing organisms include *Proteus, Pseudomonas, Staphylococcus aureus,* and *Streptococcus faecalis.*

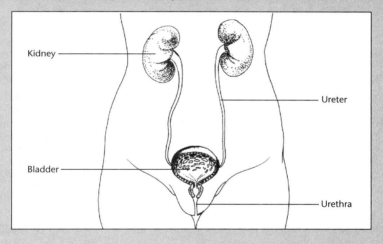

ease — may result from failure to observe treatment guidelines. And without vigilance and treatment, other kidney damage may occur from chronic UTIs — especially if the patient has a neurogenic bladder, which permits urine retention and consequent infection.

WARNING: Caution the pregnant patient that careful compliance with treatment is

necessary because her UTI can progress to pyelonephritis. This can pass on to the fetus and cause hypertension, eye infections, and decreased motor activity.

DIAGNOSTIC WORKUP

Discuss scheduled tests, beginning with laboratory tests, such as urinalysis and culture, smear and stain of urethral discharge, and a complete

Reviewing risk factors for urinary tract infection

Inform your patient that certain factors increase the risk for urinary tract infection (UTI). They include natural anatomic variations, trauma or invasive procedures, urinary tract obstruction, urine reflux, and other conditions.

Natural anatomic variations

Explain that women are more prone to UTIs than men because the female urethra is shorter — about 1" to 2" (2.5 to 5 cm), compared with about 7" to 8" (18 to 20 cm) in men. The female urethra is also closer to the anus than the male urethra. Naturally, bacteria survive longer by traveling shorter distances to colonize.

Point out that pregnant patients are especially prone to UTIs — because of hormonal changes and because the enlarged uterus exerts greater pressure on the ureters. This restricts urine flow, allowing bacteria to linger in the urinary tract.

In men, the release of prostatic fluid serves as an antibacterial shield. However, men lose this protection after about age 50, when the prostate gland begins to enlarge. In turn, this enlargement may promote urine retention.

Trauma or invasion

Inform the patient that fecal matter, sexual intercourse, and instruments (for example, catheters and cysto-scopes) can introduce bacteria into the urinary tract to trigger infection.

Obstruction

Tell the patient that a narrowed ureter or calculi (stones) lodged in the ureters or the bladder can obstruct urine flow. Slowed urine flow allows bacteria to remain and multiply, risking damage to the kidneys.

Reflux

Inform the patient that vesico-urethral reflux results when pressure inside the bladder (caused by coughing or sneezing) pushes a small amount of urine from the bladder into the urethra. When the pressure returns to normal, the urine flows back into the bladder, bringing bacteria from the urethra with it.

In vesicoureteral reflux, urine may flow back from the bladder to one or both ureters. Normally, the vesicoureteral valve shuts off reflux. Damage, however, can prevent the valve from doing its job.

Other risk factors

Advise the patient that stasis of urine in the bladder can promote infection, which, if undetected, can spread to the entire urinary system. Because urinary tract bacteria thrive on sugars, diabetes is also a risk factor.

---

blood count. Tell the patient that urinalysis involves examination of a urine specimen for signs of infection, such as a cloudy appearance and a foul odor; bacteria, pus, and proteins; red and white blood cells; and alkaline pH. A urine culture, which requires a urine specimen, can identify the disease-causing agent. If the patient collects the specimen at home, advise her to store it in the refrigerator to keep bacteria from multiplying, and then to take it to the laboratory within 1 hour to ensure accurate results.

If appropriate, discuss radiographic tests, such as kidney-ureter-bladder (KUB) radiography, excretory urography, and voiding cystourethrography. Point out that KUB radiography — an abdominal X-ray study — identifies the position of the kidneys, ureters, and bladder and helps to detect any abnormalities. Depending on KUB

Treating and preventing urinary tract infections

Dear Patient:
Here's some advice to help you treat your urinary tract infection (UTI) and prevent it from occurring again.

Treatment guidelines
●Take your prescribed medicine exactly as your doctor directs. Do not stop taking your medicine just because you feel better. Finish the prescription to kill all infection-causing germs. Otherwise, you run the risk that the infection will come back.
●Lay a warm heating pad on your abdomen and sides to soothe any pain and burning sensations you may have. Try a warm sitz bath, or ask your doctor to prescribe a pain reliever.

Diet tips
●Drink 10 to 14 glasses of fluid a day to increase urine flow and flush out germs.
●Eat foods and drink fluids with a high acid content. This will acidify your urine. Acid urine inhibits urinary tract germs.

High-acid foods include meats, nuts, plums, prunes, and whole-grain breads and cereals. High-acid drinks include cranberry and other fruit juices.

Here's a note of caution: If you're taking a sulfonamide drug (such as Gantrisin or Gantanol) to treat your infection, *avoid* cranberry juice because its high acid content can interfere with the action of the drug.
●Limit your intake of milk and other products with a high calcium content.
●Avoid caffeine, carbonated beverages, and alcohol because these substances irritate the bladder.

Prevention tip
●Practice sensible hygiene. For ex-

ample, wipe from front to back each time you go to the bathroom. This reduces the chance that germs from bowel movements will enter your urinary tract.
●Change your underpants daily.
●Wear cotton undergarments because cotton "breathes." This enhances ventilation, which deters germ growth.
●Avoid tight slacks that prevent air circulation. Inadequate ventilation encourages germs to multiply and grow.
●Take showers instead of baths because germs in the bath water can enter your urinary tract.
●Avoid bubble baths, bath oils, perfumed vaginal sprays, and strong bleaches and cleansing powders in the laundry. These products can irritate your perineal area, which may trigger germ growth and infection.
●Urinate frequently (every 3 hours) to completely empty your bladder.
●Use the bathroom as soon as you sense you need to. Delayed urination is a major cause of UTIs.
●Urinate after sexual relations. This will help rid your urinary tract of any germs.

When to call the doctor
●Call your doctor right away if you suspect you have a new or repeated UTI.
●Also, call the doctor if you notice such symptoms as an increased urge to urinate, increased urination (especially at night), pain when you urinate, or bloody or cloudy urine.

findings, the patient will usually have other studies, too. (See *Teaching patients about renal and urologic tests,* pages 302 to 309.)

TREATMENTS
Tell the patient that the major treatment goals are relieving pain and urinary frequency, urgency, and hesitancy and teaching about preventive measures and ways to avoid complications.

Discuss the primary treatment for UTI — drug therapy. Then describe lifestyle changes that may prevent recurrent UTIs, mild activity restrictions, dietary measures, and surgery (if indicated).

Activity guidelines
Tell the patient that she needn't restrict most activities. She should, however, avoid prolonged bicycling, motorcycling, and horseback riding. These activities may promote urine reflux and may damage the urinary tract.

Dietary modifications
Advise the patient to consume additional fluids — up to 14 glasses of water daily — to flush out bacteria. However, caution her to avoid coffee, tea, colas, and alcohol. Encourage her to increase her acid intake — especially meats, nuts, fruit juices, and other high-acid foods. Give her a copy of the patient teaching aid *Treating and preventing urinary tract infections,* page 321.

Medications
When culture results identify the causative microorganism, the doctor will prescribe the single-dose or short-term drugs most likely to kill or control the infection. An effective drug rapidly sterilizes the urine and relieves symptoms. Urge the patient to have her urine reanalyzed 1 to 3 days after treatment starts to judge the drug's effectiveness. If she has frequent UTIs, tell her that she may require long-term, low-dose antibiotic prophylaxis.

Explain that other antibiotics, such as sulfonamide and urinary tract antiseptics, may be used to treat UTIs. Mention that the doctor may prescribe a nonnarcotic analgesic to treat pain related to the UTI.

Surgery
If appropriate, inform the patient that surgery may be recommended to correct an obstruction that causes recurrent UTIs. Explain that common obstructive disorders include calculi, tumors, and benign prostatic hyperplasia.

Other care measures
Suggest lifestyle changes to help the patient fight recurrent UTIs. Such changes include improved hygiene habits — for example, wiping the perineum from front to back after using the bathroom to prevent fecal contamination and avoiding tight or synthetic underpants. Recommend taking showers instead of baths, and advise the patient to avoid products that can irritate the perineum. Also advise the patient to urinate after sexual intercourse.

 TIPS AND TIMESAVERS: Encourage the patient to urinate more frequently — every 2 to 3 hours during the day — and to completely empty her bladder each time. Explain that this prevents bladder overdistention and compromised blood supply to the bladder wall (risk factors for UTI).

11

Reproductive conditions

Benign prostatic hyperplasia

Because benign prostatic hyperplasia (BPH) progresses slowly, a patient may not recognize its symptoms right away. Eventually, though, he'll notice a frequent urge to urinate, difficulty starting his urine stream, and waking throughout the night to urinate.

Besides helping your patient identify these and other warning symptoms of BPH, your teaching must explain why prostatic enlargement causes these symptoms. You'll need to discuss what will happen if the patient doesn't have BPH corrected, which tests he'll have to evaluate it, and which treatments he'll undergo, such as surgery to remove prostatic tissue and relieve pressure on the urethra.

BPH most commonly affects elderly men. With this in mind, be prepared to overcome age-related learning barriers, such as impaired vision and memory, hearing loss, and other physical limitations.

Before teaching a patient about BPH, make sure you are familiar with the following topics:
• male genitourinary system, including its normal structure and function
• explanation of nonmalignant tissue overgrowth in the prostate
• signs and symptoms of BPH
• importance of treatment to prevent such complications as renal damage
• diagnostic tests, including physical examination, laboratory studies, and radiologic and endoscopic tests
• experimental drug treatments and balloon dilatation
• transurethral resection of the

prostate (TURP) or open prostatectomy
• at-home catheter care, if appropriate
• referral for sexual counseling, if indicated.

ABOUT THE DISORDER
Explain the normal structure and function of the male genitourinary system. If possible, use an anatomic drawing to point out the prostate gland at the base of the bladder surrounding the urethra.

Tell the patient that BPH is a nonmalignant overgrowth of prostatic tissue. As the gland size increases, it presses inward, compressing the urethra and obstructing urine flow. Eventually, he'll notice symptoms of obstruction — an urgent desire to void, frequent urination (day and night), difficulty starting the urine stream, decreased size and force of the urine stream, dribbling of urine, incontinence, incomplete bladder emptying, urinary tract infection, and acute urine retention.

Inform the patient that BPH is related to aging and that by age 70 most men have some degree of prostate enlargement. Explain that the cause of BPH is unknown, but researchers suspect a metabolic or hormonal condition.

Complications
Caution the patient that BPH may lead to serious complications if it remains untreated. For instance, the patient may notice a decreasing ability to empty his bladder as the enlargement causes resistance to urine flow. This residual urine may lead to urinary tract infection. Ultimately, he

may be unable to void. Then he'll experience acute urine retention and increased bladder pressure, which can result in renal damage if untreated.

DIAGNOSTIC WORKUP

Explain the physical examination to the patient. Tell him that the doctor will examine the prostate gland by inserting a gloved finger into the patient's rectum. He'll also evaluate the rectal sphincter, which indirectly reflects bladder innervation. The doctor will observe the patient as he voids to determine the size and force of his urine stream. He'll be catheterized immediately after urination to measure postvoiding residual volume.

Next, explain the blood and urine tests that evaluate BPH. Tell the patient that blood samples will be drawn to measure blood urea nitrogen, serum creatinine, and acid phosphatase levels. Urine specimens will also be collected for urinalysis and to check for infection. As ordered, teach the patient about radiologic tests such as excretory urography and endoscopic tests such as cystourethroscopy. (See *Teaching patients about reproductive system tests,* pages 337 to 342.)

TREATMENTS

Tell the patient that surgery is the primary treatment for BPH. However, researchers are investigating medications and balloon dilatation to provide long-term relief.

Surgery

Describe two types of surgery — TURP and open prostatectomy — to remove some or all prostatic tissue. (See *Surgical correction of BPH.*) For either operation, explain that the patient may be placed on a low-residue diet before surgery and that the night before surgery he may receive a cleansing enema. The doctor typically prescribes antibiotics, usually erythromycin 500 mg and neomycin 1 g every 4 hours for 24 hours before surgery.

If the patient is having a *transurethral resection,* tell him that the surgeon passes a small tubular instrument into the urethra to visualize the obstructing prostatic tissue. Then he passes an electric cutting loop through the instrument to trim away the tissue. Explain that TURP typically takes less time, requires a shorter hospital stay, and produces less postoperative pain than an open prostatectomy. If the prostate gland is extremely large, however, TURP isn't feasible and an open procedure is usually necessary.

During an *open prostatectomy,* the surgeon makes one of three incisions to expose and remove the obstructing prostatic tissue: suprapubic, retropubic, or perineal. The patient will have an indwelling catheter for several days after surgery. The catheter is connected to a continuous fluid irrigation system to ease the passage of blood clots. Tell him to expect blood in his urine for several days afterward.

Inform the patient that once the bleeding subsides, the catheter will be removed. Warn him that bladder spasms may occur while the catheter is in place, but that medication can be given to provide relief. Following catheter removal, he may experience a sensation of heaviness in the pelvic region, urinary urgency, burning during urination, difficulty controlling urination, and the reappearance of some blood in the urine. Tell him that these effects subside with time.

Medications

Discuss the drugs leuprolide acetate (Lupron) and nafarelin acetate (Synarel), which hold promise for patients who aren't candidates for surgery. Tell the patient that leuprolide acetate reduces prostate volume and improves such signs and symptoms as urinary frequency and urgency and diminished urine stream.

Explain that nafarelin acetate is used to block testosterone production. This drug causes impotence,

Surgical correction of BPH

Inform the patient facing surgery for benign prostatic hyperplasia (BPH) that the operation he'll have depends on several factors, including the extent of prostatic enlargement and the doctor's preferred technique. Describe which operation the surgeon will perform: a transurethral resection or a suprapubic, retropubic, or perineal prostatectomy.

Transurethral resection of the prostate

Explain that transurethral resection is the most common surgical procedure for BPH. After the surgeon inserts a transurethral rectoscope, he excises prostatic tissue under direct visualization, removing it through the urethra as shown here. He uses cautery to control any bleeding during the surgery. Tell the patient that he'll probably have a spinal anesthetic because it achieves better relaxation than a general anesthetic and prevents postoperative nausea and vomiting.

Suprapubic prostatectomy

If the prostate is too large for transurethral removal, inform the patient that the surgeon may perform a suprapubic prostatectomy. In this procedure, the doctor incises the bladder to reach the prostate; then he enucleates the enlarged gland by blunt dissection.

Retropubic prostatectomy

Like the suprapubic approach, a retropubic prostatectomy removes a prostate that's too large for transurethral removal. The surgeon incises the abdomen below the bladder, allowing him to see the prostatic bed and control bleeding.

Perineal prostatectomy

Inform the patient that in perineal prostatectomy the surgeon makes a curved incision behind the scrotum and in front of the anus. This perineal approach permits removal of extensive intraurethral lateral lobe hyperplasia. However, because this method may damage nerves that stimulate erection, it may cause sexual dysfunction. The surgeon probably won't use it if the patient has severe arthritis or chronic obstructive pulmonary disease that prevents the required exaggerated lithotomy position.

Transurethral resection

Penis
Bladder
Scrotum
Prostate
Rectum
Urethra

which persists until therapy is discontinued.

Balloon dilatation
Inform the patient that balloon dilatation, currently being investigated, aims to relieve obstruction by using a saline-filled balloon to dilate the part of the urethra that passes through the prostate.

Other care measures
If the patient will be discharged with an indwelling catheter in place, make sure he knows how to care for the catheter. Tell him when to return to

the health care facility for catheter removal.

Rarely, a patient experiences temporary or permanent impotence after surgery. More commonly, a patient may still be able to have an erection but will become sterile because his semen is expelled backward into the bladder instead of being ejaculated. Reassure the patient that seminal fluid in the bladder does no harm; it's simply eliminated in the urine. If he has problems adjusting sexually, refer him and his partner to a reputable counselor or organization. (See Appendix 2.)

Dysfunctional uterine bleeding

Dysfunctional uterine bleeding can be frightening and puzzling to a patient. Her first questions, "What's happening to my body?" and "Do I have cancer?" will challenge you to provide not only information but also emotional support.

You'll need to review the disorder's many causes, explain how the menstrual cycle works, and discuss appropriate tests and treatments. Most importantly, you'll need to reassure her that dysfunctional uterine bleeding is common and treatable. And if treatment includes a hysterectomy, you'll need to help her accept her altered body image and cope with possible depression or moodiness.

Before teaching a patient about dysfunctional uterine bleeding, make sure you are familiar with the following topics:
• explanation of the disorder
• description of a normal menstrual cycle
• classifications and causes of dysfunctional uterine bleeding
• diagnostic procedures and tests, including dilatation and curettage (D & C), endometrial biopsy, and laparoscopy
• hormonal therapy and adverse reactions
• hysterectomy, if appropriate

• home care after surgery
• sources of information and support.

ABOUT THE DISORDER
Explain to the patient that dysfunctional uterine bleeding is characterized by excessive and irregular uterine bleeding for which no organic cause can be found. Inform her that bleeding is judged abnormal based on its amount, time of occurrence, and duration.

Tell the patient that the disorder can be classified as true dysfunctional or pseudodysfunctional uterine bleeding. *True dysfunctional uterine bleeding* results from a disruption in the hormones that regulate the menstrual cycle and estrogen-progesterone secretions, which, in turn, causes endometrial abnormalities and abnormal bleeding. Explain that this hormonal disruption has several variations. Either the body produces no progesterone (resulting in nonovulatory dysfunctional uterine bleeding), too little progesterone (resulting in irregular endometrial ripening), too much progesterone or slow withdrawal of progesterone (resulting in irregular endometrial shedding), or too little estrogen and no progesterone (resulting in endometrial atrophy).

Pseudodysfunctional uterine bleeding, on the other hand, results from local disorders; endocrine disorders, systemic diseases, or both; and certain drugs. Local disorders include uterine fibroids, cervicitis, pelvic inflammatory disease (PID), and ovarian tumors. Endocrine disorders and systemic diseases include adrenal dysfunction, diabetes mellitus, hypothalamic or pituitary disorders, thyroid dysfunction, idiopathic thrombocytopenic purpura, leukemia, systemic lupus erythematosus, renal or hepatic disease, and obesity. Anticoagulants, oral contraceptives, and possibly digitalis glycosides can also cause abnormal uterine bleeding.

Complications
Emphasize that untreated dysfunc-

tional uterine bleeding can cause anemia. Urge the patient to report changes in breathing rate, dizziness, faintness, fatigue, and sweating to her doctor. Point out that hemorrhage from dysfunctional uterine bleeding can be life-threatening.

DIAGNOSTIC WORKUP
Tell the patient to expect a thorough physical and gynecologic examination. Forewarn her that because dysfunctional uterine bleeding can stem from many causes, the doctor may order several diagnostic tests, including D & C.

Blood and urine tests
Inform the patient that blood and urine tests may provide clues about her health. For instance, they can tell whether she has anemia or abnormal levels of follicle-stimulating hormone, luteinizing hormone, prolactin, or testosterone. Thyroid function and glucose tolerance tests can determine whether a systemic disease is causing the bleeding.

Other tests may include a complete blood count, platelet count, prothrombin time, activated partial thromboplastin time, lupus erythematosus preparation (to rule out systemic lupus erythematosus), and an antinuclear antibody test (to rule out a connective tissue disease). An SMA-12 and a urinalysis may be done to rule out renal and hepatic disease.

Diagnostic procedures
Besides D & C, the doctor may perform endometrial biopsy, hysterosalpingography, hysteroscopy, laparoscopy, or transvaginal ultrasonography. (See *Teaching patients about reproductive system tests,* pages 337 to 342.)

TREATMENTS
Explain that once the doctor determines the cause of uterine bleeding, appropriate treatment can start. For true or PID-induced dysfunctional uterine bleeding, drug therapy is customarily used, unless the patient has

cancer or is pregnant. For bleeding caused by fibroids, uterine cancer, or uterine prolapse, a hysterectomy may be performed.

Medications
If the patient has true dysfunctional uterine bleeding, explain that the doctor commonly prescribes hormonal therapy. If she has pseudodysfunctional uterine bleeding from a disorder such as PID, the doctor may prescribe other drug therapy.

Hormonal therapy
Various hormonal combinations and amounts are used depending on the underlying disorder. For nonovulation or irregular ovulation, estrogen and progesterone may help the endometrium develop normally and stimulate ovulation. Estrogen supplements stimulate the endometrium during the menstrual cycle's proliferative phase. Progesterone supplements, such as medroxyprogesterone (Provera) or norethindrone (Micronor), promote secretory development of the endometrium. If the doctor orders medroxyprogesterone, tell the patient to take it for 10 days, beginning on day 16 of her menstrual cycle. If norethindrone is prescribed, tell her to start the drug on day 5 of her cycle and discontinue it on day 25. She should expect bleeding 3 to 7 days after discontinuing either drug.

For irregular endometrial ripening, the doctor may prescribe progesterone cautiously because if the patient is in the first 4 months of pregnancy, fetal abnormalities may result. For irregular endometrial shedding, the doctor may prescribe a monophasic, biphasic, or triphasic oral contraceptive. Explain that a monophasic drug supplies the same hormonal formula for 21 days, a biphasic drug supplies two different formulas for 21 days, and a triphasic drug supplies three different formulas for 21 days.

For endometrial atrophy, indicating both estrogen and progesterone deficiencies, the doctor usually prescribes an oral contraceptive such as estro-

What happens in abdominal hysterectomy

The patient facing an abdominal hysterectomy will have many questions about the surgery and its aftermath. To answer her questions, review the surgery with her. Begin by describing, as appropriate, the three types of hysterectomies: total (removal of the entire uterus); subtotal (removal of part of the uterus, leaving the cervical stump intact); and radical (removal of the uterus, upper vagina, cervix, and parametrial tissue).

Depending on the surgeon and the operation, the patient may have a midline (vertical) incision, from the umbilicus to the symphysis pubis, or a Pfannenstiel (horizontal, or bikini line) incision.

Once the surgeon makes the incision and identifies major organs and structures, the diseased portions are carefully removed. The incision is then closed and a pad or dressing is applied.

Reassure the patient that the incision usually heals rapidly and the scar fades over time.

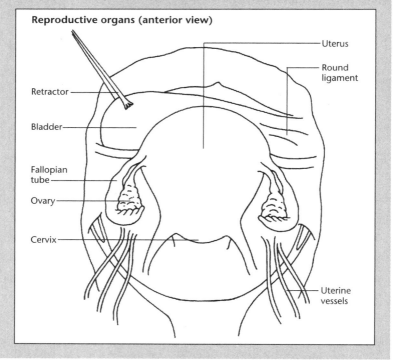

Reproductive organs (anterior view)

Uterus
Round ligament
Retractor
Bladder
Fallopian tube
Ovary
Cervix
Uterine vessels

gen with progestin (Enovid, Ovulen). Reinforce the doctor's instructions on how to take the drug and what to do if she misses a dose. Be sure to explain that withdrawal bleeding similar to a normal menstrual period should occur after she takes the last tablet.

Other drugs
If the patient has PID-induced bleeding, the doctor may prescribe antimicrobial therapy.

Surgery
Explain that surgery involves removing the uterus either abdominally or vaginally, depending on the causative disorder. (See *What happens in abdominal hysterectomy*.)

Preoperative teaching
Inform the patient that she won't be allowed any food or fluids after midnight before surgery and that she'll need to shower with an antibacterial soap and may have to douche. She may also be given a cleansing enema. The morning of surgery, an indwelling urinary catheter is inserted, and an I.V. line is started. The catheter stays in place for 24 hours. Shortly before surgery, the patient receives a sedative.

Postoperative teaching
Tell the patient that she'll return from surgery with a perineal pad in place. Inform her that she can expect some abdominal pain; advise her not to wait until the pain is intense to ask for medication. Show her how to do leg exercises to prevent thromboembolism, and explain that she'll need to get out of bed and walk several times a day. Let her know that she'll still have an I.V. line in place and will be allowed nothing by mouth until she has bowel sounds and is passing flatus; then her diet will progress from clear liquids to solid foods, as tolerated.

Home care instructions
Before the patient leaves the hospital, review home care measures with her. Discuss signs of complications to report to her doctor, and how to clean her wound to prevent infection.

Instruct her to check vaginal discharge daily, explaining that small spots of blood or brownish staining are normal and may last about a week. Instruct the patient to report bleeding that resembles a menstrual period, severe cramping, or hot flashes.

Emphasize that she shouldn't use a tampon, douche, or insert anything into her vagina for 6 weeks. To prevent constipation, suggest a diet high in fiber and tell her to drink plenty of fluids.

 WARNING: Caution the patient not to exercise vigorously, lift any heavy objects, or have sexual intercourse for 6 weeks after surgery. However, urge her to walk or exercise regularly and as tolerable.

Other care measures
The patient may feel depressed or discouraged, especially if the cause of her bleeding has been difficult to diagnose. If she needs a hysterectomy, she might feel even more depressed after surgery because of abrupt hormonal fluctuations.

Reassure her that depression and irritability are common and are only temporary. Encourage her to express her feelings about her altered body image and to feel free to ask questions. Counsel her family about possible mood swings, encouraging them to respond calmly and with understanding. As appropriate, refer the patient and her family to a source of support and information.

Endometriosis
If you've taught patients about endometriosis, you know that apprehension and misunderstanding are common responses to this disease. For instance, a patient may justifiably fear that endometriosis will cause infertility, yet she may wrongly believe that it can cause cancer or even death. By clearly explaining the disease, its possible complications, diagnostic tests, and the impact of treatment options on childbearing, you can correct her misunderstandings and help her make informed decisions about her care.

Before teaching a patient about endometriosis, make sure you are familiar with the following topics:
• pathophysiology of endometriosis and its possible causes

• importance of treatment to prevent or postpone such complications as infertility and endometrioma rupture
• description of an internal pelvic examination and abdominal palpation
• preparation for diagnostic laparoscopy
• medications to relieve pain
• rationale for using oral contraceptives and other hormonal therapies
• surgery, including therapeutic laparoscopy, total hysterectomy and bilateral salpingo-oophorectomy, and presacral neurectomy
• concerns related to the disease, including the effects of pregnancy on endometriosis, dyspareunia relief, and dietary prevention of anemia
• sources of information and support.

ABOUT THE DISORDER

Start by reassuring the patient that endometriosis isn't life-threatening or cancerous (although, rarely, an endometrial mass becomes malignant). Explain that it's a benign growth of endometrial tissue outside the uterus.

Tell the patient that tissue growths, also known as endometrial implants, are usually confined to the pelvic area but can appear anywhere in the body. Explain that hormones secreted during the menstrual cycle influence this misplaced tissue, causing profuse menstrual bleeding and, sometimes, pain in the lower abdomen, vagina, posterior pelvis, and back. Typically, the patient feels suprapubic pain that begins several days before menses and lasts possibly throughout menstruation. Associated symptoms include dyspareunia and painful bowel movements. As the tissue grows and spreads, it irritates and scars surrounding structures, leading to fibrosis, with adhesions and blood-filled cysts.

Inform the patient that the definitive cause of endometriosis is unknown, although several theories exist. (See *Possible causes of endometriosis*.) Tell her that although the causes of endometriosis are controversial, the risk factors are indisput-

able. Women with short menstrual cycles (fewer than 27 days) and long menstrual periods (more than 7 days) are prone to the disease. So are women who have a family history of the disease, have children late in life, and have a retroflexed (tilted) uterus.

Complications

Urge the patient to comply with prescribed treatment because this may help prevent or postpone complications, such as infertility, ruptured endometrioma, and anemia. Explain that endometrial implants cause inflammation. Consequently, fibrosis (scar tissue and adhesions) usually involves the fallopian tubes, ovaries, uterus, bladder, and intestine, binding these organs and contributing to infertility. Also inform her that excessive bleeding during menstruation may lead to anemia.

 WARNING: Tell the patient that sudden, excruciating abdominal pain may signal a ruptured endometrioma (an ovarian cyst composed of endometrial cells) with possible peritonitis. Emphasize that this is a life-threatening complication. Instruct her to go to the hospital emergency department immediately if such pain occurs. To prevent a misdiagnosis of acute appendicitis, advise her to alert the emergency department doctor that she has endometriosis.

DIAGNOSTIC WORKUP

Teach about diagnostic procedures to detect and confirm endometriosis, including a pelvic examination, abdominal palpation, and laparoscopy. (See *Teaching patients about reproductive system tests,* pages 337 to 342.)

Inform the patient that the doctor will take her history and then perform an internal pelvic examination to look for endometrial implants — small bluish areas on the cervix and in the vagina. He'll check the uterosacral ligaments and cul-de-sac for nodules and tenderness, the ovaries for enlargement and tenderness and

Possible causes of endometriosis

If appropriate, discuss the possible causes of endometriosis with the patient. Tell her that the most widely held explanation is retrograde menstruation. According to this theory, some blood "backs up" during every menstrual cycle, flowing up through the fallopian tubes and spilling into the pelvic cavity instead of flowing out through the cervix. Endometrial cells from this menstrual flow attach to structures in the pelvic cavity (for example, the ovaries), where they grow and respond to monthly hormonal changes, causing bleeding into the pelvic cavity.

Alternative theories

Explain that another theory proposes that endometrial cells spread through the lymph and circulatory systems and become implanted throughout the body.

A third theory purports that some endometrial cells are misplaced outside the uterus during embryonic development; after puberty, they respond to cyclic hormonal activity.

Another theory now under scrutiny views endometriosis as an autoimmune disease.

---

the adnexa for fullness and nodules. He will also palpate over the uterus to check its position and, if necessary for accuracy, will perform a digital rectal examination.

Other tests

Inform the patient that the doctor occasionally orders other tests, such as a barium enema, cystoscopy, or cul-de-sac aspiration, to pinpoint sites of endometrial tissue growth.

TREATMENTS

Advise the patient that treatment for endometriosis depends on her age, her desire for childbearing, the disease stage, and the severity of symptoms. Explain that treatment usually begins conservatively, then progresses to more aggressive measures as needed.

Common treatments include medications to relieve pain, reduce inflammation, and suppress ovulation or surgery to remove endometrial implants and adhesions. Or the doctor may recommend combined therapy: medication to shrink the implants, allowing easier surgical removal. This

treatment may also prevent adhesions.

Medications

Tell the patient that the doctor may prescribe analgesics and anti-inflammatory drugs to relieve symptoms and reduce inflammation. Examples include ibuprofen (Advil, Motrin), mefenamic acid (Ponstel, Ponstan), and naproxen (Anaprox). Inform her that hormonal agents may be the primary treatment.

Oral contraceptives

Point out that oral contraceptives treat endometriosis, not just its symptoms. Explain that suppressing ovulation with oral contraceptives has the same effect as pregnancy, which helps resolve endometriosis or cause remission.

Tell the patient that the doctor usually prescribes low-dose oral contraceptives for 6 to 9 months, depending on her response, to reduce menstrual flow and endometrial implants. Mention that this therapy may improve her condition only temporarily.

WARNING: Because oral contraceptives may cause breast tenderness, dizziness, headache, and nausea, advise the patient to take safety precautions. For example, if she feels dizzy, she shouldn't drive a car.

Androgens

Explain that danazol (Danocrine), a synthetic androgen, stops ovulation and menstruation, which induces pseudomenopause. As a result, endometrial cells atrophy, improving endometriosis. The patient can start this therapy immediately after a menstrual period. Tell her that she'll probably take danazol twice a day for 6 to 9 months.

Make sure she understands danazol's possible adverse effects, including acne, decreased breast size, edema, flushing, mild hirsutism, sweating, voice deepening, and weight gain. Explain that these effects result from the drug's androgenic (male hormone) effects and that some effects may be irreversible. She may also experience depression, dizziness, fatigue, and light-headedness.

Gonadotropin-releasing hormone analgesics

If the doctor prescribes nafarelin (Synarel) or a similar drug to reduce circulating estrogen levels, tell the patient that reduction of circulating estrogen levels induces pseudomenopause. Nafarelin is thought to be as effective as danazol in halting the progression of endometrial implants. Be sure the patient understands how this drug works, and warn her about adverse effects related to low estrogen levels, including bone loss, decreased libido, hot flashes, and vaginal dryness.

Surgery

Explain that the goal of surgery is to remove as many endometrial implants, adhesions, or endometriomas as possible and still preserve healthy, functioning tissue. Answer questions about anesthesia, and tell the patient how to follow preoperative and postoperative procedures to prevent complications and ensure recovery.

Therapeutic laparoscopy

Inform the patient that the doctor may remove endometrial implants found during diagnostic laparoscopy. Then explain how the surgeon may combine laparoscopy with such procedures as electrocautery, cryosurgery, or laser surgery to remove the implants. (See *Describing procedures for implant removal.*)

Laparotomy

If the doctor finds an ovarian cyst that contains endometrial implants, he may remove it. After making an abdominal incision to open the pelvic cavity, the surgeon aspirates the cyst, palpates the ovary to determine the cyst's depth, and cuts the cyst from the ovarian cortex. Explain that cyst removal typically relieves dysmenorrhea, abnormal bleeding, and dyspareunia and preserves normal tissue. This helps to maintain reproductive function, with minimal scarring and adhesions.

Hysterectomy and bilateral salpingo-oophorectomy

For widespread endometriosis in a patient who doesn't want to become pregnant, the doctor may recommend total hysterectomy and bilateral salpingo-oophorectomy. Explain that this surgery prevents recurrent endometriosis by removing the uterus, cervix, fallopian tubes, and ovaries. Discuss the aftereffects of surgery, including decreased estrogen levels leading to bone loss, decreased libido, hot flashes, and vaginal dryness. Then, if appropriate, discuss possible treatments, such as estrogen replacement therapy, which reduces the severity of these effects.

Presacral neurectomy

For severe pain with endometriosis, the doctor may perform a presacral neurectomy. Make sure the patient understands that this procedure re-

Describing procedures for implant removal

Tell your patient that during laparoscopy, the surgeon may remove endometrial implants and adhesions without using a knife. This spares healthy tissues, causes little or no bleeding, decreases the risk of infections and swelling, and reduces pain by sealing nerve endings.

Laser surgery

Laser energy can destroy deep-seated, widespread implants and adhesions. The surgeon may use an argon laser beam directed through a fiber-optic wave guide. This beam penetrates 1 to 2 mm but causes minimal scarring. For shallow implants or adhesions, the surgeon may use a carbon dioxide laser. Focused through the laparoscope, this beam travels only 0.1 to 1.2 mm into the target tissue as it raises the tissue's intracellular water temperature to the flash point. In turn, the tissue vaporizes, and the intense heat coagulates blood vessels. Suctioning through the laparoscope removes the vapor.

Cryosurgery

To destroy tissue by freezing, the surgeon uses the laparoscope to introduce a probe into the target area. Then he instills a refrigerant (such as liquid nitrogen or Freon) through an insulated tube to the probe's uninsulated tip. This causes intracapillary thrombosis and tissue necrosis as a frozen tissue ball forms around the tip.

Electrocautery

The surgeon uses laparoscopy to apply a small, wire loop heated by a steady, direct electrical current to implants. This destroys a small amount of tissue on contact. The intense heat coagulates vesicular blood.

---

lieves pain by removing a nerve, but that it doesn't cure endometriosis. Also explain that after this operation she may have constipation and heavier menstrual periods because of vasodilation. If appropriate, teach bowel and bladder retraining techniques.

Other care measures

If you're teaching a young woman with mild endometriosis who wants to have children, tell her that pregnancy may not always cure endometriosis, but it does delay its progression. Explain that the hormonal changes associated with pregnancy cause the implants to soften and atrophy. More than 50% of patients with mild-to-moderate endometriosis are able to become pregnant. However, caution the patient who wants to have children not to postpone pregnancy because infertility is a common complication of endometriosis.

 TIPS AND TIMESAVERS: If your patient has dyspareunia, suggest that she take an analgesic or apply a vaginal lubricant before sexual intercourse. Also suggest that she use a superior or side-lying position for greater control over pressure exerted during intercourse to help prevent dyspareunia.

If the patient feels exceptionally weak and tired or has other symptoms suggesting anemia, urge her to discuss this with her doctor. Advise her to include iron-rich foods, such as liver and soybeans, in her diet and to get adequate rest.

Finally, help the patient cope with endometriosis by acquainting her with a support group. (See Appendix 2.) If she asks for help in dealing with endometriosis-related infertility, refer her to a support group such as Resolve for infertile couples.

Fibrocystic breast changes

In teaching about fibrocystic breast changes, your first priority is to reassure the patient that this condition isn't cancerous. Emphasize that the vast majority of women with fibrocystic breast changes have no increased risk of breast cancer. In fact, many medical experts don't consider fibrocystic breast changes a disorder at all. Because of the condition's benign nature, they've dropped the use of pathologic terms, such as "fibrocystic breast disease," to describe it.

Even so, the patient's symptoms must be taken seriously. If she has lumpy breasts, prepare her for diagnostic tests, such as mammography, ultrasonography, and needle aspiration or biopsy. If she has breast discomfort, review treatment measures, including dietary changes and medications.

Although the patient with fibrocystic breasts may be no more prone to breast cancer than other women, her lumpy breasts may make it harder to detect a malignant tumor. Therefore, be sure to emphasize the need to perform monthly breast self-examinations.

Before teaching a patient about fibrocystic breast changes, make sure you are familiar with the following topics:

• signs and symptoms of fibrocystic breast changes and their relation to the menstrual cycle
• differences between benign and malignant breast lumps
• preparation for diagnostic tests, such as mammography, ultrasonography, and breast biopsy
• dietary modifications, including salt reduction and, possibly, avoidance of methylxanthines
• medications to relieve breast discomfort, such as analgesics, diuretics, danazol or bromocriptine, and hormones
• importance of monthly breast self-examinations
• sources of information and support.

ABOUT THE CONDITION

Tell the patient that fibrocystic breast changes are various differences in the breasts that occur during the menstrual cycle. (See *Cyclical changes in breast tissue.*) Above all, emphasize that the condition is benign. Also stress how common it is: About 50% of all women have signs and symptoms of fibrocystic breast changes, and 90% of all women have tissue changes characteristic of the condition.

Explain that signs and symptoms differ among patients. The most common complaints are lumpy, tender, and painful breasts, but cysts or nipple discharge also may be present. Point out the cyclical nature of most signs and symptoms and their close relationship to the menstrual cycle. Mention that they usually worsen just before the menstrual period and improve afterward.

Tell the patient that estrogen levels increase during the follicular phase of the menstrual cycle, causing fluid retention and glandular tissue proliferation. As breast tissue stretches to accommodate the excess fluid, the patient may experience breast discomfort, often described as a full, aching feeling. Breast discomfort may also result from nerve irritation and inflammation associated with edema and fibrocystic breast changes. Typically, the upper, outer quadrants of both breasts become painful in the week before menstruation. Reassure the patient that this discomfort usually subsides with the start of her menstrual period.

Explain that fibrocystic breast changes may be associated with the formation of one or more lumps called cysts, which are fluid-filled sacs that form in one or both breasts. Cysts tend to enlarge and become tender just before menstruation, then shrink or disappear afterward. Reassure the patient that fibrocystic breast tissue is rarely cancerous.

Inform the patient that an increase in fibrous tissue also may cause breast lumpiness — but again, this change

INSIGHT INTO ILLNESSES

Cyclical changes in breast tissue

Reassure your patient that some lumpiness of the breasts is normal. To help dispel her fears about fibrocystic lumps or swelling, describe the different breast tissues and their sensitivity to cyclical ovarian hormones.

Inside the breast
Tell the patient that the inside of the breast is made up primarily of fat and milk-producing mammary tissue. Explain that the mammary glands produce the milk, and the mammary ducts transport it to the nipple. Tell her that the mammary glands and ducts are sandwiched between layers of fat. These breast structures are held together by fibrous connective tissue.

Fibrocystic breast changes
Teach the patient that cyclical increases in estrogen underlie most benign breast symptoms, although exactly how this happens isn't clear. Just before menstruation, the

breasts may retain water, causing painful swelling. During the same time, two other changes may make the breasts lumpier: One or more cysts may form, and the amount of fibrous breast tissue may increase.

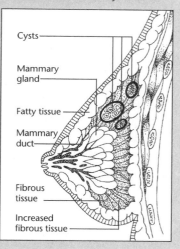

Cysts

Mammary gland

Fatty tissue

Mammary duct

Fibrous tissue

Increased fibrous tissue

---

does not indicate breast cancer. In some patients, fibrocystic breast changes are associated with nipple discharge. If so, advise the patient to see her doctor, particularly if the discharge is spontaneous, persistent, or unilateral.

Discuss how symptoms typically change with age. (See *Fibrocystic breast changes over the life span,* page 336.)

Inform the patient that the cause of fibrocystic breast changes is unknown. However, most researchers agree that ovarian hormones are involved. Fibrocystic breast changes may result from abnormal hormone production or from hypersensitive breast tissues that overrespond to

normal hormone levels. Mention that fibrocystic breast changes are more common in women with early menarche, late menopause, and irregular or anovulatory cycles. Women with fibrocystic breast changes also are more likely to have symptoms of premenstrual syndrome.

Complications
Tell the patient that fibrocystic breast changes seldom cause complications, although the signs and symptoms may progress. Rarely, a patient who undergoes biopsy for a benign breast lump is found to have atypical hyperplasia. This clinical finding, combined with a family history of breast cancer, does increase the risk of

Fibrocystic breast changes over the life span

If your patient has fibrocystic breast changes, explain how the symptoms are likely to change as she ages.

● During the late teens to early 30s, common signs and symptoms of fibrocystic breast changes are breast tenderness and fullness with minimal lumpiness in the week before menstruation.

● During the late 30s to mid-40s, breast pain typically increases and lasts longer during the menstrual cycle. Increasing breast nodularity prompts many women to seek medical evaluation.

● During the late 40s and 50s, a woman may experience increasing discomfort and the sudden onset of painful, solitary, or multiple lumps.

breast cancer. If the patient has atypical hyperplasia, advise her to seek close follow-up care.

DIAGNOSTIC WORKUP

Teach the patient that the diagnostic workup begins with a medical history and physical examination. Explain that the doctor will examine her breasts for lumps, tenderness, and other signs and symptoms. Other tests may include mammography, ultrasonography, needle aspiration, and breast biopsy. (See *Teaching patients about reproductive system tests*, pages 337 to 342.)

TREATMENTS

Reassure the patient that much can be done to relieve her signs and symptoms. Discuss dietary changes and the use of mild analgesics to minimize breast discomfort. Emphasize the importance of performing monthly breast self-examinations to detect suspicious breast changes.

Dietary modifications

Advise the patient to cut down on salt in the week before her menstrual period. Explain that reducing salt intake can help prevent the fluid retention that causes breast discomfort. Instruct her not to add salt to foods during cooking or at the table. Also caution her to avoid the many processed foods with hidden salt.

 TIPS AND TIMESAVERS: List the salt-laden foods that the patient should avoid, such as canned soups, pickles, bacon, baked goods, and commercially prepared foods.

Mention that some patients notice that their signs and symptoms subside when they avoid foods and medications containing caffeine and other methylxanthines. If the patient wants to try this treatment, recommend dietary changes to eliminate methylxanthines. However, point out that this treatment is medically unproven.

Medications

Explain that medication use varies for each patient, depending on her signs and symptoms. Drug therapy may include analgesics, mild diuretics, danazol, bromocriptine, and hormonal therapy. Vitamin E also has been prescribed by some doctors for fibrocystic breast changes.

Analgesics and diuretics

If the patient suffers breast discomfort, suggest that she talk to her doctor about taking aspirin or acetaminophen during the week before her menstrual period. The doctor also may prescribe a mild diuretic, such as chlorothiazide (Diuril) or hydrochlorothiazide (HydroDIURIL), during this time. Explain that the diuretic relieves breast fullness by reducing the amount of fluid in the body. Caution

(Text continues on page 342.)

Teaching patients about reproductive system tests

TEST AND PURPOSE	TEACHING POINTS

Breast biopsy
• To determine if a breast lump is malignant
	• If the patient will have a *needle biopsy,* tell her that the doctor uses a needle to remove a tissue sample from a breast lump. Inform her that this simple procedure is commonly performed in the doctor's office. Tell her that she need not restrict food or fluids and that she will probably receive a local anesthetic. Mention that the procedure may take only 5 to 10 minutes.
	   If the patient will have a *surgical biopsy,* tell her that she may receive either general or local anesthesia. If she's having general anesthesia, instruct her to fast from midnight before the test.
	• Describe what happens during a *needle biopsy:* The doctor cleans the skin of the breast with an antibacterial solution. Then he inserts a needle into the breast lump. Using a syringe, he aspirates a tissue or fluid sample, which he sends to the laboratory for evaluation. Warn the patient that she'll feel some pressure during the procedure.
	   If the patient is scheduled for a *surgical biopsy,* tell her that after she receives a general or local anesthetic, the doctor makes an incision in the breast to expose the mass. He may then incise a portion of tissue or excise the entire mass. Then he sends the specimen to the laboratory for evaluation. The wound is sutured, and an adhesive bandage is applied.
	• Explain what happens after a *needle biopsy:* Once the anesthetic wears off, the breast may feel sore or tender for a while. Advise the patient that the doctor will recommend a mild analgesic for pain relief. Instruct her to watch for and report bleeding, redness, or tenderness at the biopsy site.
	   After a *surgical biopsy,* tell the patient that her vital signs will be checked frequently and she'll receive an analgesic to relieve postsurgical pain. Instruct her to watch for and report bleeding, tenderness, or redness at the biopsy site.

Breast needle aspiration • To determine if a breast lump is a cyst	• Explain that this procedure is used to determine if a lump contains fluid and is, therefore, a cyst. Tell the patient that the procedure involves inserting a needle into the lump to remove any fluid that may be present. Assure her that it's quick, safe, almost always painless, and won't leave a scar.

(continued)

Teaching patients about reproductive system tests

(continued)

TEST AND PURPOSE	TEACHING POINTS
Breast ultrasonography • To help differentiate a cyst from a solid tissue mass	• Inform the patient that this test provides an image of the inside of her breasts and can help detect and evaluate breast lumps. Mention, though, that it can't distinguish whether or not a lump is cancerous. • Explain that, before the test, the patient will probably not need to restrict her diet, medications, or activities. Tell her that she will be asked to remove her clothes from the waist up and put on a hospital gown. Advise her to rest quietly during the test so the operator can concentrate on the images. Reassure her that the test is usually painless. • Describe what happens during the test: In most facilities, the patient is asked to lie on her back. Then a water-soluble gel is applied to her breast. The test operator glides a hand-held transducer back and forth over the breast. Mention that the patient will probably be able to see images of her breast on the monitor, but they'll look obscure. • Tell the patient that she can resume her normal activities immediately after the test.
Colposcopy • To visualize the cervix and vagina • To evaluate vaginal or cervical lesions • To confirm malignancy after a positive Papanicolaou test	• Explain that this test allows close study of the vagina and cervix, and thus provides more information than a routine pelvic examination. Tell the patient that it's safe and painless and takes 5 to 10 minutes. • Describe the procedure: The patient is placed in the lithotomy position. Next, the doctor inserts a vaginal speculum and swabs the cervix to remove any mucus. After viewing the cervix and vagina with the colposcope, he may biopsy areas that appear abnormal. • If a biopsy is performed, tell the patient to abstain from intercourse and not to insert anything into the vagina until the biopsy site heals.
Cystourethroscopy • To diagnose and evaluate urinary tract disorders	• Tell the patient that this 20-minute test permits visualization of the bladder and urethra and helps evaluate the degree of prostatic enlargement and urinary obstruction. Inform him that if a local anesthetic is ordered, he may receive a sedative before the test to help him relax. If a general anesthetic is used, he must fast for 8 hours before the test. • Tell the patient what happens during the test: He lies supine on an X-ray table with his hips and knees flexed. His genitalia are cleaned with an antiseptic solution, and he's draped. The doctor ad-

Teaching patients about reproductive system tests

(continued)

TEST AND PURPOSE	TEACHING POINTS
Cystourethroscopy *(continued)*	ministers a local anesthetic, if appropriate, and introduces the cystourethroscope through the urethra into the bladder. Next, he fills the bladder with irrigating solution and rotates the scope to inspect the entire bladder wall surface. If the patient receives a local anesthetic, warn him that he may feel a burning sensation when the cystourethroscope passes through the urethra. He may also feel an urgent need to urinate as the bladder fills with irrigating solution. • Describe what happens after the test: If the patient received a general anesthetic, his blood pressure, heart rate, and respirations will be monitored every 15 minutes for the first hour after the test, and then hourly until stable. Instruct him to drink plenty of fluids and to take prescribed analgesics. Advise him to avoid alcohol for 48 hours after the test. Reassure him that urinary burning and frequency will soon subside. Instruct him to take antibiotics, as ordered, to prevent bacterial infection. Tell him to report flank or abdominal pain, chills, fever, or decreased urine output to the doctor immediately. Also advise him to notify the doctor if he doesn't void within 8 hours after the test or if bright red blood continues to appear after three voidings.
Dilatation and curettage (D & C) • To obtain tissue samples from reproductive organs to investigate the cause of bleeding • To detect the spread of cancer into the endometrium	• Inform the patient that a D & C takes about 1 hour. Explain that the doctor will obtain tissue samples from the uterus, cervix, endometrium, and other sites for laboratory analysis. If the patient has endometriosis, tell her that a D & C serves as both a test and a treatment and that it may determine the cause of abnormal bleeding and may also correct it. • If the patient will have a general anesthetic, tell her not to eat or drink anything for 8 to 10 hours before the procedure. If she'll be an outpatient, caution her to arrange for transportation home. • Review what happens during the procedure: The patient lies on her back with feet in stirrups. Then she receives local or general anesthesia. The doctor dilates her cervix and scrapes the uterine lining with a curette. Then he sends tissue samples to the laboratory for microscopic evaluation. • Tell the patient that she can go home about 2 hours after the procedure.

(continued)

Teaching patients about reproductive system tests

(continued)

TEST AND PURPOSE	TEACHING POINTS
Excretory urography (intravenous pyelography) • To determine the size, shape, and position of the kidneys, their internal structures, and perirenal tissues • To evaluate and localize urinary obstruction and abnormal accumulation of fluid • To assess and diagnose complications following kidney transplantation	• Explain to the patient that this test evaluates the kidneys and urinary tract. Tell him that it takes about 1 hour. • Discuss pretest preparation: The patient should drink plenty of fluids and then fast for 8 hours before the test. Inform him that he may receive a laxative or other bowel preparation before the test. • Explain what happens during the test: The patient is placed in a supine position on an X-ray table. After injection of a contrast medium, X-rays are taken at specific intervals. Mention that a belt may be placed around his hips to keep the contrast medium at a certain level. Warn him that the X-ray machine will make loud, clacking sounds as it exposes films. Also advise him that he may experience a transient burning sensation and metallic taste when the contrast medium is injected; tell him to report these and any other sensations to the doctor. • After the test, instruct the patient to report symptoms of delayed reaction to the contrast medium, such as itching, hives, and light-headedness.
Hysterosalpingography • To confirm tubal abnormalities, such as adhesions and occlusion • To confirm uterine abnormalities, such as fistulas, adhesions, and the presence of foreign bodies	• Explain to the patient that this test confirms uterine and fallopian tube abnormalities. Tell her that it takes about 15 minutes. • Describe what happens during the test: The patient is placed on her back with her feet in the stirrups. Then the doctor inserts a vaginal speculum and swabs the cervix to remove any mucus. Next he inserts a cannula into the uterus and slowly injects a radiopaque dye. If this triggers cramping, the doctor temporarily stops the injection until the cramps subside. After the dye is injected, the uterus and fallopian tubes are viewed fluoroscopically, and radiographs are taken. Inform the patient that the test may increase the likelihood of pregnancy; as the dye flows through the tubes, it may break up adhesions, stimulate cilia that promote passage of the ovum, or alter cervical mucus to be more receptive to sperm. • After the test, tell the patient to report signs of infection, such as fever, pain, increased pulse rate, malaise, and muscle ache.

Teaching patients about reproductive system tests
(continued)

TEST AND PURPOSE	TEACHING POINTS
Laparoscopy • To visualize the pelvic organs • To determine the extent of endometrial tissue growth and classify the severity of endometriosis • To remove endometrial implants	• Tell the patient that this procedure allows the doctor to view the pelvic organs through a tubelike apparatus. Mention that it may be done with either a local or general anesthetic and that it takes about 1 hour. • Describe what happens during the test: The doctor makes a small abdominal incision through the umbilicus and inserts the laparoscope through it. If minor surgery is necessary (such as to remove an endometrioma or small fibroid tumors), the doctor performs it by passing instruments through the laparoscope. He may inject air into the abdominal cavity to see the internal structures better. • After the test, warn the patient who has had air injected into her abdominal cavity that she might experience shoulder pain from air irritating her diaphragm. Suggest that she lie in a prone position with a pillow under her abdomen to relieve this. Instruct her to watch for signs of infection, such as redness, warmth, or increased tenderness at the incision site.
Mammography • To screen for breast cancer • To investigate palpable and unpalpable breast masses, breast pain, or nipple discharge • To help differentiate benign breast changes and breast malignancy	• Explain to the patient that this test is simply an X-ray of the breast. It can be used to screen for breast cancer or to diagnose the cause of a breast complaint. Assure her that, although the test uses radiation, the amount is negligible. • Advise the patient to tell her doctor if she might be pregnant or is breast-feeding. Also tell her to ask the doctor if she should avoid using deodorant on the test day (some deodorants contain substances that may interfere with test results). Instruct her to avoid lotions, which may make the breast slippery. Tell her that she'll be asked to take off her clothing above the waist, put on a gown, and remove jewelry from her neck. • Describe what happens during the test: The patient may be asked to sit, stand, or lie still for the test. A technician will help her position her breast on an X-ray plate. Then another plate will be pressed down toward the first one to flatten the tissue. Warn the patient that she'll probably feel a cold sensation where her breast touches the plate and that the compression may cause some discomfort. Tell her that she may be asked to lift her arm or use her hand to hold her other breast out

(continued)

Teaching patients about reproductive system tests

(continued)

TEST AND PURPOSE	TEACHING POINTS
Mammography *(continued)*	of the way. While the X-ray is being taken, she'll be told to hold her breath for a few seconds. Then the procedure will be repeated for the other breast. • After the test, tell the patient that she may resume her normal diet and activities.
Pelvic ultrasonography • To detect foreign bodies and distinguish between cystic and solid masses (tumors)	• Describe the test to the patient, and tell her that it takes about 30 minutes. Reassure the pregnant patient that the test won't harm the fetus. • Instruct the patient to drink 6 to 8 glasses of fluid 1½ to 2 hours before the test. Tell her *not* to void before the test because a full bladder serves as a landmark to define other pelvic organs. • Explain what happens during the test: The patient is positioned on her back and her abdomen is coated with mineral oil. Then the technician guides a transducer over the abdomen to visualize the uterus, vagina, and adjoining organs. • Tell the patient that she will be allowed to empty her bladder immediately after the test.

the patient about the potential effects of fluid and electrolyte imbalance.

Danazol

If the patient has severe breast pain that can't be relieved by conservative measures, the doctor may prescribe the synthetic androgen danazol (Danocrine). Danazol reduces hormonal stimulation of the breast, thereby helping to reduce breast pain and nodularity.

 WARNING: Caution the patient that danazol can cause harsh adverse reactions, including acne, increased clitoris size, decreased breast size, edema, hot flashes, increased facial hair, menstrual irregularities, voice changes, and weight gain. Also point out that her symptoms may return, necessitating another course of therapy.

Bromocriptine

A prolactin blocker, bromocriptine mesylate (Parlodel) helps some women, but it also causes adverse reactions. Caution the patient that possible adverse reactions include dizziness, headache, and nausea. Like danazol, bromocriptine is usually reserved for patients with severe pain.

Hormonal therapy

Oral contraceptive use (estrogen-progestin combinations) or progesterone therapy helps to relieve breast tenderness in some patients. For example, medroxyprogesterone acetate (Provera) blocks estrogen's effects on the breast. If the doctor prescribes Provera, reinforce instructions on when to take it — typically on days 15 through 25 of the menstrual cycle. Inform her of potential adverse effects.

Surgery
As a last resort, the patient may need to have a cyst surgically removed. Usually, this operation is necessary only if a cyst can't be aspirated or if a solid mass remains after aspiration. Tell the patient that the procedure is usually done under local anesthesia in an outpatient unit.

Other care measures
Encourage the patient to perform monthly breast self-examinations. Advise her to examine her breasts at the same time during each menstrual cycle — ideally, 2 or 3 days after her menstrual period — so she doesn't become confused by her normal cyclical fibrocystic changes. Instruct her to contact her doctor if she notices any new or unusual lumps or increased tenderness.

Advise the patient to wear a support bra — even while sleeping — when she experiences breast discomfort. Point out that a support bra is especially important during exercise.

To help her cope with the condition, refer her to an agency or organization that can provide further information and support. (See Appendix 2.)

Vulvovaginitis and cervicitis

A patient with vulvovaginitis and cervicitis needs information to help limit contagion as well as to avoid the complications of cervicitis. But you may need to overcome emotional obstacles before you can teach effectively. After all, the patient may feel hesitant about describing her symptoms. Or she may be too embarrassed to discuss treatment and preventive measures.

Once you establish a rapport with the patient, your teaching will focus on promoting compliance with treatment. You'll also encourage regular gynecologic checkups, especially if the patient is sexually active, and

prompt treatment for new or recurring symptoms of infection.

Before teaching a patient with vulvovaginitis and cervicitis, make sure you are familiar with the following topics:
• types of vulvovaginitis and cervicitis
• predisposing factors
• signs and symptoms
• sexually transmitted diseases (STDs) that resemble vulvovaginitis and cervicitis
• complications such as pelvic inflammatory disease
• diagnostic workup, including blood tests, pelvic examination, and smears
• medications, such as antifungals, antiprotozoals, antibiotics, and conjugated estrogen
• how to administer an intravaginal medication
• importance of sexual abstinence or modification of sexual activity during treatment
• treatment of sexual partners
• hygiene and comfort measures
• sources of information and support.

ABOUT THE DISORDER
Tell the patient that vulvovaginitis and cervicitis are inflammations of the vulva, vagina, and cervix that cause vaginal discharge. Discuss the patient's type of vulvovaginitis: candidiasis, trichomoniasis, nonspecific vaginitis, or atrophic vaginitis. In these disorders, discharge originates in the vagina. If appropriate, explain that the two major types of cervicitis are *Chlamydia* and gonorrhea; in these disorders, discharge originates from the cervix.

The disorders are caused by various microorganisms or conditions. They may be episodic and easily treated, or they may be chronic, requiring recurrent treatment.

Except for candidiasis, nonspecific vaginitis, and atrophic vaginitis, the inflammations may be sexually transmitted. (See *Distinguishing among types of vulvovaginitis and cervicitis,* pages 344 and 345.) As appropriate,

INSIGHT INTO ILLNESSES
Distinguishing among types of vulvovaginitis and cervicitis

TYPE AND DESCRIPTION	PREDISPOSING FACTORS	SIGNS AND SYMPTOMS
VULVOVAGINITIS		
Candidiasis (moniliasis or yeast vaginitis) A change in the vaginal environment permits an overgrowth of *Candida albicans,* a common inhabitant of the vagina.	Pregnancy, oral contraceptives, antibiotic use, obesity, douching, diabetes, excessive carbohydrate intake, and constrictive clothing with poor ventilation (girdles and tight nylon clothing, for example)	Tell the patient that she may have a thick, white, curdlike vaginal discharge and vaginal itching, slight burning, and erythema.
Trichomoniasis (Trichomonas vaginitis) *Trichomonas vaginalis* bacteria are sexually transmitted to the vagina.	Multiple male sexual partners	Inform the patient that she may have profuse, thin, foul, yellow and, possibly, frothy vaginal discharge; vaginal spotting; vaginal and vulvar erythema; hemorrhagic spots on the cervix; and vaginal burning. Additional symptoms may include perineal irritation, dysuria, and urinary frequency.
Nonspecific vaginitis (*Gardnerella* vaginitis *or Haemophilus* vaginitis) By an unclear mechanism, vaginal microorganisms, predominantly *Gardnerella vaginalis,* multiply, creating bacterial overgrowth.	Vaginal tissue trauma, sexual intercourse	Tell the patient that she may have moderately increased, thin, gray-white, fish-scented vaginal discharge.
Atrophic vaginitis Decreased estrogen levels in menopause cause atrophy of the vaginal mucosa. Because the vagina can't maintain a correct acid pH, the	Menopause	Inform the patient that she may have scant, thin vaginal discharge; vaginal spotting; dryness on sexual intercourse; vaginal burning; pruritus; thin labia or less pubic hair;

Distinguishing among types of vulvovaginitis and cervicitis *(continued)*

TYPE AND DESCRIPTION	PREDISPOSING FACTORS	SIGNS AND SYMPTOMS
Atrophic vaginitis *(continued)* vagina becomes thin and fragile.		fissuring of the vulva; or smooth, red, shiny vaginal walls.

CERVICITIS

TYPE AND DESCRIPTION	PREDISPOSING FACTORS	SIGNS AND SYMPTOMS
Gonorrhea *Neisseria gonorrhoeae* bacteria are sexually transmitted to the vagina.	Multiple male sexual partners	Tell the patient that she may or may not have symptoms, including profuse, yellow, purulent vaginal discharge; dysuria; cervical erythema; and cervical edema and tenderness. Add that other possible symptoms include vulvovaginal irritation and pharyngitis, proctitis, or pelvic involvement. Mention that her male sexual partners may have urethritis.
Chlamydia **cervicitis** *Chlamydia trachomatis* bacteria are sexually transmitted to the vagina.	Multiple male sexual partners	Explain to the patient that she may or may not have symptoms. For example, she may have mild, mucoid, clear to creamy vaginal discharge; dysuria; and cervical erythema and edema. Add that her male sexual partners may experience urethritis.

discuss STDs that may coexist with or mimic these infections.

Complications

Stress that strict compliance with treatment is the best way to avoid complications. Although vulvovaginitis rarely causes complications, fissures and adhesions may develop from inflammation and scarring in chronic atrophic vaginitis.

Inform the patient that cervicitis complications are more severe because of the infection's type and the proximity to the upper reproductive tract. Both *Chlamydia* and gonorrhea can cause pelvic inflammatory disease, which can lead to infertility.

What's more, *Chlamydia* can be passed from a mother to a neonate during birth. Inclusion conjunctivitis will result if the bacteria come in contact with the neonate's eyes. The neonate may contract pneumonia if bacteria infect the upper airways.

In the same way, gonorrhea can be transmitted to the neonate, causing ophthalmic infection and, rarely, disseminated infection — if the pregnancy reaches term. Explain that pregnant patients with gonorrhea have a higher incidence of spontaneous abortion and premature births.

Additional complications of untreated gonorrhea include arthritis-dermatitis syndrome and, rarely, meningitis, endocarditis, or pericarditis. Adult conjunctivitis may result from autoinoculation with purulent discharge. Even more serious are the epidemic complications caused by disease spread. For example, the microorganisms *Chlamydia trachomatis* and *Neisseria gonorrhoeae* are transmitted sexually from partner to partner. Untreated *Chlamydia* may cause urethritis and epididymitis. Untreated gonorrhea in men may cause urethritis, epididymitis, urethral stricture, or disseminated gonococcal infection.

DIAGNOSTIC WORKUP
Inform the patient that the doctor will perform a pelvic examination to assess vaginal discharge and to obtain vaginal and cervical smears for analysis. He may also order a complete blood count to detect infection.

Pelvic examination
Because many patients feel apprehensive about a pelvic examination, take extra time to allay your patient's anxiety — especially if this is her first examination. Encourage her to express her feelings and to let the doctor know if she experiences discomfort during the examination. Explain that the doctor will use a speculum to examine the vulva, vagina, and cervix, and will use his hands to examine the uterus, fallopian tubes, and

ovaries. Mention that he may or may not perform a rectal examination.

Explain that the vaginal smear obtained during the examination is studied with a microscope to identify the type of vulvovaginitis. Once the type is identified, the doctor prescribes the appropriate drug therapy. If the doctor suspects cervicitis, he'll send the smear to the laboratory for culture and sensitivity studies and a Gram stain to detect gonorrhea or for other analysis to detect *Chlamydia*. Mention that test results will be available within 48 hours.

Inform the patient that vulvovaginitis or cervicitis may be detected if routine Papanicolaou test results indicate inflammation (white blood cells but no malignant cells). Tell her that the infectious organism may or may not be identified on the Pap test but that treatment is necessary. Instruct her to have the Pap test repeated in 3 months.

TREATMENTS
Inform your patient that medication is the primary treatment for vulvovaginitis and cervicitis. Emphasize that she and her partner require concurrent treatment to avoid reinfection and recurrent cervicitis. The doctor will also advise sexual abstinence during treatment and may recommend sitz baths to soothe perineal irritation and to minimize odor.

Medications
Explain that the doctor may prescribe medication based on an initial clinical impression. However, he may change the medication, depending on diagnostic test results. Remind the patient that effective drug therapy kills or controls the causative microorganism.

The doctor will prescribe antifungal agents to treat candidiasis, antiprotozoal agents for trichomoniasis, other antimicrobial agents for nonspecific vaginitis and both kinds of cervicitis, and conjugated estrogen for atrophic vaginitis. Add that the drugs may be administered orally or intravaginally.

WARNING: Stress that the patient must complete the prescribed medication regimen. Caution her that absence of symptoms doesn't necessarily mean absence of infection.

Other care measures
Discuss specific hygiene measures and sexual abstinence that accompany drug treatment.

Personal hygiene
Teach the patient about personal hygiene practices that minimize perineal irritation and odor. As appropriate, offer advice for soothing discomfort from vulvovaginal irritation. (See *Tips for relieving vulvovaginal irritation.*)

Sexual abstinence
Inform the patient that sexual abstinence is essential in cervicitis and in some forms of vulvovaginitis. Tell her that her partner also must be treated for and cured of STDs before he can resume sex. If appropriate, direct her to advise her sexual partners to be examined and treated by their own doctors or in a public health or STD clinic.

Caution the patient and her infected sexual partner to wait 48 hours to 1 week or longer after completing treatment before resuming sexual relations. Explain that the doctor may need to perform a follow-up examination, and that cultures may be necessary before he approves resumed sexual activity.

Point out that some patients have intercourse using condoms during treatment. However, they still risk infecting each other.

Tell the patient with gonorrhea that her name must be reported to the local public health department, and that she'll be asked to identify her sexual partners to ensure that they receive treatment.

Advise the patient with a nonsexually transmitted vulvovaginitis (candidiasis, nonspecific vaginitis, or atrophic vaginitis) that sexual absti-

Tips for relieving vulvovaginal irritation

If your patient has vulvovaginal irritation, provide the following tips to soothe the irritation and avoid recurrence.
• Shower daily. If discharge or odor seems excessive, wash between showers with soap and water. Rinse soap away thoroughly to avoid increasing irritation.
• Avoid tub baths, especially with bubbles or oils.
• Change underwear daily.
• Use unscented, white toilet tissue and sanitary napkins.
• Avoid using feminine hygiene deodorant sprays, douches, perfumes, creams, or chemicals around the perineum.
• Wear white cotton underwear.
• Avoid nylon pantyhose without a cotton crotch and tight panties made of synthetic fabrics that inhibit ventilation.
• Change a wet bathing suit promptly rather than wear it until it dries.
• Avoid contamination by remembering to wipe the perineal area from front to back each time you use the bathroom.
• Take antibiotics cautiously because some can cause candidiasis.
• Consider using alternative birth control methods if oral contraceptives cause recurrent candidiasis.

nence can minimize vulvovaginal irritation. Add that her partners don't need treatment unless she has recurrent infection.

 TIPS AND TIMESAVERS: Suggest that the patient with atrophic vaginitis use a lubricant during intercourse to enhance her comfort.

Medical checkups

Urge the patient to seek prompt evaluation and treatment for recurrent vaginal discharge or irritation. Explain that because infection — especially cervicitis — can recur with or without symptoms, she should schedule regular gynecologic checkups. Finally, refer the patient to an appropriate source of information and support. (See Appendix 2.)

12

Cancer

Bladder cancer

Bladder cancer accounts for about 40,000 new cancer cases and more than 10,000 deaths annually. Because this cancer commonly recurs after treatment, your teaching should emphasize warning signs, risk factors, and the importance of regular follow-up evaluations.

Your teaching will also cover the test and treatment procedures used initially and in ongoing care. Of course, you'll individualize your teaching to the patient's cancer stage and his particular need for encouragement and support.

Before teaching a patient about bladder cancer, make sure you are familiar with the following topics:
• where bladder cancer develops
• signs and symptoms of bladder cancer, such as hematuria and dysuria
• risk factors, including industrial exposure to carcinogens, cigarette smoking, and a high-protein, high-fat diet
• complications and the risk of recurrent bladder cancer
• diagnostic and staging studies, including laboratory tests, excretory urography, retrograde cystography, cystoscopy, bone scans, and ultrasonography
• explanation of treatments, especially chemotherapy, radiation therapy, and surgery (such as transurethral resection of the bladder, cystectomy, and urinary diversion)
• management of urinary diversion, if appropriate
• sources of information and support.

ABOUT THE DISORDER
Explain that bladder cancer usually originates in the mucosal tissue that lines the bladder wall. Disease confined to the mucosal layer is superficial (noninvasive). Once rooted in the muscular layer, the cancer is termed invasive. From there, it may metastasize, growing and replicating rapidly and erratically and then spreading when the tumor cells break away and enter the blood or lymphatic circulation.

Bladder cancer can mimic other diseases such as urinary tract infection. The patient may be asymptomatic, or he may experience episodic hematuria and accompanying dysuria, urinary frequency and urgency, tenesmus, nocturia, pelvic pressure, bladder irritability, fatigue, and weight loss.

Point out that no one knows exactly what causes bladder cancer, but certain predisposing factors have been identified. (See *Risk factors for bladder cancer,* page 350.)

Complications
Despite treatment, patients with superficial disease have a 30% to 80% chance for disease recurrence. However, only about 10% of superficial bladder cancers develop into invasive disease. With invasive disease, the chance for metastasis increases to 40% to 90%.

DIAGNOSTIC WORKUP
Explain that the patient will have a complete physical examination, including a rectal or vaginal examination to search for masses. Then the patient may undergo blood and urine tests, excretory urography, retrograde cystography, cystoscopy, and a bone scan. Other diagnostic imaging pro-

INSIGHT INTO ILLNESSES

Risk factors for bladder cancer

Bladder cancer has a higher incidence in industrialized nations, particularly in urban areas. Persons at high risk include:
- elderly patients with chronic obstructive pulmonary disease or bladder calculi
- patients who have undergone pelvic radiation therapy or drug therapy with cyclophosphamide (Cytoxan)
- patients with recurring urinary tract infections associated with indwelling catheterization

- hairstylists
- metal workers
- painters
- rubber workers
- textile workers
- leather finishers
- other laborers exposed to environmental carcinogens.

Lifestyle factors
Other risk factors for bladder cancer include cigarette smoking and a diet high in protein and fat.

cedures include a chest X-ray, a computed tomography scan, magnetic resonance imaging (MRI), and ultrasonography. (See *Teaching patients about tests to diagnose cancer,* pages 388 to 399.) Explain whether the test will confirm the diagnosis, stage the disease, or monitor the patient's progress with treatment.

Laboratory tests
Advise the patient that blood will be drawn for a complete blood count and chemistry profile. Explain that test findings can reveal conditions associated with bladder cancer, such as anemia, as well as help stage an existing disease. For example, elevated alkaline phosphatase levels suggest that the cancer has spread to the bones.

Inform the patient that he'll supply a urine specimen for analysis to detect bacteria, protein, and blood. Additional cytologic studies may reveal cancer cells in the urine.

TREATMENTS
Explain that treatment for bladder cancer varies, depending on the patient's lifestyle, other medical problems, and mental outlook. As appro-

priate, teach the patient about chemotherapy, radiation therapy, and surgery, such as transurethral resection of the bladder (TURB) or cystectomy. Investigational treatments include biotherapy, neoadjuvant chemotherapy and radiation therapy, and photodynamic therapy.

Activity guidelines
Advise the patient to alternate activity with rest periods to conserve his energy, especially while he's undergoing treatment. Encourage him, however, to continue participation in his usual activities of daily living.

Medications
Whether the patient is having systemic chemotherapy, intravesical chemotherapy, or an investigational treatment such as biotherapy, teach him about its purpose, method of administration, and potential adverse effects.

Systemic chemotherapy
Systemic chemotherapy is typically chosen for locally extensive bladder cancer and metastatic cancer. Several drugs may be given intravenously in combination. The most active agent

is cisplatin (Platinol). Other active agents include doxorubicin (Adriamycin), methotrexate sodium (Folex), and vinblastine sulfate (Velban).

Intravesical chemotherapy

Used for treating superficial tumors (especially tumors in many sites) and for preventing tumor recurrence, intravesical chemotherapy directly washes the bladder with anticancer drugs. Explain to the patient that he will lie horizontally as the drug flows through a catheter into his bladder. Then, as directed, he'll turn from side to side and onto his back to ensure complete lavage of the inner bladder wall.

Radiation therapy

Inform the patient that radiation therapy destroys the cancer cells' ability to grow and multiply. Point out that, although radiation also affects normal cells, these cells usually recover quickly.

Make sure the patient understands when and where he'll receive radiation therapy and who will administer it. Reinforce the doctor's explanations, and answer any questions.

Describe common adverse effects of radiation therapy, such as mouth sores, dry mouth, nausea and vomiting, diarrhea or constipation, stomach upset, muscle ache, weakness, numbness or tingling, hair loss, fatigue, and dry or sensitive skin. Advise the patient to notify the doctor if adverse effects persist or become especially troublesome or if fever or unusual pain develops.

Combination therapy

The patient who has a localized bladder tumor too extensive for surgical removal may be a candidate for an experimental combination of radiation and chemotherapy. This adjuvant therapy shrinks the tumor so that surgery can effectively remove it or so that the bladder can be retained.

Biotherapy

Also known as immunotherapy, this investigational treatment uses the intravesical route to instill interferonalpha and tumor necrosis factor. Explain that these agents may stimulate the patient's immune system to produce natural substances that kill abnormal cells or delay cancer cell growth.

Photodynamic therapy

Tell the patient scheduled for this treatment that it requires an I.V. injection of a photosensitizing agent called hematoporphyrin derivative (HPD). Because malignant tissue appears to have an affinity for HPD, superficial bladder cancer cells readily absorb the drug. Then the doctor uses a cystoscope to introduce a laser light into the bladder. Exposing HPD-impregnated tumor cells to light kills them.

 WARNING: Caution the patient to avoid sunlight for about 30 days after undergoing photodynamic therapy because HPD sensitizes both tumor tissue and normal tissue to light.

Surgery

As appropriate, teach the patient about bladder cancer surgery: TURB or cystectomy.

Transurethral resection of the bladder

Most commonly performed to remove superficial and early bladder cancers, TURB requires the surgeon to insert a cystoscope through the urethra and into the bladder to remove lesions under local anesthetic. Briefly explain the procedure. Inform the patient that he may receive a local anesthetic and be awake during treatment.

Reassure him that he should experience little or no discomfort and that postoperative effects, such as hematuria and a burning sensation during urination, should quickly subside. If he experiences additional discomfort with painful bladder spasms, instruct him to request pain-relieving medica-

Teaching about urinary diversions

If your patient is scheduled for a simple or radical cystectomy, he'll need a urinary diversion to substitute for his bladder. Teach him about the diversion he'll receive.

Ileal loop or ileal conduit

Also called a ureteroileostomy or urostomy, ileal loop or conduit is one of the most commonly performed supravesicular urinary diversions. The surgeon first sutures about 6" (15 cm) of the ileum closed. Next, he attaches the ureters to the ileum and pulls the ileum through the abdominal wall to form a stoma. Then he reconnects the bowel.

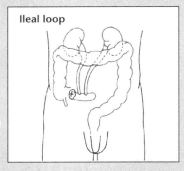

Ileal loop

Teaching points

Tell the patient that he'll awaken from surgery with a nasogastric tube in place, and he won't be allowed to eat for several days. He'll also have an ostomy bag in place. This urine-collecting bag won't be changed for several days. Warn him that initially after surgery, his urine will contain blood. Also explain that he may see catheters or stents protruding from the stoma and into the urine-collecting bag. These devices, which assist healing, will be removed a few days after surgery. Urge the patient to move carefully to avoid dislodging them.

Possible complications

Review possible problems, such as anuria from edema or obstruction at the ureterointestinal anastomosis; urine or fecal leakage at the anastomosis; abdominal distention or a dusky stoma from vascular infarction of the conduit site; stomal stenosis; pyelonephritis; renal calculi; and skin problems such as stomal ulceration.

Ureterosigmoidostomy or ureteroileosigmoidostomy

If the surgeon will perform ureterosigmoidostomy or ureteroileosigmoidostomy, tell the patient that his ureters will be diverted into his sigmoid colon so that he will void through his anus. He won't need to wear an ostomy bag. This procedure is performed only if the patient has good anal sphincter tone.

Teaching points

Advise the patient to sit or stand frequently after surgery to avoid urine reflux. Also warn him that this diversion may produce urinary incontinence when he passes flatus. Add that following a diet low in gas-forming foods may help to allay this problem. Teach the patient to avoid possible electrolyte imbalances related to this diversion by following a diet low in chloride and salt and by taking potassium supplements.

Possible complications

Explain that anuria — resulting from ureteral obstruction, stricture, edema, or fecal matter and mucus — can lead to kidney failure. Also, urine leakage from the anastomosis, pyelonephritis, electrolyte imbalances, and renal calculi may complicate ureterosigmoidostomy.

Ureterostomy

Teach the patient that ureterostomy involves diverting the ureters

Teaching about urinary diversions *(continued)*

through an opening on the abdominal wall. Depending on the procedure, one or more stomas will be created. For example, the patient will have one stoma if the surgeon performs a transureteroureterostomy, which directs one ureter into the other so that only one tube opens to the outside.

The patient will have two stomas if the surgeon performs a double-barrel ureterostomy, which brings the two ureters side by side to the abdominal surface. Because this procedure can be completed quickly, the surgeon may perform it in a patient with low tolerance for anesthesia.

Teaching points
Tell the patient that he will need to wear an ostomy bag — an external urine-collecting bag — after surgery. However, because the stoma created by this diversion rises very little above skin level, the ostomy bag may adhere poorly. Recommend using an adhesive-backed ostomy bag for better results.

Possible complications
Warn the patient that a dusky (cyanotic) stoma may signal vascular insufficiency, which can lead to stenosis.

tion. Point out that the operation shouldn't interfere with normal genitourinary function. Potential complications can include hematuria, urine retention, bladder perforation, and urinary tract infection.

Review care after TURB. Inform the patient that he'll have an indwelling urinary catheter for 1 to 5 days to ensure urine drainage and that he may need continuous bladder irrigation for 24 hours or more. Advise him that slight hematuria may last for several weeks after the resection. However, he should promptly report bleeding or hematuria that lasts longer than several weeks, fever, chills, or flank pain.

Encourage him to drink plenty of water — about 10 glasses (80 oz [2.8 L]) daily — and to void every 2 to 3 hours. Explain that a high fluid intake reduces the risk of urinary tract infection, clot formation, and urethral obstruction. Stress that he shouldn't ignore the urge to urinate.

To promote healing and reduce the risk of bleeding from increased intra-abdominal pressure, advise the patient to refrain from sexual and other strenuous activity, not to lift anything heavier than 10 lb (4.5 kg), and

to continue taking a stool softener or other laxative until the doctor orders otherwise.

Emphasize the importance of regular follow-up examinations to assess the need for further treatment. Point out that early detection and removal of bladder tumors through transurethral resection may prevent the need for cystectomy.

Cystectomy
If the patient has advanced bladder cancer, removal of the bladder and surrounding structures may be necessary. Cystectomy may be partial (segmental), simple (total), or radical. For a single, easily accessible tumor, the patient may have a partial cystectomy to remove the diseased portion and preserve bladder function. For multiple tumors or extensive cancer, he may have a simple cystectomy to remove the entire bladder, preserve surrounding structures, and create a permanent urinary diversion. (See *Teaching about urinary diversions*.)

For muscle-invasive primary bladder cancer, the surgeon may recommend a radical cystectomy to remove the bladder and all surrounding diseased tissues and structures and to create a permanent urinary diversion.

Provide encouragement and support to the patient having this operation. Radical and simple cystectomy can cause psychological problems related to an altered body image and to loss of sexual or reproductive function. The surgery typically produces impotence in men, although sometimes the surgeon can preserve the nerves needed for ejaculation. In women, the surgery may change the vaginal structure, which may cause discomfort or pain with intercourse.

Reassure the patient that, with adequate support services, he can continue most of his usual activities. Arrange for him to consult an enterostomal therapist, who can provide additional instruction and support.

Other care measures

Stress the importance of complying with follow-up appointments to assess healing and detect recurrent disease. The rate of bladder cancer recurrence is high for patients who retain their bladders. Even those who have undergone cystectomy can still develop metastatic disease.

Advise the patient to report dysuria, frequency, and hematuria to the doctor as soon as possible. Point out that he'll need regular yearly physical examinations and diagnostic tests. As appropriate, refer him to sources of information and support. (See Appendix 2).

Breast cancer

Although all women are vulnerable to breast cancer, several factors, such as early onset of menarche and a family history of the disease, increase the risk for some. Nevertheless, earlier detection, more accurate staging, improved treatment, and better long-term follow-up care have lengthened disease-free periods.

Teaching about breast cancer can save or lengthen lives. If your patient suspects breast cancer, your first teaching priority may involve help-

ing her to voice her concerns about the disease and its treatment. Other priorities include informing her about the disease, correcting misconceptions, and providing emotional support.

Specifically, you'll describe a diagnostic workup that may include mammography, biopsy, and a body scan. If test results confirm breast cancer, you'll explain treatment options and recommend ways to reduce or eliminate the adverse effects of treatment. Finally, because the patient is at risk for recurrent breast cancer and for metastasis, you'll emphasize the benefits of complying with follow-up care, performing breast self-examination, and recognizing signs and symptoms of cancer elsewhere in the body. Throughout your teaching, you'll be challenged to ease the patient's anxiety and to maintain a positive focus.

Before teaching a patient about breast cancer, make sure you are familiar with the following topics:
• risk factors and warning signs
• description of breast structure and tumor sites
• breast cancer stages
• diagnostic tests, such as blood tests, mammography, and biopsy
• chemotherapy, hormonal therapy, and radiation, including how to combat adverse effects
• types of breast cancer surgery and perioperative considerations, such as preparation for surgery, pain after surgery, and coping with emotional distress
• breast prosthesis and reconstruction
• postmastectomy care, including lymphedema and infection prevention, strengthening exercises, and tips for dressing
• follow-up care
• sources of information and support.

ABOUT THE DISORDER

Explain that the cause of breast cancer is unknown, although researchers recently found a gene that may predispose some women to a certain form of the disease. Women with a statistically higher risk for breast cancer include those with a history of the disease (a close relative with breast cancer) and those who have experienced an early menarche (before age 12) or late menopause (after age 50). Nulliparity or first childbirth after age 30 is also a risk factor. However, most women who develop breast cancer have no significant risk factors.

Describe normal breast anatomy, including lobes, lobules, acini, and ducts. Also discuss possible tumor sites. (See *Explaining breast structure and tumor sites*, page 356.)

Review cancer's warning signs: any breast lump or mass; a change in breast symmetry or size; a change in breast skin, such as thickening, dimpling, swelling, ulceration, reddening, or warming in spots; nipple discharge in a nonlactating woman; or nipple itching, burning, erosion, or retraction.

Complications
Inform the patient that cancer in one breast increases the risk of cancer developing in the other breast or spreading to another site. Be discreet, though, in deciding when and how to teach about potential complications, and try not to increase the patient's anxiety. Stress that early detection of cancer recurrence carries a greater chance for control or cure.

DIAGNOSTIC WORKUP
Tell the patient that she may undergo extensive testing to help confirm cancer, select and monitor treatment, predict prognosis, and check for recurrence.

Understandably, the patient may feel fearful and powerless as she endures these tests and awaits the results. Your teaching can support her through this difficult time. Help her maintain a sense of control by clearly explaining the test procedures and encouraging her to voice her questions and concerns. Finally, support her efforts to make informed decisions based on diagnostic findings.

Testing may begin with blood studies and mammography. Other tests may include a chest X-ray, a needle

or excisional biopsy, and bone, brain, or liver scans. (See *Teaching patients about tests to diagnose cancer,* pages 388 to 399.)

Blood tests
Tell the patient that blood chemistry studies to check electrolyte balance and kidney function and a complete blood count to detect anemia and infection are routinely performed in suspected breast disease. In addition, arterial blood gas analysis is done to check for blood oxygenation, and prothrombin time and partial thromboplastin time are used to check clotting times. Explain that specialized blood tests, such as radioimmunoassays to detect tumor markers, provide important information about the extent of cancer and treatment effectiveness.

TREATMENTS
First, help the patient cope with the breast cancer diagnosis; then help her explore treatment options. Surgery is usually the initial treatment, with chemotherapy or radiation therapy performed postoperatively. Hormonal therapy may be another option if cancer recurs. Emphasize how the patient can participate in posttreatment care by practicing breast self-examination and scheduling regular follow-up examinations and mammograms after surgery.

Medications
Drug treatment for breast cancer falls into two groups: chemotherapy and hormonal therapy.

Chemotherapy
Explain that chemotherapy uses certain drugs or drug combinations to kill cancer cells, to keep cancer cells from replicating, or to decrease the tumor's effects. The patient may have chemotherapy postoperatively or receive it along with radiation therapy, or as primary therapy. Discuss how and where the patient will receive chemotherapy — in specific cycles and sequences, so that her body can

INSIGHT INTO ILLNESSES

Explaining breast structure and tumor sites

Once the doctor diagnoses breast cancer, help the patient understand the disease by describing breast structure, supporting structures and related lymph nodes, and the area affected by her tumor.

Breast structures

Inform the patient that the breast is a glandular organ composed of lobes, lobules, acini, and ducts. These structures are arranged like spokes on a wheel, with the lobes (15 to 20 in each breast) branching into lobules and terminating in the acini, where milk is produced. The ducts direct the milk toward the lactiferous sinuses in the nipple. These sinuses have external openings through which the milk flows.

Supporting structures

Composed mostly of fat (adipose tissue), the breast is enclosed by a membrane of fascia and supported by ligaments. Ligaments lie over the pectoral muscles, which cover the ribs and aid in arm movement.

Lymphatics

Each breast has an elaborate lymphatic system that drains primarily into the axilla. Lymph nodes also lie within the breast, between the pectoral muscles, and above and below the clavicle. All these nodes may be sites for metastasis. The preponderance of axillary lymph nodes, however, accounts for the axillary node enlargement common in breast cancer.

Tumor sources and sites

Tell the patient that about 90% of breast tumors arise from the epithelial cells that line the ducts. About half of all breast cancers develop in the breast's upper outer quadrant, the section containing the most glandular tissue. The second most common cancer site is the nipple, where all the breast ducts converge. The next most common site is the upper inner quadrant, followed by the lower outer quadrant and then the lower inner quadrant.

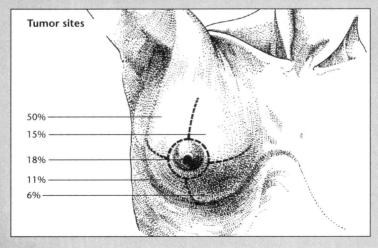

Tumor sites

50%
15%
18%
11%
6%

recover during the drug-free period.
Then prepare the patient for possible adverse effects and discuss ways to manage them. Provide nutritional information and tips for appetite stimulation.

 TIPS AND TIMESAVERS: Inform the patient that chemotherapy may cause her to tire easily. Suggest that she pace her activities and rest frequently to help conserve her energy.

Hormonal therapy
If the patient is having hormonal therapy, explain that this treatment decreases levels of estrogen and other hormones suspected of nourishing breast cancer cells. For example, anti-estrogen therapy, specifically tamoxifen, is used in postmenopausal women and is most effective against estrogen-receptor positive tumors. Or the patient may receive anti-androgen therapy (aminoglutethimide) or androgen (fluoxymesterone), estrogen (diethylstilbestrol), or progestin (megestrol acetate) therapy. Discuss drug administration and possible adverse effects, such as abnormal bleeding, hirsutism, menstrual irregularities, mental depression, and weight gain.

Radiation
Radiation therapy may be given after several types of breast cancer surgery, but it's typically used after lumpectomy and for recurrent cancer or metastatic disease. Let the patient know that before surgery, radiation therapy may help to shrink the tumor. After surgery (and sometimes given along with chemotherapy), radiation may prevent remaining cancer cells from growing, thus preventing recurrent disease.

Inform the patient that radiation therapy is typically given 5 days a week for about 6 weeks. Tell her that the actual treatment takes only 30 minutes, although consultation and planning may take 1 hour or longer.

Depending on which type of radiation the patient is receiving (external or internal), describe the procedure and equipment. Then discuss adverse effects, such as hematuria, urinary urgency and frequency, and diarrhea, and suggest ways to manage these problems. Also, explain that radiation therapy, like chemotherapy, may cause her to tire easily.

Surgery
A woman with breast cancer may fear mastectomy — the primary treatment — almost as much as cancer itself, perhaps because mastectomy threatens her self-image more than any other surgery. To relieve your patient's fears, you'll need to do considerable teaching before and after surgery.

Preoperative considerations
Discuss the particular operation the surgeon plans (if known), and answer any questions. Make sure the patient understands exactly what the surgery involves.

If the patient is having a *lumpectomy,* explain that the surgeon removes the breast lump and a margin of normal tissue around it. He may also remove some axillary lymph nodes to screen for disease.

In a *simple mastectomy,* the surgeon removes the entire breast as well as some of the axillary lymph nodes if cancer has spread beyond the breast. In a *modified radical mastectomy,* he removes the breast, axillary lymph nodes, and the lining over the chest muscles. In a *radical mastectomy,* rarely performed now, the breast, the chest muscles under the breast, and all the axillary lymph nodes are removed, leaving a hollow chest area.

Inform the patient that before surgery, she'll be given a sedative to calm her. Once in the operating room, she'll receive a general anesthetic. Describe the dressing and surgical drain she'll have after the operation.

Warn the patient that she'll have some breast-area pain after surgery and may have pain or paresthesia in her shoulder, upper arm, axilla, and

Recommended schedule for breast cancer screening

Tell the patient that breast cancer can occur in any woman at any age. The American Cancer Society recommends breast self-examination and cancer screening as part of every woman's routine health regimen. Urge your patient to follow these guidelines for breast cancer screening.

At any age

See your doctor immediately if you discover a breast lump, notice a discharge from your nipple, or have any other signs of breast cancer. Comply with your doctor's recommendations for follow-up breast examinations and mammograms.

Beginning at age 20

Examine your own breasts monthly, 2 to 3 days after your menstrual period begins if you're over age 20.

Beginning at age 35

Schedule an appointment for a baseline mammogram if you're between ages 35 and 40. Continue to perform monthly breast self-examinations.

Beginning at age 40

Visit your doctor for a yearly breast examination if you're between ages 40 and 49, and schedule mammography every 1 to 2 years. Continue to perform monthly breast self-examinations.

Beginning at age 50

Visit your doctor for a yearly physical examination, and have a yearly mammogram. Perform monthly breast self-examinations. (Postmenopausal women should examine their breasts on the same date each month.)

other parts of her chest. Depending on her operation, also mention that she may have lymphedema and phantom breast pain (temporary tingling or pins-and-needles sensation in the area of the removed breast tissue). Reassure her that she'll receive adequate pain-relief medication.

Postoperative support

After the operation, answer the patient's questions and discuss new concerns. Discuss available resources for recovering patients, and if she agrees, arrange for her to meet with another breast cancer patient from the American Cancer Society or the Reach for Recovery Foundation.

Self-care tips

Point out that effective self-care after surgery can speed recovery and prevent surgical complications such as infection. If the patient will be discharged with a drain in place, show

her how to care for it. Stress ways to minimize lymphedema by elevating the affected arm frequently, avoiding restrictive clothing, and massaging the affected arm to increase circulation.

Exercise guidelines

Discuss postoperative physical activity with the patient. Advise her that ordinarily she can return to her regular activities within several weeks. However, tell her to check with the doctor before undertaking strenuous exercise.

Instruct the patient to exercise the arm and shoulder of her affected side to prevent muscle shortening, maintain muscle tone, and improve blood and lymph circulation. Once she has permission to start these exercises, show her how to perform them.

Breast prosthesis and breast reconstruction

Assist the patient in dealing with an altered body image. Tell her that after the breast area heals (2 to 6 months after surgery), she can wear a breast prosthesis or explore breast reconstruction options. If she decides to use a breast prosthesis, describe the temporary, light-weight products that are available for the immediate postoperative period (4 to 6 weeks). Add that after she heals completely, she can select a ready-made permanent prosthesis or have one custom designed.

If the patient has questions about breast reconstruction, explain that the surgeon rebuilds the breast using muscle and tissue from the patient's chest, back, and abdomen. In some instances, he may implant a manufactured prosthesis, or he may work with both body tissues and manufactured materials. Inform the patient that the usual waiting period for reconstruction is 6 to 9 months after mastectomy. Depending on the circumstances, however, the procedure may be performed sooner or even along with the initial surgery.

Warn the patient that the reconstructed breast won't be exactly like her natural breast. Add that reconstruction outcomes vary. Urge her to discuss her concerns with the doctor.

Sexual activity

The patient may voice concerns about sexual activity after mastectomy. In particular, she may wonder if she and her partner will feel the same about having sex. Tell her that she may resume sexual activity as soon as she feels ready, but encourage her and her partner to discuss their feelings about the patient's breast surgery. If appropriate, refer the couple for counseling to a psychiatrist, clinical specialist, social worker, or social agency.

Other care measures

Stress that effective home care and regular follow-up examinations after breast cancer surgery are essential in preventing complications and detecting any new or recurrent cancer. Discuss the benefits of breast self-examination and show the patient how to perform it. Urge her to examine her breasts monthly — about 2 or 3 days after her menstrual period. If she's postmenopausal, suggest that she examine her breasts on the same date each month.

Also review the patient's follow-up care schedule. A typical plan is to see the doctor every 3 to 4 months for 2 years after surgery; then every 6 months for another 3 years; then yearly thereafter. She'll also need to schedule a yearly mammogram, a chest X-ray, routine blood work and, possibly, a bone scan. (See *Recommended schedule for breast cancer screening.*)

Finally, refer the patient to a local or national organization for further information and support. (See Appendix 2.)

Cervical cancer

The best time to teach a woman about cervical cancer is before it's ever diagnosed. Inform patients that regular Papanicolaou tests can detect this cancer in its earliest stages, before signs and symptoms appear. Explain that the disease usually can be cured if detected early. If your patient has an abnormal Pap test, counsel her about the need for further procedures, such as colposcopy, conization, or dilatation and curettage (D & C).

If your patient has invasive cervical cancer, clarify the disorder's stage and recommended treatment. Teach her how to minimize the adverse effects of therapy, and provide psychological support. Above all, emphasize the need for long-term follow-up care to monitor disease recurrence or progression.

Before teaching a patient about cervical cancer, make sure you are familiar with the following topics:
• explanation of the disease and predisposing factors

• importance of Pap tests for early detection
• staging and diagnostic procedures, such as biopsy, colposcopy, and conization
• chemotherapeutic agents and external and internal radiation therapy, including radiation implants
• surgery, such as abdominal hysterectomy or pelvic exenteration
• need for follow-up care to monitor disease recurrence or progression
• sources of information and support.

ABOUT THE DISORDER
Inform the patient that cervical cancer affects the lower portion of the uterus that protrudes into the vagina. This cancer occurs when normal cells begin to divide and grow at an uncontrolled rate.

Point out that, although the cause of cervical cancer is unknown, several predisposing factors have been linked to its development. These include intercourse before age 18, multiple sexual partners, multiple pregnancies, history of carcinoma in situ, and herpes simplex virus type 2 or other sexually transmitted diseases. Although the incidence of cervical cancer increases in low socioeconomic groups, women in all groups are at risk.

Explain that preinvasive carcinoma, the earliest stage of cervical cancer, produces no symptoms or other clinically apparent changes. Untreated, this cancer progresses to invasive cervical cancer, with malignant cells spreading beyond the cervical epithelial lining. Discuss the symptoms of early invasive cancer, including spotting after sexual intercourse, bleeding between menstrual periods, or unusually heavy menstrual bleeding. Advancing cancer may cause a yellowish or foul-smelling vaginal discharge (commonly tinged with blood), pelvic pain, rectal bleeding, hematuria, and anemia accompanied by extreme fatigue.

Complications
Emphasize that early treatment may cure cervical cancer or prevent metastasis. With early treatment, the 5-year survival rate is 80% to 90%. By the time the disorder produces symptoms, the survival rate drops sharply. With delayed treatment, the survival rate drops still further.

DIAGNOSTIC WORKUP
Stress that regular Pap tests can detect cervical cancer in its earliest stages. If your patient's Pap test reveals an abnormality, advise her that this doesn't necessarily mean she has cancer. Point out that the Pap test serves only as an indicator. She'll need to undergo further tests, such as cervical biopsy and colposcopy, conization, and D & C. (See *Teaching patients about tests to diagnose cancer,* pages 388 to 399.)

Other tests
If the patient has invasive cancer, inform her that additional tests may be done to determine whether cancer has spread to other organs. She'll have blood studies to assess her hemoglobin level and white blood cell and platelet counts and to evaluate kidney and liver function. Discuss tests to detect metastasis to the bones, liver, pelvis, abdomen, and chest.

Explain that the diagnostic workup aims to determine the stage of cancer. Tell the patient that tumor staging helps to direct treatment.

TREATMENTS
Emphasize the need for a joint evaluation between a gynecologist and an oncologist to determine the best course of treatment. Discuss the need for internal or external radiation therapy. Explain chemotherapeutic agents, if appropriate, and alert the patient to possible adverse effects. Review modifications related to sexual intercourse after therapy. Also discuss douching to reduce foul discharge resulting from treatment.

Medications
If the patient has advanced disease, chemotherapy may be recommended. Explain that chemotherapeutic drugs interfere with the replication of

Teaching about radiation implants

If your patient is scheduled to have an internal radiation implant, explain that this therapy treats cervical cancer by temporary insertion of a radioisotope (contained inside a special holder) in her vagina. Once in place, the implant destroys cancer cells in her cervix while at the same time exposing healthy tissues to minimal radiation.

Tell the patient that she can expect to stay in the hospital about 3 to 4 days, with the implant in place for about 2 to 3 days. Then review the following teaching topics.

Before the implant procedure

Inform the patient that the day before or the morning of the implant procedure, she will be admitted to the hospital and given a private room. Once the implant is in place, she'll be isolated from other patients and the hospital staff to protect them from unnecessary radiation exposure.

The evening before the procedure, the patient will receive a low-fiber or liquid supper, and the doctor may order an enema to cleanse her bowels. If she is to have a general anesthetic, advise her that she won't be permitted to eat or drink after midnight before the procedure. Also inform her that before going to the operating room, she may receive a douche with an antiseptic solution.

During the implant procedure

Tell the patient that in the operating room, she will receive a local or general anesthetic, as the doctor directs. Then a catheter will be placed in her bladder to drain urine.

Next, the doctor implants the holding device for the radioisotope, then adds packing to secure it in place. This may take 20 minutes. X-rays are taken to confirm that the holder is in the right position.

Inform the patient that parts of the holder will be visible outside the vagina.

In the recovery room, the nurse will check the patient's temperature, blood pressure, heartbeat, and breathing for an hour or two until she recovers from the anesthesia. Tell her that when she returns to her room, the doctor will insert the radioisotope into the holder. Assure her that this takes only a few minutes and doesn't hurt.

Advise the patient that the doctor or nurse may draw markings on her inner thighs. They'll check these landmarks periodically to make sure that the implant doesn't move out of place. Next, the nurse may put support stockings on the patient's legs to improve circulation while she is confined to bed.

Safety precautions

Once the radioisotope is in the holder, the hospital staff implements safety measures to avoid exposure to unnecessary radiation. Tell the patient she'll notice that:
● all hospital workers who come into her room wear a film badge to measure their radiation exposure.
● hospital staff members and visitors limit their visits to her room because radiation exposure increases with time.
● lead shields may surround her bed to protect the staff from radiation.
● staff members may stand some distance away from her bed while talking to her. The farther away they stand, the less radiation they receive.

While the implant is in place

For the next 2 to 3 days, the patient will lie on her back while the implant does its work. Caution her not to move too much because of the risk of dislodging it.

(continued)

Teaching about radiation implants *(continued)*

The head of the bed may be raised slightly at mealtimes, and she may receive a liquid or a low-fiber diet. Explain that this will help prevent her from having gas and bowel movements. She also may take medicine to prevent bowel movements and diarrhea.

Forewarn the patient to expect some discomfort. Advise her to ask the nurse for medicine if she feels sick to her stomach or if she has pain.

Inform the patient that the vaginal packing causes pressure and a sensation of having to void. Tell her that she will have a urinary catheter in place.

She should also expect to have vaginal drainage while the implant is in place. Tell her that pads will be placed beneath her and changed frequently to keep her dry and clean. The bed linens won't be changed, though, because the movement might dislodge the implant.

Recommend that the patient practice breathing deeply and coughing hourly while awake. Advise her to exercise her feet and ankles to stimulate the circulation.

After the implant is removed
Explain that the patient will probably go home the day the doctor removes the implant. A nurse will remove the urinary catheter.

To help the patient cope with adverse effects as she recuperates, provide these tips:
- Try to rest frequently during the day because you may feel tired for several weeks.
- Douche once a day with a solution of 2 tbs of vinegar (or Betadine, available at the drugstore) to 1 quart (1 liter) of water. This helps minimize the odor from vaginal discharge, which may last for 2 or more weeks.
- Follow a low-fiber diet. Eat small, frequent meals, and avoid coffee, tea, and cocoa. These measures may relieve diarrhea, which may continue for about 2 weeks.
- As comfort permits, resume regular sexual intercourse to counteract a narrowed vagina that may result from scar tissue. Ask the doctor or the nurse about using a dilator.

When to call the doctor
Tell the patient to call the doctor right away if she experiences any of the following signs or symptoms:
- inability to urinate within 6 to 8 hours of having the catheter removed
- burning when she urinates
- bloody urine
- bowel problems, such as constipation, diarrhea, or rectal bleeding
- extreme nausea or vomiting
- temperature over 100° F (37.7° C)
- persistent or unusual pain.

cancer cells. After determining the type and sequence of drugs the patient will receive, review how the drugs will be administered — intravenously or intra-arterially, for example — and alert the patient to possible side effects. Instruct her to report burning, itching, or pain around the I.V. site to help prevent extravasation and damage to surrounding tissues.

Radiation therapy
Tell the patient that radiation therapy is the treatment of choice for cervical cancer. Explain that she may receive external or internal radiation or both.

External radiation
Delivered by a large machine that beams X-rays at the tumor, external radiation destroys cancer cells and some healthy cells. Assure the patient that normal tissues recover quickly. Before therapy begins, explain that the radiation oncologist will define

the exact treatment areas with a waterproof marking pen. Remind the patient not to remove these markings from her skin until she completes therapy.

Tell the patient that during the therapy session, she will lie flat on her back on a treatment table in the radiation room. Explain that the doctor determines the radiation dose and duration, depending on the cancer stage. Afterward, she may return to her room or to her home if she's an outpatient.

Because external radiation can dry the skin around the target site, discuss measures to prevent skin breakdown. Instruct the patient to keep her skin clean and dry, especially where the skin creases. If she needs a skin lubricant, ask your facility's radiation department to recommend a lotion.

Internal radiation
Explain that internal radiation involves placing a radioactive source inside the body in one of two ways. In the *interstitial approach,* the radiation oncologist inserts radioactive needle- or bead-like devices into the tumor or surrounding tissues. These devices may remain in place temporarily or permanently. In the *intracavitary approach,* the oncologist inserts a special holder that is later filled with a radioactive source into the vagina. (See *Teaching about radiation implants,* pages 361 and 362.)

Before the patient consents to an intracavitary implant, make sure she understands that she'll be confined to bed for 2 to 3 days. Inform her that the full benefit of internal or external radiation may not be evident for several months. Support her efforts to cope with long-term adverse effects. For example, vaginal narrowing caused by scar tissue may be managed by regular sexual intercourse, dilation, or both. Also explain that pelvic radiation may decrease female hormone levels, causing infertility and amenorrhea.

Surgery
Explain that surgery for cervical cancer depends on the stage of cancer. Operations range from total abdominal hysterectomy (with or without lymphadenectomy) to pelvic exenteration.

Abdominal hysterectomy
Inform the patient having an abdominal hysterectomy that her uterus will be removed through an incision in the abdomen. Then discuss the type of hysterectomy she'll have. In a *total hysterectomy,* the surgeon excises the body of the uterus and the cervix, leaving the ovaries and fallopian tubes intact. In a *radical hysterectomy,* he removes the reproductive organs, including the ovaries and the fallopian tubes.

Explore the patient's expectations about her menstrual and reproductive status after surgery. If she's premenopausal, warn her that hot flashes, night sweats, vaginal dryness, insomnia, and headaches may follow removal of the ovaries. Although average recovery time lasts 6 to 8 weeks, suggest that she resume activities at her own pace. Advise her to ask the doctor for instructions about resuming sexual activity and, if appropriate, using tampons or douches.

Pelvic exenteration
Inform the patient scheduled for pelvic exenteration that the surgeon will remove all of her reproductive and pelvic structures, including the vagina, urinary bladder, and rectum. Explain ileal conduit, and discuss possible colostomy. Outline the rigorous presurgical bowel and skin preparation she'll undergo to minimize any infection risk. Prepare her for postoperative considerations, such as I.V. therapy, a central venous pressure catheter, a blood drainage system, and an unsutured perineal wound with gauze packing.

Other care measures
If the patient has advanced disease, explain that tumor drainage may cause a heavy, foul vaginal discharge.

Identifying colorectal cancer risk factors

Although you can't tell your patient exactly what causes colorectal cancer, you can discuss the following risk factors linked to its development:
• high-fat, low-fiber diet — explain that fats produce bile acids, which are converted to chemical carcinogens by colon bacteria; then, if too little dietary fiber slows bowel motility, these carcinogens make prolonged contact with the bowel mucosa, increasing the opportunity for cancer development.

• age (increased incidence over age 40)
• adenomatous intestinal polyps
• familial polyposis, Gardner's syndrome, or a family history of cancer
• personal cancer history
• inflammatory bowel disease (ulcerative colitis or Crohn's disease)
• colon injury or surgery
• sedentary lifestyle
• occupational exposure to carcinogens, such as organic dyes, solvents, or abrasives.

To help control the odor, advise her to douche with a solution of povidone-iodine (Betadine) and water or vinegar and water.

Explore how the patient feels about possible lifestyle changes resulting from treatment, and urge her to comply with recommended follow-up visits to her gynecologist or oncologist once she completes initial therapy. Stress the value of follow-up examinations in detecting disease recurrence or controlling progression. If appropriate, urge her to contact an organization for information and support. (See Appendix 2.)

Colorectal cancer

Diagnosis of colorectal cancer is certain to evoke myriad emotions in a patient — and pose a twofold challenge for you. First you'll need to support him as he confronts his fears about death, cancer, and treatment. Then you'll need to ensure that he and his family have accurate and adequate information for making decisions about treatment. You'll also want to encourage him to participate in care throughout his treatment and to maintain a positive attitude.

Initially, you'll prepare the patient for diagnostic tests. Then you may need to clarify the results, explaining how the tumor type and location, its

stage, and the patient's overall health help determine the most effective therapy. You'll discuss treatments, which may include surgery, radiation, and chemotherapy, and you may teach about stoma care.

Before teaching a patient about colorectal cancer, make sure you are familiar with the following topics:
• explanation of colorectal cancer
• risk factors, such as age and a high-fat, low-fiber diet
• signs and symptoms, including rectal bleeding and a change in bowel habits
• complications, such as intestinal obstruction and anemia
• diagnostic tests, including fecal occult blood test, barium enema, colonoscopy, and sigmoidoscopy
• chemotherapy and radiation therapy
• explanation of surgery, such as low anterior resection, Hartmann's procedure, and loop colostomy
• postoperative care
• colostomy care and lifestyle changes
• sources of information and support.

ABOUT THE DISORDER
Tell the patient that colorectal cancer is one of the most common cancers affecting men and women. Point out that about 95% of colorectal tumors are adenocarcinomas. Review the risk

factors for this disease. (See *Identifying colorectal cancer risk factors.*)

Inform the patient that most colorectal cancers grow slowly and cause few, if any, symptoms until the disease is well advanced. Review the symptoms of colorectal disease with the patient and his family:
• rectal bleeding
• change in bowel habits (diarrhea or constipation)
• thin, pencil-like stools
• persistent fatigue
• abdominal cramps or bloating
• fecal urgency
• sensation of incomplete defecation (tenesmus)
• weight loss
• pain (a late symptom).

Explain that tumors can spread by direct invasion, or they can infiltrate the blood or lymphatic system. Mention that tumor size doesn't necessarily correlate with the extent of metastasis.

Complications
Untreated, colorectal cancer is invariably fatal. Explain that as the tumor grows and encroaches on abdominal organs, abdominal distention and intestinal obstruction occur. Untreated rectal bleeding can lead to anemia.

DIAGNOSTIC WORKUP
Prepare the patient for serial tests to diagnose and stage colorectal cancer or to monitor its recurrence or progress. In addition to a digital rectal examination and fecal occult blood test, he may have a barium enema or a double contrast barium enema, sigmoidoscopy or colonoscopy, excretory urography or computed tomography scan, and specific blood tests. (See *Teaching patients about tests to diagnose cancer,* pages 388 to 399.) Inform the patient that preoperative test results are used to determine which surgical procedure he'll undergo.

Digital rectal examination
Tell the patient that a digital rectal examination can detect suspicious rectal and perianal lesions. Explain that this test is an essential part of every GI workup and takes only a few minutes.

Tell the patient that the doctor will apply a lubricant to a gloved finger to minimize discomfort and possible bleeding. Then he'll insert the finger into the rectum and palpate for masses and enlarged lymph nodes.

Fecal occult blood test
Tell the patient that the fecal occult blood test is a simple test that detects occult blood in the stool. Explain that rectal bleeding, a warning sign of colorectal cancer, isn't always visible in the stool.

Depending on the doctor's orders, tell the patient how to use a home test kit to analyze a stool sample or how to collect the sample and deliver it to the doctor's office (or laboratory) for analysis. Give him a copy of the patient teaching aid *Testing for blood in your stools,* page 366.

Blood tests
Inform the patient that blood tests, including a complete blood count, may be ordered to detect anemia, evaluate liver function, and monitor recurrence or metastasis.

Liver function studies are used to monitor liver function and disease progression (colorectal cancer commonly metastasizes to the liver). Explain that elevated liver enzyme levels may prompt the doctor to order a liver scan and biopsy.

Inform the patient that blood levels of carcinoembryonic antigen (CEA), a biological tumor marker, increase in colorectal cancer before treatment. Explain further that CEA levels usually decline after the tumor is removed. A postoperative increase in CEA levels may suggest disease recurrence or metastasis.

TREATMENTS
Because surgical tumor resection is the mainstay of treatment for colorectal cancer, your teaching will focus on preparing the patient to undergo and recover from surgery and, as appropriate, continue treatment

Testing for blood in your stools

Dear Patient:

A home fecal occult blood test is an easy, inexpensive way to detect blood in your stool. For accurate results, follow the directions given by the nurse or doctor, read the instructions included with the test kit, and review these steps.

How to get ready

Don't eat red meat or raw fruits and vegetables for 3 days before you take the test or during the test period. Also avoid diet supplements containing iron or vitamin C and painkillers containing aspirin or ibuprofen (for example, Advil or Nuprin) for 3 days before the test or during the test period. All of these substances can affect test results.

Increase your intake of high-fiber foods, such as whole-grain breads and cereals. Your doctor may also ask you to eat popcorn or nuts.

How to perform the test

1. Make sure all your supplies are in one place. They may include your test cards (or slides), a chemical developer, a wooden applicator, and a watch with a second hand.
2. Obtain a stool sample from the toilet bowl. Use the applicator to smear a thin film of the sample onto the slot marked "A" on the front of the test card. Smear a thin film of a second sample from a *different area of the same stool* onto the slot marked "B" on the same side of the card.
3. *If the doctor or a laboratory* will be analyzing the test samples, close slots A and B. Put your name and the date on the test kit, and return the card (or slide) to the doctor or lab as soon as possible.

If you're doing the test yourself, turn the card over and open the back

window. Apply 2 drops of the chemical developer to the paper covering each sample. Wait 1 minute, then read the results.

If either slot has a bluish tint, the test results are positive for blood in the stool. If neither slot looks blue, the test results are normal. Write down the results.

4. Repeat the test on your next two bowel movements. Report the results of all of the tests to the doctor. Even if only one of the six test results is positive, the doctor may recommend other tests.

Discard any unused supplies when you've completed all tests.

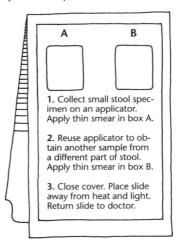

1. Collect small stool specimen on an applicator. Apply thin smear in box A.

2. Reuse applicator to obtain another sample from a different part of stool. Apply thin smear in box B.

3. Close cover. Place slide away from heat and light. Return slide to doctor.

through chemotherapy, radiation therapy, or both.

Medications

Explain that when surgery isn't possible or successful, chemotherapy with fluorouracil (5-fluorouracil) may bring about remission or improvement. Other cytotoxic drugs may be tried as well.

Describe the common adverse effects of fluorouracil I.V. administration: nausea and vomiting soon after treatment, and diarrhea, mouth soreness, and swallowing difficulties 5 to 8 days later.

 WARNING: Instruct the patient to watch for and report such adverse effects as stomatitis and ecchymoses, petechiae, and easy bruising. Also tell him that other adverse effects of chemotherapy may include hair loss, hyperpigmentation of the face and hands, hypotension or weakness, itchy eyes, leukopenia, and rash.

Discuss measures for reducing discomfort. For instance, advise the patient that he may receive an antiemetic before receiving fluorouracil. This will minimize nausea. Also explain that he'll have frequent blood tests to ensure that he can take the drug safely.

Radiation therapy

Inform the patient that radiation therapy may be recommended before surgery to shrink a tumor or after surgery (and perhaps combined with chemotherapy) to halt any remaining cancer cell growth and to prevent recurrence. Explain that bombarding cancer cells with high-level radiation destroys their ability to grow and multiply. Point out that radiation also affects normal cells, but they usually recover quickly. Mention that diarrhea and skin rash are common adverse effects that subside about 2 to 3 weeks after radiation therapy ends.

Tell the patient that the duration of preoperative radiation therapy depends on the dose. For instance, if he receives low-dose radiation (500 rads), he may have a single treatment. If he receives moderate-dose radiation (2,000 to 2,500 rads), treatment may occur over 2 weeks, with surgery following 2 weeks later. If he has high-dose radiation (4,500 to 5,000 rads), therapy may last 4 to 6 weeks, with surgery following in 6 weeks. Postoperative radiation therapy usually begins about 1 month after surgery.

Surgery

Inform the patient that surgery — the treatment of choice for colorectal cancer — aims to remove the tumor and surrounding tissue, including regional lymph nodes (to aid staging). Explain that the type of surgery depends on the tumor's location. Point out that an end-to-end anastomosis is created whenever possible; if not, a colostomy may be necessary. If appropriate, discuss colostomies. Answer the patient's questions about colostomy types, permanence, placement, and care.

Preoperative considerations

Tell the patient that he'll need to follow a low-residue diet for 3 to 5 days before surgery. Then he'll consume only clear liquids for 1 to 3 days. Explain that the doctor may prescribe an antibiotic to decrease the bacterial count in the colon. Inform him that he'll probably receive enemas or saline lavage for 4 to 5 days before surgery to ensure thorough cleansing of the GI tract.

Postoperative instructions

Because postoperative complications may not develop until after the patient's discharge, caution him to contact the doctor should he suspect or have anastomotic leaks, hemorrhage, irregular bowel function, phantom rectum, ruptured pelvic peritoneum, stricture, urinary dysfunction, or wound infection.

If the patient has a colostomy, focus your teaching on stoma care. Initially, discuss the stoma's function and appearance (large, protruding,

(Text continues on page 371.)

Irrigating your colostomy

Dear Patient:

Irrigating your colostomy at about the same time each day can help you establish a regular bowel pattern and avoid the inconvenience of unexpected bowel movements.

Choose a time (about 1 hour) when you won't be rushed or interrupted — preferably after a meal. Follow the instructions given by the nurse or doctor. Also read the directions that come with the irrigation kit, and review the procedure below.

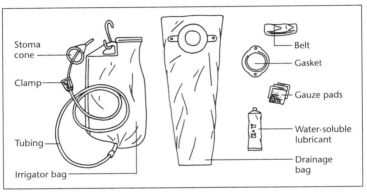

1. Lay out your supplies in one handy place. You'll need gauze pads, a water-soluble lubricant, a drainage bag (often called a drainage sleeve), an irrigator bag, a stoma cone (optional), tubing, a clamp, a gasket, and a belt (if the drainage bag isn't self-adhering). Also make sure you have an irrigation solution and a clean colostomy pouch to replace your used one.

2. Now, sit on the toilet or on a chair next to the toilet. Remove your colostomy pouch. If your system has more than one piece, make sure you leave the wafer or faceplate on.

3. Next, connect the drainage bag and the gasket. Then attach one end of the belt to the gasket on the drainage bag. Hold the gasket with one hand while you wrap the belt around your waist with your other hand. Then attach the other end of

the belt to the gasket.

4. Carefully encircle the stoma with the gasket (as shown here), adjust the belt to fit, and dangle the bottom end of the drainage bag into the toilet.

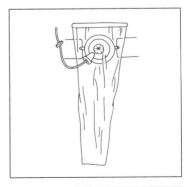

This teaching aid may be photocopied only by an individual health care professional for use in his or her clinical practice. Photocopying by hospitals, home care agencies, or other institutions requires a licensing agreement from the publisher. © 1998 Springhouse Corporation.

Irrigating your colostomy *(continued)*

5. If you're using a stoma cone, gently twist together the end of the cone's tube and the end of the tube leading to the irrigator bag until you hear a snap.
6. Fill the irrigator bag with about 1 qt (1 L) of lukewarm water or irrigation solution, as the doctor orders. Hang the filled bag on a towel rack or a hook placed next to the toilet. During irrigation, the bag should be above your stoma at shoulder level.
7. Hold the end of the irrigator tube over the toilet. Open the control clamp and allow a small amount of water or irrigation solution to flow through the tubing. This will force any trapped air out of the tubing. Then close the control clamp.
8. Next, squeeze a small amount of water-soluble lubricant onto a gauze pad and roll the first 3" (7.5 cm) of the tube in the lubricant. Now slowly slide the tube through the open top of the drainage bag and into your stoma. About 2" (5 cm) of tube should be in the stoma. If you meet resistance, don't force the tube. Instead, try to relax, and pull the tube out slightly.

Unclamp the flow control and allow a small amount of water or irrigation solution to flow into the colon. Wait about 5 minutes and then try again to insert the tube. If you repeatedly have trouble inserting the tube, notify the doctor.

If the doctor wants you to irrigate your colostomy with a stoma cone instead of a tube, first lubricate the tip of the cone. Then insert the lubricated tip through the open end of the drainage bag and into your stoma until it fits snugly.

To prevent backflow, always hold the cone in place against the stoma during irrigation.
9. Open the flow clamp of the irriga-

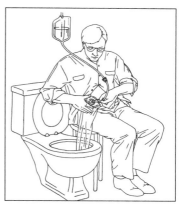

tor bag, and let the water or irrigation solution run slowly into your colon. This should take about 10 to 15 minutes. If you get stomach cramps, reduce the flow or stop the procedure until the cramps go away. After the fluid has entered your colon, slowly remove the tube or cone from your stoma.
10. After the initial surge of water or irrigation solution returns, you can fold the drainage bag back, clamp it shut, and do whatever you want to until all the fluid and stool have returned. It will take about 30 minutes for the colon to empty completely.
11. After the colon empties, return to the toilet. Unhook the belt and remove the drainage bag. Then clean the area around your stoma with warm water, dry the area gently, and apply a clean colostomy pouch. Finally, wash the irrigation equipment with warm (not hot) water and mild dish detergent, rinse it, and hang it to dry. Then store the irrigation equipment for reuse.
Important: Don't irrigate if you have diarrhea. If diarrhea lasts more than 72 hours, call the doctor or nurse.

Dietary recommendations after colostomy

If your patient has undergone a colostomy, pass on these tips for eating sensibly.

Staying regular

• To promote regularity, eat three meals of about the same size and at the same time daily. Avoid between-meal or late-night snacks.

• Increase your fiber intake, such as by eating more fresh fruits and vegetables, whole-grain cereals, nuts, and prunes.

• To relieve constipation, become more active or increase your fluid intake to at least eight full (8-oz) glasses daily. Eliminate constipating medicines, such as iron preparations or narcotic-containing pain relievers.

• If you must take an occasional laxative, ask the doctor to recommend a mild one, such as docusate salts (Colace, Surfak). If you're taking a bulk-forming laxative such as psyllium (Metamucil) or methylcellulose (Cologel), avoid bowel impaction by drinking at least eight full glasses of fluid daily.

Caution: To avoid upsetting your fluid and electrolyte balance, take laxatives (and diuretics) only as recommended by the doctor. If you become mildly dehydrated, drink such liquids as bouillon, tea, or fluid electrolyte replacement (such as Gatorade) to promote rehydration.

Controlling flatulence

• Eat slowly and chew food well to prevent swallowing air and subsequent bloating.

• To identify foods that cause gas, keep a daily record of the foods you eat and your reaction to them. Gas-producing foods include apple juice, beer, broccoli, cabbage, carbonated beverages, dairy products, dried beans, and onions. You may want to eat such foods only at home.

• Consider using odor-proof pouches, pouch deodorants, or a vented stoma plug to control odor. If gas builds up in the pouch, "burp" the pouch rather than pierce it.

• Talk to the doctor about taking simethicone (Mylicon, Phazyme) after meals and at bedtime to relieve belching or bloating. If you're taking tablets, chew them thoroughly.

Dealing with diarrhea

• To relieve occasional diarrhea, eat applesauce, bananas, or rice.

• Be aware that some medications such as antibiotics can cause diarrhea. Consult the doctor for an alternative medication if a prescription drug causes diarrhea.

• If the doctor recommends an anti-diarrheal preparation, take *only* this medication. Occasional diarrhea usually responds to a nonprescription product, such as kaolin and pectin (Kaopectate), bismuth subsalicylate (Pepto-Bismol), or loperamide (Imodium). Or the doctor may prescribe diphenoxylate (Lomotil) or paregoric. Be aware that paregoric usually relieves severe diarrhea but is habit-forming; take it only as directed.

• If you have an ascending or right transverse colostomy, expect semiliquid to soft stools. You'll need to routinely empty your pouch several times each day. If you must empty the pouch more often, you may have diarrhea. Consult the doctor if you experience diarrhea for more than a day.

• If you have a descending or sigmoid colostomy, expect to have semiformed to formed stools. You'll probably have one or two bowel movements at predictable times each day. Consult the doctor about more frequent bowel movements that persist for more than 2 days.

and swollen after surgery). Explain that swelling will subside over 6 to 9 weeks. Then tell the patient that the stoma won't hurt when touched because it has no nerve endings capable of detecting sharp pain. Add that the stoma should appear red, moist, and soft. Explain further that he won't be able to control the stoma at will because it has no muscles. However, he can learn to control his bowel movements by irrigating his colostomy. Give him a copy of the patient teaching aid *Irrigating your colostomy*, pages 368 and 369.)

Reassure the colostomy patient that his pouch shouldn't show under most garments. Caution him to avoid tight belts or tight underwear because they can irritate the stoma and block stool drainage.

Discuss ways to adapt the patient's lifestyle during recovery. Tell the patient to limit activity and to avoid heavy lifting or strenuous exercise until he's fully recovered (about 6 weeks). Point out that he'll need the doctor's permission to return to work.

 TIPS AND TIMESAVERS:
Reassure the patient that having a colostomy usually does not change the desire or capacity for a fulfilling sex life. Suggest that he empty the pouch before sexual intercourse or that he use a stoma plug.

Mention that some men experience temporary impotence after a colostomy. If the patient encounters such a problem, suggest that he talk with the doctor, enterostomal therapist, or a professional counselor.

However, after an abdominoperineal resection that results in a colostomy, nearly all men and many women experience sexual dysfunction. In men, partial or complete dysfunction depends on whether the nerve fibers controlling erection remain intact. In women, dysfunction may result from scarring or contracture at the surgical site.

Give the patient tips for eating sensibly. Inform him that he'll probably follow a low-residue diet for 1 to 2 weeks after surgery. He'll be able to resume a normal diet after his bowel heals. (See *Dietary recommendations after colostomy*.)

Other care measures

Stress the importance of regular physical examinations. For patients over age 40, emphasize the need for colorectal cancer screening, including annual sigmoidoscopy and rectal examinations. Discourage smoking, which contributes to altered bowel motility. Help the patient establish a regular bowel routine.

Finally, encourage the patient recovering from colorectal cancer to use support services offered by community and national organizations. (See Appendix 2.)

Laryngeal cancer

Few challenges are greater than helping a cancer patient learn to cope with his diagnosis, treatment, and aftercare. The patient's fears about cancer and its effects are usually uppermost in his mind, and this can distract him from learning.

When the patient has laryngeal cancer, your challenge grows because the primary treatment — laryngectomy — will dramatically affect his lifestyle and self-image. If surgery involves removal of all or part of the larynx, he will be temporarily or permanently unable to speak after surgery. If it involves removal of the upper trachea, he'll have to breathe through a tracheostomy. If it also involves removal of the epiglottis, he'll have difficulty swallowing.

As a result, the patient may be especially concerned about how he'll sound, look and, in some cases, eat after surgery. His concerns may increase if he requires a radical neck dissection, which may disfigure his face and neck and interfere with muscle function.

Besides emotionally preparing the patient for laryngectomy and its aftermath, you'll need to prepare his family. For example, they'll need to know how to perform such daily procedures as tracheal suctioning and stoma care. And they may need to learn how to respond positively to the patient, helping him to adapt successfully.

Before teaching a patient about laryngeal cancer, make sure you are familiar with the following topics:
• explanation of the type of laryngeal cancer — glottic or supraglottic carcinoma
• description of affected laryngeal structures
• diagnostic tests, including indirect or direct laryngoscopy
• preparation for chemotherapy or radiation therapy
• preparation for partial or total laryngectomy or radical neck dissection
• self-care measures, such as tracheal suctioning, stoma care, and exercises after surgery
• new ways to speak and to swallow
• emergency measures, such as mouth-to-stoma resuscitation
• sources of information and support.

ABOUT THE DISORDER

Distinguish the patient's type of laryngeal cancer: *glottic carcinoma,* which involves the structures around the glottis; or *supraglottic carcinoma,* which involves structures above the glottis, such as the epiglottis and false vocal cords.

If your patient has *glottic carcinoma,* tell him that hoarseness (an early cancer sign) stems from one or more tumors impinging on the true vocal cords, which prevent the cords from coming close together during speech. Explain that these tumors occur in the earliest stage of this type of laryngeal cancer. Typically, they remain localized. However, if they spread, the cancer usually involves only the local structures higher in the neck or the regional lymph nodes.

Inform the patient with *supraglottic carcinoma* that this type of cancer originates in some laryngeal structure other than the true vocal cords. Discuss its sometimes vague symptoms, such as coughing, difficulty swallowing, the sensation of a lump in the throat, changes in voice pitch,

a long-lasting sore throat (more than 6 weeks), pain in the laryngeal prominence, and a burning sensation after drinking hot liquids. Hoarseness is a late sign. If appropriate, mention that this type of laryngeal cancer grows more aggressively than glottic carcinoma and metastasizes more rapidly to associated structures and to lymph nodes in the neck — a reason not to delay treatment.

Complications

Emphasize that laryngeal cancer will spread and cause death if it remains untreated. Explain that with glottic carcinoma, the patient will experience difficulty swallowing and pain as the tumor grows. With untreated supraglottic carcinoma, swallowing will become increasingly difficult also. Hoarseness and severe pain accompany the tumor's spread to the true vocal cords.

DIAGNOSTIC WORKUP

Prepare the patient for tests to confirm laryngeal cancer and determine its extent. Explain that diagnosis may begin with indirect laryngoscopy, usually an office procedure. If this examination reveals a suspicious lesion, the doctor will order direct laryngoscopy and perform a biopsy for a definitive diagnosis. (See *Teaching patients about tests to diagnose cancer,* pages 388 to 399.)

Subsequent tests

If biopsy confirms laryngeal cancer, the doctor may order tests to gauge the extent of the cancer. These may include various scans, neck radiography, tomography, and contrast studies. Be sure to explain each test's purpose, preparation, procedure, and aftercare to the patient.

TREATMENTS

Explain that treatment has two goals: to eliminate the cancer and to preserve as much normal speech as possible. The most common treatment is partial or total laryngectomy. The doctor may recomend other treatments, including chemotherapy, radi-

How to suction a tracheostomy tube

If your patient has a tracheostomy, explain that the nurse will show him how to suction his tracheostomy to remove secretions that accumulate there. Then provide the following instructions to help him or his caregiver remember the steps.

1. Gather the following equipment:
- suction machine
- connecting tubing
- basin
- water
- suction catheter
- gloves.

You can sterilize normal tap water by boiling it for 5 minutes. As the water cools, put a lid on the pot so the water stays germ-free. Keep a supply of sterile water in a glass jar that has been sterilized by boiling. You can also buy sterile water. Keep a bulb syringe nearby, in case the suction machine malfunctions or there's a power failure.

Wash your hands thoroughly. Then fill the basin with sterile water and set it aside.

2. Turn on the suction machine, and adjust the regulator dial to the proper setting. Usually, the setting should be between – 80 and –120 mm Hg, but no higher than –120 mm Hg.

3. Open the wrapper of the suction catheter or container and apply gloves. After gloving, remove the suction catheter from its wrapper or airtight container.

4. Now, attach the suction catheter to the control valve on the suction tubing.

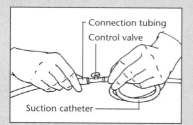

Connection tubing
Control valve
Suction catheter

5. Dip the loose tip of the catheter into the sterile water. This will help the catheter glide more easily.

6. Take a few deep breaths and gently insert the moist catheter between 5" and 8" (12.7 and 20.3 cm) into the trachea through your tracheostomy tube or stoma until you feel resistance.

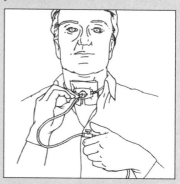

Caution: Take care not to injure yourself. Also be careful not to cover the catheter's suction port during insertion. The suction pressure that results will damage the tissues that line the trachea.

7. With your thumb, alternately cover and uncover the catheter's suction port to start and stop the suction. As you do this, slowly withdraw the catheter from the trachea, rolling it between your thumb and finger as you go. This should take no more than 10 seconds. (Longer than that steals oxygen from your lungs.)

8. Put the catheter tip in the sterile water to clean the suction catheter and the connection tube. Then turn off the suction machine and disconnect the catheter from the connection tubing. Discard the disposable catheter in a plastic-lined wastebasket.

If you're using a reusable catheter, sterilize it according to the manufacturer's instructions.

ation therapy, or a combination of these.

Medications
If the patient will receive chemotherapy, explain how these drugs affect the cancer, how he'll receive them, how often he must take them, and what adverse effects he can expect.

Radiation therapy
If the patient has a localized cancer in an early stage, the doctor may recommend radiation therapy as the primary treatment instead of surgery. Radiation therapy may also be used before surgery to shrink large laryngeal tumors or after surgery to prevent metastasis or treat recurrent cancer.

Discuss why the patient needs radiation therapy and how it will affect the disease. Then describe the procedure. Discuss the adverse effects and how to manage them. For instance, explain that most patients experience taste changes, decreased salivation, and skin changes.

Surgery
Inform the patient that laryngoscopic surgery may eliminate early localized glottic tumors. Tell him that his speech won't be affected and that he can return to his usual activities shortly afterward. To remove more extensive tumors, the surgeon may perform partial laryngectomy (laryngofissure, vertical hemilaryngectomy, horizontal supraglottic laryngectomy) or total laryngectomy. For advanced disease, he'll perform a total radical neck dissection. Make sure the patient and his family understand the extent of the planned surgery.

Explaining communication
Encourage the patient to express his concerns if surgery will cut off vocal communication. Help him choose an alternative means of communication, such as writing, sign language, or a communication board. Offer to arrange a meeting with another laryngectomee to discuss the patient's concerns.

If the patient is having a partial laryngectomy, explain that he can speak when his doctor determines that he can use his voice, usually 2 to 3 days after surgery. Then, caution him to whisper until his throat heals. If he's having a total laryngectomy, reassure him that speech rehabilitation can help him talk again.

Discussing suctioning
Inform the patient that when he awakens from surgery, he'll have a tracheostomy tube in place. Advise him that secretions accumulating in the tube will be removed by suctioning. Tell him that he and his nurse will decide on a signal that he can use to tell her that he needs suctioning. Assure him that his breathing will be monitored frequently.

Reviewing feeding
Explain that the patient will have a nasogastric tube in place and that he'll receive food through this tube until the surgical site heals.

If the patient is scheduled for a total laryngectomy, mention that he'll start eating again (thick, easy-to-swallow foods, such as gelatin or ice cream) about a week after his surgery, when he can swallow normally.

Discussing swallowing
If the patient is undergoing a supraglottic laryngectomy, he will receive instruction in the new swallowing technique he'll use after the operation. Inform him that this swallowing technique requires a lot of energy and patience. What's more, it can leave him feeling frustrated and frightened for a while. After surgery, continue to encourage him.

Although the patient won't experience much discomfort at the incision site, tell him that he may feel pain when he first attempts to swallow. Encourage him to request pain medication early, before the pain becomes unbearable. Reassure him that the pain will diminish with time.

Reinforcing discharge instructions
If the patient will be going home

Caring for a tracheostomy tube

Explain to your patient that as part of his laryngectomy, the doctor created a permanent tracheostomy — a small opening, or stoma — in the throat. Point out that inserting a tube into the tracheostomy makes breathing easier because the tube keeps the windpipe open.

Inform the patient that a tracheostomy tube, commonly called a trach, features three parts: an inner cannula, an outer cannula, and an obturator.

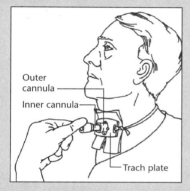

Outer cannula

Inner cannula

Trach plate

Explain that the inner cannula fits inside the outer cannula, which the patient inserts with the obturator.

Then provide the patient or his caregiver with the following instructions on caring for the tracheostomy tube.

How to clean the inner cannula

To prevent infection, remove and clean the inner cannula regularly, as the doctor orders.
1. Gather this equipment near a sink: a small basin, a small brush, mild liquid dish detergent, a gauze pad, a pair of scissors, and clean trach ties (twill tape).

Or open a prepackaged kit that contains the equipment you need. Now wash your hands and apply gloves. Position a mirror so that you can see your face and throat clearly.
2. Unlock the inner cannula and remove it by pulling steadily outward and downward. Prepare to clean the soiled cannula immediately for reinsertion. (Or put this soiled cannula aside and slip a clean inner cannula inside the outer cannula.) If you start to cough, cover your stoma with a tissue, bend forward, and relax until the coughing stops.
3. Next, clean the soiled cannula. Here's how: Soak the cannula in mild liquid dish detergent and water. Then clean it with a small brush. If your cannula is heavily soiled, try soaking it in a basin of diluted hydrogen peroxide solution. You'll see foaming as the solution reacts with the secretions coating the cannula. When the foaming stops, clean the cannula inside and outside with the brush. (*Note:* You can obtain a special trach tube brush at a medical supply company or pharmacy. However, the small brushes used to clean coffee pots or baby bottles work just as well. They're inexpensive and available at hardware stores. Just make sure to use the brush only for your trach tube.)
4. Rinse the inner cannula under running water. Make sure you've removed all of the cleaning solution. Shake off the excess water and reinsert the clean, moist cannula immediately. Don't dry it; the remaining water drops help lubricate the cannula, making reinsertion easier. Remove soiled gloves and apply a clean pair.
5. After you lock the clean inner cannula in place, replace the soiled trach ties that secure the trach plate.

(continued)

Caring for a tracheostomy tube *(continued)*

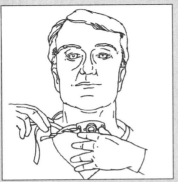

Use scissors to carefully clip and remove one trach tie at a time. Knot the end of each clean trach tie to prevent fraying, then cut a ½" (1.3 cm) slit in each tie. Thread the end that isn't knotted through the opening on the trach plate. Then, feed the end through the slit, and gently pull the tie taut. Do the same for the other tie.

6. Secure the ties at the side of your neck with a square knot. Leave enough room so you can breathe comfortably. You should be able to slip two fingers between the side of your neck and the knot.

7. Finally, place a 4" × 4" gauze bib behind the tube to protect your neck. To make the bib, cut a slit down the middle of the gauze pad until you reach the center. Next, cut a hole in the center just big enough to go around the trach tube. Carefully insert the gauze bib under the trach plate and gently around the stoma site.

How to reinsert the trach tube
Suppose you accidentally cough out your trach tube. *Don't panic.* Follow these simple steps to reinsert it.

1. Remove the inner cannula from the dislodged trach tube. If you're using a cuffed tube, be sure you deflate the cuff first.

2. Insert the obturator into the outer cannula. Then, use the obturator to reinsert the trach tube into your stoma.

3. Hold the trach plate in place and immediately remove the obturator. Then insert the inner cannula into the trach tube. Next, turn the inner cannula clockwise until it locks in place. Chances are you'll cough or gag while you're doing this, so be sure to hold onto the trach plate securely.

4. Insert the tip of a syringe into the tube's pillow port. Inflate the cuff, as your doctor orders. The inflated cuff will help prevent the tube from accidentally being dislodged again.

5. After inflating the cuff, secure the trach ties and tuck a gauze pad under the trach plate.

with a tracheostomy tube, teach him and his family how to suction and care for the tube. (See *How to suction a tracheostomy tube*, page 373, and *Caring for a tracheostomy tube*.)

After a radical neck dissection, stress the importance of exercising to support the patient's shoulders and to strengthen his back muscles. Tell him to notify the doctor if he experiences wheezing, stridor, fever, or milky drainage from the stoma (especially after meals).

If the patient has had a total laryngectomy or radical neck dissection, help him find ways to cope with the effects surgery will have on his lifestyle and functioning. A social worker can direct the patient and his family to available community resources and help them obtain or rent equipment and supplies.

Other care measures
As you assist the patient in adapting to a new lifestyle, be prepared to answer questions on a wide range of

issues, especially stoma care. Also cover preventing infection, humidifying the air, and other precautions. Finally, discuss how to deal with emergencies.

Preventing infection
Caution the patient that bacteria can now reach his lungs more easily, making him more susceptible to colds and other respiratory infections. Advise him to check with his doctor before taking over-the-counter cold medicines containing ingredients that could dry his mucous membranes.

 TIPS AND TIMESAVERS: Stress the importance of maintaining good oral hygiene to prevent infection. Advise the patient to rinse his mouth several times a day with mouthwash or a solution of 3% hydrogen peroxide and water.

Humidifying the air
Advise the patient to keep his home and workplace (if possible) well humidified. Tell him to cover his stoma with a scarf made of cotton or other porous material if he must be out in the cold. Stress that breathing cold, dry air can be especially irritating to the lungs.

Other precautions
Mention that heavy lifting and strenuous activity will be difficult after surgery because the patient won't be able to hold his breath to increase the pressure in his chest when straining. Discuss specific restrictions ordered by his doctor.

Also explain to the patient that he won't be able to hold his breath and bear down to have a bowel movement. Advise him to eat foods with high-fiber content to prevent constipation. Or suggest that he ask his doctor about using a stool softener.

Dealing with emergencies
Tell the patient who's had a total laryngectomy to notify his doctor immediately if he has pain, difficulty swallowing, or bloody or purulent sputum. Suggest that he obtain a medical alert tag and carry an identification card with these instructions: "In case of emergency, open my collar. I breathe through my neck."

Show members of the patient's family how to perform mouth-to-stoma resuscitation. If the patient lives alone, suggest that he and a friend or a neighbor arrange a "buddy" system so that he has daily contact with another person who can summon help if needed.

Emphasize that despite a tracheostomy, the patient can lead a full and healthful life. Refer him and his family to the appropriate organizations for further information and support. (See Appendix 2.)

Leukemia
When you teach about leukemia, a cancer of the blood-forming tissues, you'll be dealing with patients who are understandably frightened and depressed about their condition. Try to establish a trusting relationship with the patient, helping to calm his fears and encourage communication. Because many leukemia patients are children, you must be especially sensitive to their emotional needs and those of their families.

Once you've established rapport, teach the patient (or his parents if he's too young to understand) about leukemia's different types. Help him to understand his particular type and its treatment. Inform him about diagnostic tests, chemotherapy, possible radiation therapy, dietary changes, activity restrictions and, if appropriate, bone marrow transplantation.

Above all, encourage the patient to comply with therapy. Emphasize that therapy aims to achieve and maintain remission and to minimize complications.

Before teaching a patient about leukemia, make sure you are familiar with the following topics:
• how leukemia develops
• major types of leukemia
• preparation for diagnostic tests, such as bone marrow aspiration or biopsy

- activity restrictions and the need for adequate rest
- foods to eat and avoid
- chemotherapy
- ancillary treatments such as radiation therapy
- preparation for bone marrow transplantation, if necessary
- risk of graft-versus-host disease
- tips to prevent bleeding and infection
- sources of information and support.

ABOUT THE DISORDER

Tell the patient that leukemia refers to a group of disorders in which certain blood cells grow and multiply uncontrollably. Leukemia usually involves the white blood cells (WBCs), or leukocytes. Rarely, it involves the red blood cells (RBCs), or erythrocytes.

Explain that leukemia can originate in the bone marrow or the lymph nodes, leading to the growth of functionally impaired, immature cells called blasts. These cells multiply, accumulate in the bone marrow, and inhibit the normal growth of WBCs, RBCs, and platelets. As a result, the production of normal blood cells diminishes, leading to anemia, leukopenia, and thrombocytopenia — known collectively as pancytopenia.

Inform the patient that leukemic cells also spill into the bloodstream, where they travel throughout the body. They may infiltrate and cause complications in the spleen, lymph nodes, central nervous system (CNS), kidneys, testes, skin, tonsils, and gums.

Although the precise cause of leukemia is unknown, tell the patient that exposure to certain chemicals (such as benzene) or large doses of radiation may play a role. Other possible factors include viral infections, immunologic defects, and genetic abnormalities.

Types of leukemia

Teach the patient about his specific type of leukemia. (See *How leukemia develops.*) In *acute leukemia,* symp-

toms arise suddenly and progress rapidly. In *chronic leukemia,* symptoms appear gradually. Explain that both acute and chronic leukemia are further divided into subclasses, depending on which type of WBC has become cancerous. In either form of leukemia, treatment can prolong life and help to prevent complications, such as infection, hemorrhage, and pain.

Acute leukemia

The two main types of acute leukemia are *acute myelocytic leukemia,* in which granulocytes or monocytes proliferate, and *acute lymphocytic leukemia* (ALL), in which lymphocytes grow unchecked. Acute leukemia produces immature, undifferentiated WBCs.

Acute leukemia is most common in young children. Its incidence declines after adolescence but then increases again in later adulthood. Also, it is more common among people with certain genetic conditions such as Down syndrome.

Chronic leukemia

Explain that the two types of chronic leukemia are *chronic myelocytic leukemia* (CML) and *chronic lymphocytic leukemia.* Chronic leukemia produces relatively more mature and competent cells than does acute leukemia.

Explain that chronic leukemia most commonly strikes people over age 20. Incidence increases with age, peaking among those age 60 to 70.

If your patient has CML, tell him that this disease may be characterized by an abnormal chromosome called the Philadelphia chromosome. This genetic abnormality may result from exposure to radiation or carcinogenic chemicals.

Complications

Point out that acute leukemia, if untreated, typically causes death within a few months. Emphasize that in either acute or chronic leukemia, treatment can help to prevent such com-

INSIGHT INTO ILLNESSES

How leukemia develops

Tell your patient how bone marrow cells may give rise to four major leukemia types. Explain that all white blood cells (WBCs) derive from pluripotent stem cells. As the pluripotent cells mature, they differentiate into lymphoid stem cells and myeloid stem cells.

These stem cells normally develop into mature WBCs: lymphoid stem cells become lymphocytes, and myeloid stem cells become granular leukocytes. In leukemia, either type of stem cell begins to grow uncontrollably. The disorder may be acute or chronic.

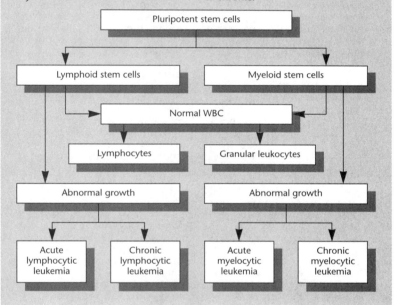

plications as infection, hemorrhage, and pain, and may prolong life. In many patients with chronic leukemia, life expectancy exceeds 5 years.

DIAGNOSTIC WORKUP

Teach the patient about blood tests to detect leukemia, including a complete blood count and blood urea nitrogen (BUN) and creatinine analyses. Explain that an elevated WBC count may indicate leukemia or infection. Elevated BUN and creatinine levels suggest that leukemia cells

have invaded the kidney and caused renal insufficiency.

Inform the patient about other tests to confirm the diagnosis, including cerebrospinal fluid analysis, computed tomography scan, and bone marrow aspiration or biopsy. (See *Teaching patients about tests to diagnose cancer,* pages 388 to 399.)

TREATMENTS

Inform the patient that chemotherapy — the major treatment for leukemia — aims to induce remission by killing leukemic cells and restoring normal blood cell production. Other treatments include radiation therapy and possibly bone marrow transplantation. During treatment, the patient may have activity restrictions and dietary changes.

Activity guidelines

Advise the patient to limit activities and to plan rest periods throughout the day. Explain that fatigue may result from stress related to his leukemia or from such treatments as chemotherapy or radiation. Suggest that he sleep at least 8 hours at night and take naps during the day, if possible. Tell him that he may need to shorten his workday or stop working during treatment.

Dietary modifications

Encourage the patient to eat foods high in calories and protein to help him maintain his strength and prevent body tissues from breaking down.

 TIPS AND TIMESAVERS: If the patient loses his appetite, recommend eating frequent, small meals. If he complains of a bitter or metallic taste, advise him to drink more fluids, such as water, apple juice, or tea.

Because the patient is at risk for developing mouth ulcers, advise him to eliminate alcohol, extremely hot or spicy foods, and acidic beverages, such as orange or tomato juice, from his diet. Suggest that he eat soft, bland foods, such as soft-boiled or poached eggs and oatmeal, and soothing foods, such as ice pops or pudding. If his WBC count is below normal, instruct him to avoid fresh, unpeeled fruit, salads, unwashed vegetables, raw meat, and uncooked eggs to prevent infection.

Medications

Explain that a combination of drugs is usually necessary to control the disorder. Inform the patient that he may receive different drugs during various treatment stages. He may also receive a prophylactic antibiotic to prevent infection caused by lowered resistance. During remission, he may receive the same drugs in different dosages.

Procedures

For some patients, radiation therapy and leukapheresis may be used as ancillary treatments.

Radiation therapy

Inform the patient with ALL that treatment may call for brain irradiation for 2 to 3 weeks, usually with chemotherapy, to treat effects on the CNS. Local radiation also may be used in chronic leukemia. It attempts to shrink organs enlarged or impaired by leukemic cells.

Leukapheresis

Explain that leukapheresis is a supportive measure used to treat CML that involves removing and separating abnormal or excessive WBCs. Inform the patient that his blood will go through a cell sorter that removes abnormal cells. Then his filtered blood will be reinfused into him.

Surgery

Inform the patient undergoing bone marrow transplantation that this procedure replaces diseased marrow with healthy cells. The new bone marrow may come from a donor or from the patient (after treatment to eliminate cancer cells). Tell him that the healthy bone marrow forms new blood cells in the marrow.

Bone marrow transplants

Review the three types of bone marrow transplants. In an *autologous transplant,* the patient receives his own marrow. In a *syngeneic transplant,* bone marrow comes from a twin with identical tissue. In an *allogeneic transplant,* the most common procedure, the patient receives marrow from a fully or partially matched donor, such as a sibling, parent, or unrelated donor.

Before and during transplantation

Inform the patient that before the

Teaching about graft-versus-host disease

If your patient will undergo a bone marrow transplant, make sure he understands the risk of developing graft-versus-host disease (GVHD). Explain that this immune system disease occurs when white blood cells attack and destroy foreign bone marrow cells from a donor. GVHD affects the skin, liver, intestinal mucosa, and lymph system. It may be acute or chronic.

Acute GVHD

Tell the patient to report any signs or symptoms immediately because GVHD can occur as soon as 1 week after transplantation or, more commonly, between 30 and 50 days after transplantation. An erythematous rash appears first, followed by green, watery diarrhea, abdominal cramps and, in severe disease, right upper quadrant pain, hepatosplenomegaly, jaundice, and enlarged lymph nodes. With severe infection, mortality is 85%.

Diagnosis and treatment

Inform the patient that the doctor may order a skin biopsy and blood tests to detect elevated liver enzyme and bilirubin levels.

Explain that treatment includes high-dose corticosteroids, lymphocyte immune globulin, or cyclosporine. Experimental treatment involves monoclonal antibodies to destroy donor T lymphocytes.

Chronic GVHD

A patient may experience chronic GVHD without first having acute GVHD. Signs and symptoms appear about 100 days after transplantation and resemble autoimmune collagen vascular disorders such as systemic lupus erythematosus. Chronic GVHD is characterized by scleroderma-like skin fibrosis and sicca syndrome, in which the mucosa and tear ducts become abnormally dry. The patient may also experience pulmonary changes and muscle wasting.

Diagnosis and treatment

Explain that skin and mucosal tissue biopsies confirm chronic GVHD. Localized skin involvement may resolve without therapy. Early systemic involvement is usually treated with immunosuppressive drug combinations, which are still investigational.

Prevention

Inform the patient that he may undergo GVHD preventive therapy. Immunosuppressive therapy against donor T lymphocytes is one preventive measure.

However, the most common treatment is methotrexate, an antimetabolite that inhibits synthesis of deoxyribonucleic acid and has a cytotoxic effect on rapidly dividing cells. Irradiation of blood products before they're administered may also help prevent T-lymphocyte replication.

Still experimental is the removal of T lymphocytes from the marrow before it's transplanted. This is done by treating the marrow with monoclonal antibodies or by binding the T lymphocytes to plant substances called lectins.

Teaching tips

If your patient already has GVHD, teach him ways to prevent infection. Also advise him that drinking plenty of fluids and eating a well-balanced diet will help to counter fluid and electrolyte losses caused by diarrhea and vomiting. If he has thrombocytopenia, urge him to report signs of gastrointestinal blood loss, such as bloody vomit or black, tarry stools. Also tell him to notify his doctor or nurse if he has sore skin lesions, abdominal cramps, or other unusual or persistent symptoms.

Preventing infection

Reinforce what the doctor and nurse have told your patient about his increased risk of getting an infection. Then describe these simple steps he can take to protect himself.

Follow the doctor's directions
- Be sure to take all medications exactly as prescribed. Don't discontinue any medicine unless your doctor tells you to do so.
- Keep all medical appointments so that your doctor can monitor your progress and drug effects.
- If you need to go to another doctor or to a dentist, be sure to explain that you're receiving an immunosuppressant drug.
- Wear a medical alert tag identifying you as taking an immunosuppressant drug.

Avoid sources of infection
- To minimize your exposure to infections, avoid crowds and people who have colds, flu, chickenpox, shingles, or other contagious illnesses.
- Don't receive any immunizations — especially live-virus vaccines such as poliovirus vaccines — without first checking with your doctor. These preparations contain weakened but living viruses that can cause illness in anyone who's taking an immunosuppressant drug. Similarly, avoid contact with anyone who has recently been vaccinated.
- Wash your hands thoroughly before preparing food. To avoid ingesting harmful organisms, thoroughly wash and cook all food before you eat it.
- Examine your mouth and skin daily for lesions, cuts, or rashes.
- Avoid vaginal or anal intercourse while your resistance to infection is decreased.

Recognize hazards
- Learn to recognize early signs and symptoms of infection: sore throat, fever, chills, or a tired or sluggish feeling. Call your doctor immediately if you think you're coming down with an infection.
- Treat minor skin injuries with triple antibiotic ointment. If the injury is a deep one, or if it becomes swollen, red, or tender, call your doctor at once.

Perform routine hygiene
- Practice good oral and personal hygiene, especially hand washing. Report any mouth sores or ulcerations to your doctor.
- Don't use commercial mouthwashes because their high alcohol and sugar content may irritate your mouth and provide a medium for bacterial growth.

procedure, he may receive chemotherapy and total-body radiation to remove all traces of leukemia and prevent rejection of the new bone marrow. Explain that the new bone marrow will be infused through a central venous catheter or an I.V. line. The transplanted cells will circulate in his bloodstream and eventually lodge in the bone marrow space, where healthy blood cells begin forming in 2 to 4 weeks.

After transplantation
Inform the patient that he'll receive antibiotics. Then he'll be placed in a sterile environment or a room with laminar airflow to reduce the risk of infection. For 3 to 4 weeks after the transplant, he may need packed RBC transfusions to prevent anemia and platelet transfusions to prevent bleeding. Advise him to plan to return to work or school between 9 months and 1 year after the transplantation.

Make sure the patient understands the risks involved in bone marrow transplantation. Explain that the most serious complication is graft-versus-host disease. (See *Teaching about graft-versus-host disease,* page 381.) Urge the patient to report any signs of infection. Also instruct him to notify the doctor if he notices any bleeding — for example, from his nose or gums.

Other care measures

Inform the patient that because of his lowered resistance to disease, he must take special care to prevent infection. (See *Preventing infection.*) Advise him to avoid contact with pet or human feces and to avoid cleaning cat-litter boxes and fish tanks. Direct him to call the doctor if he has chills, fever, or a nonhealing wound with drainage, redness, and tenderness.

Also explain that he must take care to prevent bleeding because his blood may not have enough platelets for proper clotting. Urge him to report excessive bleeding or bruising to his doctor immediately.

 WARNING: Caution the patient to avoid rough or hazardous activities, such as football or carpentry, and to be extra careful while gardening or handling pets that might scratch or bite. Suggest other precautions to avoid bleeding, such as using a soft toothbrush and an electric shaver instead of a razor. Advise him not to wear tight clothing, which could impair his circulation.

Throughout your care, provide emotional support. Refer the patient and his family to appropriate sources of information and support. (See Appendix 2.)

Lung cancer

Teaching your patient and his family about lung cancer will pose a challenge because the diagnosis is frightening. Lung cancer is the leading cause of cancer death; few patients live 5 or more years after diagnosis.

Despite these grim statistics, you can help your patient adjust to the diagnosis by educating him about the disease and his treatment options so that informed decisions can be made. He will need your support and instruction throughout treatment to derive the greatest benefit from therapy and learn to manage adverse effects.

You'll also help your patient and his family form realistic expectations about treatment outcomes without providing false hope. Despite lung cancer's overall poor prognosis, you'll emphasize that treatment possibilities include cure, control, or symptomatic relief.

Before teaching a patient about lung cancer, make sure you are familiar with the following topics:
• explanation of lung anatomy and disease progression
• major types of lung cancer
• complications from metastasis
• diagnostic tests, such as pulmonary function tests, bronchoscopy, and computed tomography (CT)
• treatments for lung cancer, including chemotherapy, radiation therapy, and surgery
• ways to manage or minimize treatment's adverse effects
• pain management techniques, such as relaxation and stimulation
• health promotion and lung cancer risk factors, such as smoking and industrial carcinogens
• sources of information and support.

ABOUT THE DISORDER

Inform the patient that repeated exposure to airborne carcinogens, such as cigarette smoke and asbestos, causes the epithelial cells that line the airways to lose their protective properties. This may precipitate lung cancer.

Tell the patient that lung cancer is 10 times more common in smokers than in nonsmokers; at least 85% of lung cancer patients are smokers. Air pollution and industrial carcinogens also are risk factors, especially when combined with cigarette smoking.

If appropriate, discuss the most common lung cancer types — for example, adenocarcinoma, small-cell (oat cell) carcinoma, or epidermoid (squamous cell) carcinoma. Inform the patient that a pathologist determines the cancer type after reviewing tissue samples obtained during the diagnostic workup, and that the type of treatment the patient receives depends on the cancer type and the tumor stage.

Complications
Explain that by following the treatment plan, the patient boosts his chances for cure or control and for avoiding complications from cancer spread or from the adverse effects of treatment. Nevertheless, despite compliance with treatment, the primary tumor may grow and invade neighboring tissues. Or, cancer cells may be carried to other parts of the body by the circulatory or lymphatic system. Lung cancer most commonly spreads to the brain, bones, liver, and adrenal glands.

Because early lung cancer is difficult to detect, disease complications may be the presenting symptoms.

DIAGNOSTIC WORKUP
Because so many lung cancer patients remain symptom-free while the disease advances, metastasis has occurred in about 70% of patients by the time of diagnosis. Tell the patient that diagnostic tests may include X-ray, lung tomography, pulmonary function tests, bronchoscopy, needle biopsy, thoracentesis, mediastinoscopy, CT scan, bone scan, gallium scan, and liver-spleen scan to detect a tumor and to determine its location, type and size, extent of metastasis, and appropriate therapy. (See *Teaching patients about tests to diagnose cancer,* pages 388 to 399.)

The patient may also have blood tests to monitor the disease and treatment. These tests include a complete blood count, blood chemistries, arterial blood gas studies, and liver function studies.

TREATMENTS
Inform the patient that treatment depends on the type and stage of the disease. Surgery, radiation therapy, and chemotherapy are all options. Teach him about the benefits and risks of each so that he knows what to expect.

Medications
Discuss analgesic medications to relieve pain and anticancer drugs to treat lung cancer.

Analgesics
If the patient is taking a narcotic drug, such as morphine (Duramorph) or hydromorphone (Dilaudid), advise him to avoid driving and other activities that require alertness. To help prevent constipation, suggest that he use a stool softener. Tell him to take the drug exactly as prescribed, even when his pain subsides.

 WARNING: Instruct the patient not to drink alcohol or use other central nervous system depressants while taking narcotics.

Chemotherapy
If the patient is undergoing chemotherapy, explain that this form of drug therapy kills cancer cells by interfering with their reproduction. He'll receive these drugs by mouth or by injection into his veins, muscles, or spinal fluid. Typically, they're given in specific cycles and sequences so that his body can recover during the drug-free period.

If appropriate, provide instructions for administering chemotherapy at home, including advice for taking liquids, tablets, pills, or capsules. If he'll receive chemotherapy through an implanted infusion port (such as Infus-A-Port or Port-A-Cath), explain that he'll need no dressing or special care after the incision heals.

Explain that adverse effects occur during chemotherapy because the drugs can affect any rapidly growing cells in the body — normal cells as well as cancer cells. Normal cells most likely to be affected are in the bone marrow, digestive tract, reproductive organs, and hair follicles.

Teach prophylactic measures to de-

crease the adverse effects of chemotherapy. For example, inform the patient that proper mouth care from
the start of chemotherapy can help
prevent mouth ulcers.

 TIPS AND TIMESAVERS: Advise
the patient to get lots of rest,
but caution him not to become too inactive because this may
lead to deconditioning and even
more fatigue. Help him plan his daily
routine to make the most of his limited energy.

With the dietitian, teach the patient how to balance his diet and eat
foods high in calories and protein to
promote healing. Also provide tips to
stimulate his appetite if his desire for
food lags during chemotherapy. For
easier digestion, suggest eating five or
six small meals a day instead of three
big ones. Tell him that drinking plenty of fluids will help flush the toxic
by-products produced by chemotherapy or tumor breakdown from his
body.

Radiation therapy
Explain to the patient that radiation
therapy destroys the cancer cells'
ability to grow and multiply, but also
affects normal cells. Tell him to notify the doctor if adverse effects persist
or become especially troublesome or
if he has a fever, cough, or unusual
pain. For activity and diet teaching
points during radiation therapy, refer
to the guidelines for controlling the
adverse effects of chemotherapy (see
above).

Surgery
If the patient is scheduled for surgery,
supplement and reinforce the doctor's explanation of the surgery. (See
Teaching about lung surgery.) Point out
which part of the lung will be removed.

Inform the patient that the surgeon
will perform a thoracotomy — an incision of the chest wall — to remove
the cancerous lung tissue. Show him
the area where he can expect to feel
the incision after surgery (for example, posterolateral, anterolateral, or
mediastinal).

Teaching about lung surgery

If your patient has operable lung
cancer and is scheduled for
surgery, discuss the type of operation. Explain that the surgeon
may perform one of four procedures.
- If the patient will have a *lobectomy,* inform him that the surgeon will remove a cancerous
lobe from the lung.
- If the patient is undergoing
segmentectomy, teach him that
the surgeon will remove one or
more lung segments in an attempt to preserve as much functional, healthy tissue as possible.
- Tell the patient scheduled for
wedge resection that the surgeon
will remove lung tissue without
regard to segmental planes. This
operation is reserved for small
cancers in patients with poor
pulmonary reserve.
- If the patient will undergo
pneumonectomy, explain that the
surgeon will remove an entire
cancerous lung.

Next, discuss possible complications — most notably, atelectasis and
acute respiratory failure. Explain how
lung cancer limits cardiopulmonary
reserve and increases the risk for
complications.

Reassure the patient that the health
care team will monitor his condition
after surgery to minimize atelectasis
and to reverse it promptly. Note that
significant atelectasis could prolong
his need for intubation and mechanical ventilation as well as lead to
pneumonia, sepsis, and acute respiratory failure.

Inform the patient that he'll remain intubated for 4 to 6 hours after
surgery, or perhaps overnight, to support his breathing and to clear mucus
from his lungs.

Unless the patient is scheduled for

a pneumonectomy, inform him that he'll have a chest tube in place after surgery to drain blood and fluid and to help expand his lung. Emphasize that coughing and deep-breathing exercises after surgery promote free breathing passages. Also teach segmental breathing exercises, which use biofeedback.

Pain control
Tell the patient that he'll receive analgesics postoperatively. However, explain that the dosage won't be strong enough to fully relieve pain because analgesics depress respiration and interfere with bronchial hygiene.

Mobility measures
Inform the patient that as soon as his vital signs stabilize, he'll begin taking steps to regain mobility. First he'll sit and dangle his legs over the bedside; next he'll sit in a chair, and then he'll begin walking with assistance.

Other care measures
Because both chemotherapy and radiation therapy increase susceptibility to infection, warn the patient to stay away from crowds and to avoid individuals with known infections. Also show him proper hand-washing techniques to prevent infection.

Pain-management skills are another teaching priority. Explain pain-reduction methods, such as relaxation or stimulation techniques, to help him manage anxiety, nausea, vomiting, and discomfort.

If appropriate, inform the patient and his family about hospital and community sources of support. Refer them to a social worker, psychologist, or religious or spiritual counselor, and arrange an appointment if they wish you to do so. Also refer them to the American Lung Association for further information. (See Appendix 2.)

Take the time to respond to the patient's questions about his illness, without burdening him with more information than he needs or wants to know. If he has terminal cancer,

offer advice on local counseling services and hospice or home care.

Testicular cancer
Although testicular cancer represents only 1% of cancers diagnosed in men, it's a leading cause of cancer deaths in men ages 15 to 34. The patient with testicular cancer faces difficult treatment, and he's almost certain to fear sexual impairment and physical disfigurement. The first goal of your teaching is to establish a trusting relationship with him, encouraging him to ask questions and express his fears.

Address the patient's concerns as you teach about tests to diagnose and stage testicular cancer and treatments, including surgery to remove the affected testicle and chemotherapy and radiation therapy to arrest the cancer. Reassure him that sterility and impotence aren't inevitable consequences of surgery. Finally, advise him to examine his testicles once a month to detect possible recurrence of cancer at its earliest, most treatable stage.

Before teaching a patient about testicular cancer, make sure you are familiar with the following topics:
• explanation of tumor cell types — seminoma and nonseminoma
• risk factors, including cryptorchidism, congenital abnormalities, hormone use, and traumatic injury
• early signs and symptoms, such as a lump in the testicle and swelling or a feeling of heaviness in the scrotum
• signs and symptoms of advanced cancer, such as vague abdominal pain, coughing, and dyspnea
• importance of early detection and treatment to prevent metastasis
• diagnostic tests, such as blood studies, computed tomography (CT) scan, and testicular biopsy
• staging testicular cancer
• chemotherapy and measures to combat adverse effects
• preparation for radiation therapy or autologous bone marrow transplant
• inguinal orchiectomy and postoperative care

• sexual concerns after orchiectomy
• sources of information and support.

ABOUT THE DISORDER

Tailor your teaching to the patient's form of testicular cancer — germinal or nongerminal. Explain that a *germinal* tumor stems from primitive germ cells; the relatively rare *nongerminal* tumor arises from interstitial cells. About 60% of germinal tumors are *seminomas.* Commonly detected before metastasis, these slow-growing cancers are highly curable. Most seminomas respond to radiation therapy.

Nonseminomas include embryonal tumors, teratomas, and choriocarcinomas. Yolk sac–type embryonal tumors, so named because they arise from embryonic cells, may appear in infants and children (although this tumor type also develops in young adults). Nonseminomas, especially teratomas and choriocarcinomas, spread more aggressively than seminomas. About 65% of patients with nonseminomas have metastasis by the time testicular cancer is diagnosed. As a result, survival rates for patients with this type of tumor are lower.

If appropriate, inform the patient that testicular cancer occurs more commonly in white men than in black men and rarely in Asian, Hispanic, or Native American men. Point out that the cause of this cancer isn't known; however, 1 of every 10 patients has a history of cryptorchidism. Other risk factors include congenital and chromosomal abnormalities, including gonadal aplasia, hermaphroditism, and Klinefelter's syndrome; exposure to diethylstilbestrol or other hormones; and traumatic injury. Viral diseases such as mumps may also play a role.

Explain that a small, hard, painless lump in one testicle may be the initial sign of disease. (See *Common sites of testicular tumors,* page 400.) Other signs are swelling or a feeling of heaviness in the scrotum. Pain is unlikely unless infarction or hemor-

rhage occurs. Gynecomastia and nipple tenderness may result from tumors that secrete human chorionic gonadotropin or estrogen.

Point out the signs and symptoms of late-stage cancer or metastasis: vague abdominal pain, anorexia, behavioral changes, cognitive deficits, coughing, dyspnea, hemoptysis, swelling in the supraclavicular region, and vomiting. Common sites of metastasis include the lungs, liver, bone, and brain.

Complications

Emphasize that early detection and treatment are essential to prevent metastasis. Reiterate how the tumor's proximity to inguinal and abdominal lymph nodes provides cancer cells with easy access to lymphatic circulation and vital organs, such as the lungs and brain.

DIAGNOSTIC WORKUP

Inform the patient that a complete health history and physical examination begin the diagnostic process. Mention that he'll be asked to recall injuries to the scrotum, hormone use, and viral infections such as mumps.

Explain how diagnostic tests, such as CT scans and biopsy, can stage the severity of the cancer, based on whether the tumor is confined to the scrotum or has spread to lymph nodes and secondary organs. Tell the patient that the prognosis depends on the cancer's cell type and stage. Prepare him for laboratory and radiologic studies to diagnose, stage, and monitor his condition. (see *Teaching patients about tests to diagnose cancer,* pages 388 to 399.)

Blood tests

Advise the patient that he'll undergo several routine blood tests, including a complete blood count. The doctor will also evaluate beta-subunit human chorionic gonadotropin (hCG) and alpha-fetoprotein (AFP) levels. Explain that elevated levels of these proteins (tumor markers) suggest a

(Text continues on page 400.)

Teaching patients about tests to diagnose cancer

TEST AND PURPOSE	TEACHING POINTS
Barium enema studies ● To aid diagnosis of colorectal cancer and inflammatory disease ● To detect polyps, diverticula, and structural changes in the large intestine	● Tell the patient that these radiologic studies use barium, and sometimes air, to examine the large intestine. If the study uses barium and air, tell the patient it's called a double-contrast barium enema test. The test is useful for detecting abnormalities in an obstructed colon region that can't be observed by endoscopy. ● Advise the patient to follow a low-residue diet for 1 to 3 days and then a clear liquid diet for 24 hours before the test to clean the intestine. For further cleansing, the patient will receive a laxative the afternoon before the test and cleansing enemas the evening before or morning of the test. Or the doctor may order a saline lavage. ● Describe what happens during the test: The patient may be secured to a tiltable table, and the doctor takes an X-ray to make sure the large intestine is empty. Then the patient lies on his left side while the doctor inserts a small lubricated tube into the patient's rectum. Once the tube is inserted, the barium is instilled slowly to fill the bowel while X-rays are taken. Instruct the patient to keep his anal sphincter tightly contracted against the tube to hold it in position and prevent barium leakage. Stress the importance of retaining the barium, because accurate test results depend on adequately coating the large intestine. If the doctor also will instill air through the tube, tell the patient that the table may be tilted and that he'll be assisted into various positions to aid filling. Instruct him to breathe slowly and deeply through his mouth to ease discomfort if he experiences cramps as the barium or air fills the large intestine. ● Inform the patient that after the test, he can expel the barium into a bedpan or toilet. Because barium hardens, causing intestinal obstruction or impaction, he'll receive another laxative and an enema to flush any remaining barium from the intestine. Mention that barium gives the stool a light color for up to 3 days after the test.
Bone marrow aspiration and biopsy ● To diagnose primary and metastatic tumors	● Inform the patient with leukemia that this procedure helps to confirm the diagnosis and identify which white blood cell type has become cancerous. Explain that it permits microscopic examination of a bone marrow specimen. Tell him that he will re-

Teaching patients about tests to diagnose cancer
(continued)

TEST AND PURPOSE	TEACHING POINTS
Bone marrow aspiration and biopsy *(continued)* • To aid staging of disease • To evaluate the effectiveness of chemotherapy and help monitor myelosuppression	ceive a local anesthetic and that the procedure usually takes only 5 to 10 minutes, unless additional bone marrow specimens are needed. The patient needn't restrict food or fluids before the test. • Inform the patient that before the procedure, a blood sample will be drawn for analysis. Then about 1 hour before the test, he'll receive a mild sedative. • Explain what happens during the test: For the *biopsy procedure,* tell him that, after the doctor positions him, he numbs the biopsy area with a local anesthetic before inserting a needle through the skin and into the bone marrow. Next, he inserts another needle inside the first needle and directs it into the marrow cavity to obtain a tissue plug. After withdrawing the needles, the doctor cleans the site and applies a sterile bandage. Advise the patient to remain as still as possible. Explain that for *aspiration,* the doctor inserts a needle through the skin and into the cortex of the bone. After aspirating 0.2 to 0.5 ml of marrow, the doctor withdraws the needle and applies pressure to stop bleeding at the site, then cleans the site and applies a sterile adhesive bandage. • After either aspiration or tissue biopsy, advise the patient to rest quietly for several hours and to report any bleeding.
Bone scan (bone scintigraphy) • To detect cancer that has spread to the bones	• Explain to the patient that this painless test can often detect bone abnormalities before conventional X-rays can. • Describe pretest preparation: The patient need not fast before the test. However, he should avoid eating a meal or drinking large amounts of fluids right before the test. • Explain what happens during the test: After applying a tourniquet on the patient's arm, the doctor injects a small dose of a radioactive isotope. Assure the patient that the isotope emits less radiation than a standard X-ray machine. A 2- to 3-hour waiting period follows injection of the isotope. During this time, the patient will need to drink 4 to 6 glasses of fluid. Then he'll be asked to lie supine on a table within the scanner. The scanner will move slowly back and forth, recording images for about 1 hour. Instruct him to lie as still as possible during the test. Tell him that he may be asked to assume various positions on the table. *(continued)*

Teaching patients about tests to diagnose cancer

(continued)

TEST AND PURPOSE	TEACHING POINTS

Breast biopsy
• To determine if a breast lump is malignant
	• If the patient will have a *needle biopsy,* tell her that the doctor uses a needle to remove a tissue sample from a breast lump. Inform her that this simple procedure is commonly performed in the doctor's office. Tell her that she need not restrict food or fluids and will probably receive a local anesthetic. Mention that the procedure may take only 5 to 10 minutes.
	   If the patient will have a *surgical biopsy,* tell her that she may receive either general or local anesthesia. If she's having general anesthesia, instruct her to fast from midnight before the test.
	• Describe what happens during a *needle biopsy:* The doctor cleans the skin with an antibacterial solution. Then he inserts a needle into the breast lump. Using a syringe, he aspirates a tissue or fluid sample, which he sends to the pathology laboratory for evaluation. Warn the patient that she'll feel some pressure during the procedure.
	   If the patient is having a *surgical biopsy,* tell her that after she receives a general or local anesthetic, the doctor makes an incision in the breast to expose the mass. He may then incise a portion of tissue or excise the entire mass. Then he sends the specimen to the laboratory for evaluation. The wound is sutured, and an adhesive bandage is applied.
	• Explain what happens after a *needle biopsy:* Once the anesthetic wears off, the breast may feel sore or tender for a while. Advise the patient that the doctor will recommend a mild analgesic for pain relief. Instruct her to watch for and report bleeding, redness, or tenderness at the biopsy site.
	   After a *surgical biopsy,* tell the patient that her vital signs will be checked frequently and she'll receive an analgesic to relieve postsurgical pain. Instruct her to watch for and report bleeding, tenderness, or redness at the biopsy site.

Bronchoscopy • To visually examine a possible tumor, secretions, or other obstruction demonstrated on X-ray	• Explain that this test allows direct examination of the patient's airways and takes 45 to 60 minutes. • Describe pretest restrictions: The patient must not eat or drink for 6 hours before the test. However, he should continue taking prescribed drugs unless the doctor orders otherwise. • Explain what happens during the test: If the test will be done with a local anesthetic, the patient may receive a sedative to help him relax. Prepare

Teaching patients about tests to diagnose cancer

(continued)

TEST AND PURPOSE	TEACHING POINTS
Bronchoscopy *(continued)* • To help diagnose bronchogenic carcinoma, tuberculosis, interstitial pulmonary disease, or fungal or parasitic pulmonary infection by obtaining a tissue or mucus specimen for examination	him for the unpleasant taste and coolness of the anesthetic throat spray used to suppress the gag reflex and ease bronchoscope passage. The patient will probably be placed in a supine position on a table or bed, although he may be asked to sit upright in a chair. Tell him to remain relaxed, with his arms at his sides, and to breathe through his nose during the test. Mention that the doctor will insert the bronchoscope tube through the patient's nose or mouth into the airway. Then he'll flush small amounts of anesthetic through the tube to suppress coughing and wheezing. Reassure him that, although he may experience dyspnea during the test, he won't suffocate. Also tell him that oxygen will be given through the bronchoscope. • Describe what happens after the test: The patient's blood pressure, heart rate, and breathing are monitored for about 15 minutes. He should lie on his side or sit with his head elevated at least 30 degrees until his gag reflex returns. Food, fluid, and oral drugs are withheld for about 2 hours or until his gag reflex returns. Reassure the patient that hoarseness or a sore throat is temporary. He can have throat lozenges or liquid gargle when his gag reflex returns. • Advise the patient to report bloody mucus, dyspnea, wheezing, or chest pain immediately.
Chest X-ray (chest radiography) • To detect respiratory disorders, such as pneumonia, atelectasis, pneumothorax, pulmonary bullae, and tumors • To detect mediastinal abnormalities such as tumors and cardiac disease	• Tell the patient that this test can determine if cancer has spread to the lungs. Mention that it takes only minutes, but that the technician or doctor will need additional time to check the quality of the films. • Describe pretest preparation: The patient must put on a gown without snaps, but may keep his pants, socks, and shoes on. Instruct him to remove all jewelry from his neck and chest. • Explain what happens during the test: The patient will stand or sit in front of the X-ray machine (if the X-ray is performed in the radiology department) or will be helped to a sitting position (if it's performed at the bedside). He must take a deep breath and hold it for a few seconds while the X-ray is taken. Urge him to remain still for those few seconds. Reassure him that he'll be exposed to only slight amounts of radiation.

(continued)

Teaching patients about tests to diagnose cancer

(continued)

TEST AND PURPOSE	TEACHING POINTS
Computed tomography scan (CT scan) • To detect and evaluate pathologic conditions, such as tumors and obstruction	• Inform the patient that this test uses multiple computed X-ray images to help diagnose or evaluate for cancer and other diseases. Mention that it takes 30 to 60 minutes and causes little discomfort. Reassure him that the technician will be able to see and hear him from an adjacent room. • Describe pretest preparation: If a contrast dye will be used, the patient must fast for 4 hours before the test. Just before the test, he should remove all jewelry. • Explain what happens during the test: The patient lies in a supine position on an X-ray table. To restrict movement, a strap is placed across the body part to be scanned. The table then slides into the large, tunnel-shaped machine. When the dye is injected, the patient may experience transient nausea, flushing, warmth, and a salty taste. Stress that he must not move during the test because movement may invalidate test results and require repeat testing. Urge him to relax and breathe normally. Reassure him that radiation exposure is minimal. • Tell the patient that he can resume his usual activities and diet immediately after the test.
Cystoscopy • To visualize internal bladder structures	• Explain to the patient that this 20-minute test usually is performed in the doctor's office. Tell him that he may receive a general anesthetic; if so, he should not eat for 8 hours before the test. If he'll have a local anesthetic, he may receive a sedative to help him relax before the test. (If the patient is a woman, she will not receive any anesthetic.) If the doctor plans to take bladder X-rays, describe the preparation he may receive to clean his bowels to ensure sharper, clearer X-ray images. • Describe what happens during the test: The patient lies in a supine position (with his hips and knees flexed) on an X-ray table. The genitalia are cleaned with an antiseptic solution, and he's covered with a sterile drape. Next, the doctor administers a local anesthetic, if appropriate, and introduces the cystoscope through the urethra and into the bladder. Explain that the bladder is filled with irrigating solution and the cystoscope is rotated to inspect the bladder wall surface. If a local anesthetic is used, warn the patient that he may feel a burning sensation as the cystoscope advances through the urethra. He may also feel an urgent need to void as the bladder fills with the irrigating solution.

Teaching patients about tests to diagnose cancer

(continued)

TEST AND PURPOSE	TEACHING POINTS
Dilatation and curettage (D & C) • To obtain tissue samples from reproductive organs to investigate the cause of bleeding • To detect the spread of cancer into the endometrium	• Inform the patient that a D & C takes about 1 hour and allows the doctor to obtain tissue samples from the uterus, cervix, endometrium, and other sites for laboratory analysis. • If the patient will have a general anesthetic, tell her not to eat or drink anything for 8 to 10 hours before the procedure. If she'll be an outpatient, caution her to arrange for transportation home because she'll be groggy afterward. • Describe what happens during the procedure: The patient lies on her back with feet in stirrups. Then she receives local or general anesthesia. The doctor dilates her cervix and scrapes the uterine lining with a curette. Then he sends tissue samples to the laboratory for microscopic evaluation. • Tell the patient that she can go home about 2 hours after the procedure.
Excretory urography (intravenous pyelography) • To determine the size, shape, and position of the bladder and other renal structures and perirenal tissues • To detect tumors or metastasis elsewhere in the urinary tract	• Explain to the patient that this test evaluates the kidneys and urinary tract. Tell him that it takes about 1 hour. • Discuss pretest preparation: The patient should drink plenty of fluids and then fast for 8 hours before the test. Inform him that he may receive a laxative or other bowel preparation before the test. • Explain what happens during the test: The patient will be placed in a supine position on an X-ray table. After injection of a contrast medium, X-rays will be taken at specific intervals. Mention that a belt may be placed around his hips to keep the contrast medium at a certain level. Warn the patient that the X-ray machine will make loud, clacking sounds as it exposes films. Also warn him that he may experience a transient burning sensation and metallic taste when the contrast medium is injected; tell him to report these and any other sensations to the doctor. • After the test, instruct the patient to report symptoms of delayed reaction to the contrast medium.
Gallium scan • To detect primary or metastatic neoplasms and inflammatory lesions	• Explain that this scan helps detect primary and metastatic tumors. Inform the patient that he needn't restrict food or fluids. Tell him that the test requires a total body scan (usually performed *(continued)*

Teaching patients about tests to diagnose cancer

(continued)

TEST AND PURPOSE	TEACHING POINTS
Gallium scan *(continued)* ● To evaluate malignant lymphoma and identify recurrent tumors following chemotherapy or radiation therapy	24 to 48 hours after the I.V. injection of radioactive gallium). Warn him that he may experience transient discomfort from the needle puncture during the injection. Reassure him, however, that the substance is only slightly radioactive and is not harmful. If the radiologist will use a gamma scintillation camera, assure the patient that the uptake probe and detector head may touch his skin but won't cause discomfort. If he uses a rectilinear scanner, describe the soft, irregular clicking noise it makes as it registers radiation emissions. ● Describe what happens during the test: The patient may be positioned erect or prone or in an appropriate combination of these positions, depending on his physical condition and which views (or angles) the doctor chooses. Scans or scintigraphs are then taken from anterior, posterior and, occasionally, lateral views. ● Tell the patient that he won't need any special care after the test.
Laryngoscopy, direct ● To detect lesions, strictures, or foreign bodies in the larynx ● To aid diagnosis of laryngeal cancer ● To examine the larynx when the view provided by indirect laryngoscopy is inadequate	● Inform the patient that this procedure permits direct laryngeal examination and procurement of tissue samples for histologic analysis. During the examination, the doctor can also remove small, localized lesions. Explain that the laryngoscope is a thin, hollow tube containing a light and a special lens, which is designed to pass through the patient's mouth. ● Tell the patient that the test takes place in an operating room. Instruct him to refrain from eating, drinking, and taking nonprescription drugs for 8 hours before the test. Just before the test, tell him to remove any contact lenses, dentures, and jewelry. He should also remember to use the bathroom. Inform him that he'll receive medication to help him relax and to reduce his oral secretions. ● Describe what happens during the test: If the patient will have a local anesthetic, explain that he may feel uncomfortable, but he shouldn't feel pain. Prepare him for the unpleasant taste and coldness of the anesthetic spray that suppresses the gag reflex. Explain that his head will be positioned and held in place while the doctor passes the laryngoscope through his mouth and throat and on to the larynx. Reassure the patient that he'll be able to breathe.

Teaching patients about tests to diagnose cancer

(continued)

TEST AND PURPOSE	TEACHING POINTS
Laryngoscopy, direct *(continued)*	If appropriate, mention that, besides obtaining a tissue sample, the doctor may perform minor surgery, such as endoscopic laser surgery to remove a small, localized glottic tumor. • After the test, the patient will be instructed to lie on his side or sit with his head elevated at least 30 degrees until his gag reflex returns (usually in about 2 hours). In the meantime, he should avoid food, fluids, and oral drugs. Tell him that he'll have a sore throat and hoarseness temporarily. Advise him to spit out saliva rather than swallow it for up to 8 hours after the test. During this time, he should avoid clearing his throat and coughing because these actions can dislodge blood clots at the biopsy site and possibly cause hemorrhage. Show the patient how to wear an ice collar to prevent or minimize swelling.
Liver-spleen scans • To screen for hepatic metastases and hepatocellular disease • To detect focal disease, such as tumors, cysts, and abscesses in the liver and spleen	• Inform the patient that these scans can show metastasis to the liver and spleen through pictures taken with a special scanner or camera. Inform him that he needn't restrict food or fluids before the test. Tell him that it takes about 1 hour. • Tell the patient that he will receive an injection of a radioactive isotope, ^{99m}Tc — technetium Tc 99m sulfur colloid — through an I.V. line in his hand or arm. Assure him that the injection isn't dangerous because the test substance contains only trace amounts of radioactivity. • Tell the patient what happens during the test: The radioactive isotope is injected and after 10 to 15 minutes, the patient's abdomen is scanned. The patient is placed in supine, left and right lateral, left and right anterior oblique, and prone positions to ensure optimal visualization of the liver and spleen. Tell the patient to report flushing, feverishness, light-headedness, or difficulty breathing. If the test equipment includes a rectilinear scanner, he'll hear a soft, irregular clicking noise as it moves across his abdomen. If the test equipment includes a gamma scintillation camera, he'll feel the camera lightly touch his abdomen. He may be asked to hold his breath briefly to ensure clear, high-quality pictures. • After the scintigraphs have been taken, they are reviewed for clarity before the patient is allowed to leave.

(continued)

Teaching patients about tests to diagnose cancer
(continued)

TEST AND PURPOSE	TEACHING POINTS
Mammography • To screen for breast cancer • To investigate palpable and unpalpable breast masses, breast pain, or nipple discharge • To help differentiate benign breast changes from breast cancer	• Explain to the patient that this test is simply an X-ray of the breast. It can be used to screen for breast cancer or to diagnose the cause of a breast complaint. Assure her that although the test uses radiation, the amount is negligible. • Advise the patient to tell her doctor if she might be pregnant or is breast-feeding. Also tell her to ask the doctor if she should avoid using deodorant on the test day (some deodorants contain substances that may interfere with test results). Instruct her to avoid lotions, which may make the breast slippery. Tell her that she'll be asked to take off her clothing above the waist, put on a gown, and remove jewelry from her neck. • Describe what happens during the test: The patient may be asked to sit, stand, or lie still for the test. A technician helps her position her breast on an X-ray plate. Then another plate is pressed down toward the first one to flatten the tissue. Warn the patient that she'll probably feel a cold sensation where her breast touches the plate and that the compression may cause some discomfort. Tell her that she may be asked to lift her arm or use her hand to hold her other breast out of the way. While the X-ray is being taken, she'll be told to hold her breath for a few seconds. Then the procedure will be repeated for the other breast.
Mediastinoscopy • To detect bronchogenic carcinoma, lymphoma, or sarcoidosis • To determine staging of lung cancer	• Explain that this test, which is performed in the operating room, allows the doctor to visualize the mediastinal area and obtain tissue samples for analysis, to help determine the appropriate treatment. Tell the patient that he will receive an I.V. sedative before the test and then a general anesthetic. • Describe what happens during the test: While the patient is anesthetized, the doctor inserts an endotracheal tube to ensure an open airway. Then he makes a small incision in the patient's chest and inserts a mediastinoscope to obtain tissue specimens for analysis. • Advise the patient that when he awakens in the recovery room, the endotracheal tube may remain in place for several hours or overnight. Warn him that he may have pain or tenderness at the incision site, a sore throat, and hoarseness. He may also experience nausea, vomiting, and a sense of unreality from the anesthetic.

Teaching patients about tests to diagnose cancer
(continued)

TEST AND PURPOSE	TEACHING POINTS
Pulmonary function tests • To estimate the degree of lung dysfunction resulting from lung cancer	• Explain that these tests evaluate the patient's lung function. • Describe pretest restrictions: The patient must not smoke for 4 hours before testing and must avoid eating a large meal or drinking a large amount of fluid before the test. • Discuss pretest preparation: The patient should put on loose, comfortable clothing. If he wears dentures, advise him to keep them in to help form a tight seal around the mouthpiece. Just before the test, he will be asked to void. • Explain what happens during the test: The patient sits upright and wears a nose clip. Or he may sit in a small airtight box called a *body plethysmograph* and will not need the nose clip. Forewarn him that inside the plethysmograph, he may experience claustrophobia. Reassure him that he won't suffocate and that he will be able to communicate with the technician through the window in the box. 　Tell him that he will be asked to breathe in a certain way for each test; for example, to inhale deeply and exhale completely, or to inhale quickly. Explain that he may receive an aerosolized bronchodilator and may then repeat one or two tests to evaluate the drug's effectiveness. An arterial puncture may also be performed during the test for arterial blood gas analysis. 　Emphasize that the test will proceed quickly if the patient follows directions, tries hard, and keeps a tight seal around the mouthpiece or tube to ensure accurate results. 　Tell the patient that he may experience dyspnea and fatigue during the test but will be allowed to rest periodically. Instruct him to tell the technician if he experiences dizziness, chest pain, palpitations, nausea, severe difficulty breathing, or wheezing.
Renal ultrasonography • To determine the size, shape, and position of renal organs and perirenal tissues • To distinguish a bladder cyst from a tumor	• Explain to the patient that this test helps detect cancer and other abnormalities in the bladder and other renal structures. Tell him that it takes about 30 minutes. Reassure him that the test is safe and painless. • Explain what happens during the test: The patient is placed in a prone position and the area to be scanned is exposed. Then the technician applies ultrasound jelly and guides a transducer over

(continued)

Teaching patients about tests to diagnose cancer

(continued)

TEST AND PURPOSE	TEACHING POINTS
Renal ultrasonography *(continued)*	this area. During the test, the patient may be asked to breathe deeply to assess kidney movement during respiration.
Retrograde cystography • To diagnose bladder rupture without urethral involvement, neurogenic bladder, recurrent urinary tract infections, reflux, diverticula, and tumors • To diagnose urethral strictures, laceration, diverticula, and congenital abnormalities • To examine the renal collecting system when excretory urography is contraindicated or inconclusive	• Explain to the patient that this test evaluates the structure and integrity of the bladder, renal collecting system, or urethra. Tell him that it takes about 30 minutes to 1 hour. • Describe pretest preparation: If a general anesthetic is ordered, tell the patient to fast for 8 hours before the test. • Explain what happens during the test: The patient is placed in a supine position on an X-ray table. A catheter is inserted into the bladder; then a contrast medium is instilled through the catheter. He'll be asked to assume various positions while X-ray films are taken. • Describe what happens after the test: The patient's blood pressure, heart rate, and breathing are monitored frequently until stable. His urine volume and color are also monitored. Instruct him to notify the doctor if blood continues to appear in his urine after the third voiding or if he develops chills, fever, or an increased pulse or respiration rate.
Sigmoidoscopy and colonoscopy • To diagnose malignant and benign neoplasms of the bowel • To aid diagnosis of inflammatory, infectious, and ulcerative bowel disease	• Tell the patient that sigmoidoscopy allows the doctor to see inside the lower part of the large bowel, whereas colonoscopy allows the doctor to visualize all of the large bowel. Tell him that the test takes 15 to 30 minutes. • Instruct the patient to follow a liquid diet for 48 hours before the test. He may drink clear juices without pulp, broth, tea, gelatin, and water, and usually is instructed to continue taking prescription medication. Tell him to take a laxative the evening before the test and to give himself an enema the morning of the test. If the test is scheduled for early morning, instruct him not to consume anything after midnight. Just before the test, the patient will take off his clothes and put on a hospital gown. Then he will be asked to empty his bladder. • Describe what happens during the test: An assistant helps the patient to lie on his left side with knees flexed and then drapes him with a sheet. Then the doctor inserts a lubricated, gloved finger into the patient's anus and passes an endoscope through the anus into the rectum. Warn the pa-

Teaching patients about tests to diagnose cancer

(continued)

TEST AND PURPOSE	TEACHING POINTS
Sigmoidoscopy and colonoscopy *(continued)*	tient that he may feel some discomfort and the urge to move his bowel as the endoscope passes through the rectal sphincters. Advise him to bear down gently as the endoscope is first inserted and to breathe slowly and deeply through his mouth to help him relax. Inform the patient that air may be instilled into the bowel to distend it and permit better viewing. Tell him that if he feels the urge to expel some air, he should do so and not be embarrassed. Also inform him that the doctor may remove biopsy specimens or polyps from the lining of the bowel during the test. Reassure the patient that this is painless. • Explain what occurs after the test: A nurse will monitor the patient's vital signs for about 1 hour. The patient should expect to pass large amounts of gas and may have slight rectal bleeding. Tell him to notify the doctor immediately if he experiences fever, abdominal swelling, tenderness, or heavy, bright red bleeding.
Thoracentesis (pleural fluid aspiration) • To obtain a specimen of pleural fluid for analysis • To obtain a lung tissue biopsy specimen	• Inform the patient that this test provides samples of tissue or fluid from around the lungs, helping the doctor gauge the extent of disease. • Describe pretest preparation: The patient will put on a hospital gown, and the area around the needle insertion site will be shaved. • Explain what happens during the test: The patient is positioned either sitting with his arms on pillows or lying partially on his side. The doctor cleans the needle insertion site with a cold antiseptic solution, then injects a local anesthetic. Tell the patient that he may feel a burning sensation during injection. After the patient's skin is numb, the doctor inserts the needle, obtains the sample, and withdraws the needle. Warn the patient that he will feel pressure during needle insertion and withdrawal. Instruct him to remain still and to avoid coughing, breathing deeply, or moving. Tell him to immediately report dyspnea, palpitations, wheezing, dizziness, weakness, or diaphoresis, which may indicate respiratory distress. After withdrawing the needle, the doctor applies slight pressure and then an adhesive bandage. • Describe what happens after the test: The patient's vital signs are monitored frequently for several hours. Instruct him to report any fluid or blood leakage from the needle insertion site.

INSIGHT INTO ILLNESSES

Common sites of testicular tumors

Use this illustration of a testicle and surrounding anatomic structures to teach your patient where to look for signs of testicular cancer. Because the testicles lie so close to the retroperitoneal lymph nodes, testicular cancer cells readily spread to these nodes. Instruct the patient to seek medical attention if he finds a firm, painless lump or nodule, usually about the size of a pea.

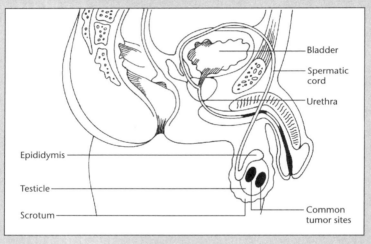

testicular tumor. The markers can also differentiate a seminoma from a nonseminoma: Elevated hCG and AFP levels point to a nonseminoma, whereas elevated hCG and normal AFP levels indicate a seminoma.

TREATMENTS
Explain that treatments for testicular cancer include surgery, radiation, and chemotherapy in various combinations. In some cases, therapy may involve autologous bone marrow transplantation. Because treatment usually begins with surgical removal of the affected testicle (orchiectomy), your initial teaching may focus on preparing the patient for surgery. Then, as

appropriate, teach about postoperative radiation or chemotherapy.

Before treatment begins, discuss the possibility of sperm banking and refer the patient to appropriate resources.

Medications
Review the purpose, dosage, and possible adverse effects of any prescribed pain medication for testicular cancer. Prepare the patient for chemotherapy, if appropriate. Emphasize that recent advances in chemotherapy offer improved prognoses for patients with testicular cancer. Educate the patient about the type and sequence of drugs he'll receive. Combination therapy is typically used because different drugs

affect cancer cells at various stages of cell division.

Review the common adverse effects of the patient's drug regimen. Tell him that adverse effects occur during chemotherapy because these drugs affect any rapidly growing cells in the body — normal or cancerous.

Procedures

If the patient has a seminoma, postoperative treatment typically involves radiation therapy of the abdominal (and possibly mediastinal) areas. Explain that this form of testicular cancer is especially responsive to radiation. If the patient's cancer has metastasized to the lymphatic system, he may undergo autologous bone marrow transplantation.

Radiation therapy

Explain that bombarding cancer cells with high-level radiation destroys their ability to grow and multiply. Point out that radiation also affects normal cells, but reassure the patient that these cells usually recover quickly. Tell him that the doctor will minimize damage to normal cells by calculating the most effective overall dose and then dividing this dose into several individual treatments.

Inform the patient that a simulated treatment session is performed before radiation therapy to determine the exact location and size of his tumor. Then the area is outlined with an ink marker.

 WARNING: Caution the patient not to wash off the ink because it's important to treat the same body area each time.

Describe standard skin care measures that the patient will take after radiation therapy. Instruct him not to apply soap, deodorant, lotion, perfume, topical medication, or extreme heat or cold to the treatment area, and caution him to avoid rubbing the skin. Suggest that he wear loose, soft clothing and avoid activities that might irritate the area. Advise him to protect the area from direct exposure

to the sun, even after radiation therapy is completed, for as long as the doctor recommends.

Autologous bone marrow transplantation

Tell the patient that this procedure involves high-dose chemotherapy coupled with removal and treatment of the patient's bone marrow to kill cancer cells. The remaining processed and healthy marrow cells are reinjected into the patient to reseed the bone marrow.

Surgery

If the patient will undergo orchiectomy, provide information about the operation and instructions for postoperative care. Address his psychological response to the surgery, and encourage him to express his concerns. Above all, reassure him that unilateral orchiectomy isn't synonymous with castration.

Describe the operation, explaining that the surgeon makes an inguinal incision to remove the testicle and the entire spermatic cord. The surgeon may also remove retroperitoneal lymph nodes or metastases in distant organs. Sometimes, the patient may have chemotherapy or radiation therapy before surgery to shrink the tumor.

Inform the patient that after surgery he'll have a urinary catheter in place. If the surgeon plans a retroperitoneal lymphadenectomy, the patient will also have a nasogastric tube. Explain that this will prevent abdominal distention. Otherwise, he'll be able to eat and drink normally as soon as his bowel resumes functioning.

To prevent respiratory complications, show the patient how to cough and deep breathe deeply at least once every hour. Assure him that he'll receive pain medication as necessary. Mention that he may also wear a scrotal supporter to minimize pain and protect the scrotum.

Other care measures

Because testicular self-examination is the best way to detect a new or recurrent tumor, ensure that the patient knows how to perform this procedure. Urge him to examine himself monthly and to report any changes to the doctor at once.

As with all cancers, recognize that testicular cancer profoundly affects the patient's emotional well-being and lifestyle. As needed, direct him and his family to appropriate sources of information and support. (See Appendix 2.)

Appendices and Index

1

Critical thinking self-test

This self-test presents critical thinking questions based on information in this book. You'll find the answers along with rationales on page 405.

---

1. When teaching a patient who's recovering from a myocardial infarction (MI), the caregiver should cover the topic of sex after an MI. Which of the following statements should guide your teaching on this topic?
a. Sex is too strenuous for most patients recovering from an MI.
b. Sex is the farthest thing from the patient's mind at a time like this.
c. After an MI, sexual activities must be drastically altered.
d. Most patients can safely resume sexual activity 3 to 4 weeks after an MI.

2. After a cerebrovascular accident (CVA), the patient must learn how to cope with neurologic deficits. Which approach would be most appropriate to use when teaching the patient how to manage activites of daily living?
a. Visiting the patient's home to assess for possible problems such as navigating stairs
b. Consulting with and supporting the teaching plans of other members of the health care team
c. Instructing the patient to rely on others' help as much as possible rather than trying to be self-sufficient
d. Suggesting teaching sessions only when the patient seems ready to learn.

3. Your patient has been diagnosed with carpal tunnel syndrome. Which teaching technique would best help her to understand the cause of her symptoms?

a. Using role playing, with the patient showing you how she uses her hand on the job
b. Showing her an illustration of the hand and wrist and explaining the related anatomy and physiology
c. Conducting a question-and-answer session so that all of her concerns are addressed
d. Requesting a return demonstration to evaluate if she understands where the surgeon will make the incision.

4. A patient with newly diagnosed diabetes mellitus asks why he needs to inject insulin rather than take a pill. Your best response would be to:
a. explain that the doctor feels the injection is best for the patient
b. inform him that he'll probably be able to switch to an oral antidiabetic drug later
c. tell him that he needs insulin because his pancreas is not producing enough of it
d. describe new developments in diabetes care.

5. You are teaching a patient, age 32, who will be discharged after treatment for an infection secondary to acquired immunodeficiency syndrome (AIDS). Which of the following points should you discuss?
a. The importance of getting adequate rest
b. The need to avoid crowds and people with known infections
c. Drinking only bottled water when traveling to foreign countries

d. Keeping air conditioners and humidifiers cleaned and repaired.

6. Your patient with cirrhosis is scheduled for a percutaneous liver biopsy. What should you tell him to help prepare him for this diagnostic test?
a. The test only takes a few minutes and won't hurt.

b. He may feel discomfort as the anesthetic is given and as the biopsy needle is inserted.
c. The procedure will be all over before he knows it.
d. He'll feel fine after the procedure.

Answers and rationales
1. d. Most patients who have had an MI can safely resume regular sexual activity a few weeks after discharge. The caregiver should inform the patient that a satisfying sex life can help speed his recovery and should explain that, in terms of physical demands, sex is a moderate form of exercise. However, it can place a strain on the heart if it's accompanied by emotional stress. To reduce the risk of such strain, the patient should choose a quiet, familiar setting for sex and use relaxing positions that allow unrestricted breathing and don't require him to use his arms to support himself or his partner. Also instruct him to ask the doctor if he should take nitroglycerin before having sex to prevent episodes of angina during or after sex.
2. b. When caring for a patient who has had a CVA, your role is to support the plan devised by the appropriate therapist. Caregivers should encourage the patient to be as self-reliant as possible rather than depending on others.
3. b. Showing the patient an illustration of the anatomic structures involved and explaining the physiology of the median nerve and carpal tunnel will help her to understand how easily the nerve can be compressed, causing swelling and inflammation leading to numbness and pain.
4. c. If you feel you're sufficiently knowledgeable about the forms of diabetes mellitus and the appropriate medications for each form to discuss these topics with the patient, explain that he must take insulin because his pancreas isn't producing enough of it in response to elevated glucose levels. If you're not comfortable answering the question, consult with the diabetes nurse educator.
5. a, b, c, and d. Getting adequate rest, avoiding crowds and people with infections, drinking only bottled water when traveling to foreign countries, and keeping air conditioners and humidifiers cleaned and in good repair (so that they don't harbor infectious organisms) are crucial to reducing the risk of infection in patients with AIDS.
6. b. Health care professionals must be truthful with patients, even when the truth isn't entirely pleasant. Percutaneous liver biopsy can cause discomfort when the anesthetic is administered and when the biopsy needle is inserted; many patients also experience pain for several hours after the procedure. Therefore, telling the patient that it won't hurt, that it will be all over before he knows it, or that he'll be fine afterwards would be dishonest.

Sources of information and support

CARDIOVASCULAR CONDITIONS

Aneurysm
American Heart Association
7272 Greenville Ave.
Dallas, TX 75231-4596
(214) 373-6300

Arrhythmias
American Heart Association
7272 Greenville Ave.
Dallas, TX 75231-4596
(214) 373-6300

Coronary Club
9500 Euclid Ave., Mailcode EE-37
Cleveland, OH 44106
(216) 444-3690

Heart Disease Research Foundation
50 Court St.
Brooklyn, NY 11201
(718) 649-6210

Arterial occlusive disease
American Heart Association
7272 Greenville Ave.
Dallas; TX 75231-4596
(214) 373-6300

Coronary artery disease
American Heart Association
7272 Greenville Ave.
Dallas, TX 75231-4596
(214) 373-6300

American Lung Association
1740 Broadway
New York, NY 10019-4374
(212) 315-8700

Deep vein thrombosis
American Heart Association
7272 Greenville Ave.
Dallas, TX 75231-4596
(214) 373-6300

Heart failure
American Heart Association
7272 Greenville Ave.
Dallas, TX 75231-4596
(214) 373-6300

U.S. Department of Health and
  Human Services
Public Health Service
Agency for Health Care Policy and
  Research
1 (800) 358-9295

Hypertension
American Heart Association
7272 Greenville Ave.
Dallas, TX 75231-4596
(214) 373-6300

High Blood Pressure Information
  Center
National Institutes of Health
4733 Bethesda Ave.
Bethesda, MD 20814
(301) 952-3260

Myocardial infarction
American Heart Association
7272 Greenville Ave.
Dallas, TX 75231-4596
(214) 373-6300

American Lung Association
1740 Broadway
New York, NY 10019-4374
(212) 315-8700; 1 (800) LUNG-USA

Valvular heart disease
American Heart Association
7272 Greenville Ave.
Dallas, TX 75231-4596
(214) 373-6300

RESPIRATORY CONDITIONS

Acute bronchitis
American Lung Association
1740 Broadway
New York, NY 10019-4374
(212) 315-8700; 1 (800) LUNG-USA

Asthma
American Lung Association
1740 Broadway
New York, NY 10019-4374
(212) 315-8700; 1 (800) LUNG-USA

Asthma Hotline
1 (800) 222-LUNG

National Institute of Allergy and
  Infectious Diseases
31 Center Dr., MSC 2520
Building 31, Room 7A 50
Bethesda, MD 2
0892-2520
(301) 496-5717

**Chronic obstructive pulmonary
  disease**
American Cancer Society (smoking
  cessation)
1599 Clifton Rd., NE
Atlanta, GA 30329
(404) 320-3333

American Lung Association
1740 Broadway
New York, NY 10019-4374
(212) 315-8700; 1 (800) LUNG-USA

Croup
American Lung Association
1740 Broadway
New York, NY 10019-4374
(212) 315-8700; 1 (800) LUNG-USA

Occupational respiratory diseases
American Lung Association
1740 Broadway
New York, NY 10019-4374
(212) 315-8700; 1 (800) LUNG-USA

National Institute for Occupational
  Safety and Health (NIOSH)
1600 Clifton Rd., NE
Atlanta, GA 30333
(404) 639-3771

National Jewish Center for
  Immunology and Respiratory
  Medicine
1400 Jackson St.
Denver, CO 80206
(303) 388-4461

Occupational Safety and Health
  Administration (OSHA)
U.S. Department of Labor
200 Constitution Ave., NW
Washington, DC 20210
(202) 219-5000

Pleural disorders
American Lung Association
1740 Broadway
New York, NY 10019-4374
(212) 315-8700; 1 (800) LUNG-USA

National Jewish Center for
  Immunology and Respiratory
  Medicine
1400 Jackson St.
Denver, CO 80206
(303) 388-4461

(continued)

Pneumonia
American Lung Association
1740 Broadway
New York, NY 10019-4374
(212) 315-8700; 1 (800) LUNG-USA

Pulmonary embolism
American Lung Association
1740 Broadway
New York, NY 10019-4374
(212) 315-8700; 1 (800) LUNG-USA

GASTROINTESTINAL CONDITIONS

Chronic pancreatitis
Alcoholics Anonymous World
   Services
475 Riverside Dr.
New York, NY 10163
(212) 870-3400

American Diabetes Association
   National Service Center
P.O. Box 25757
1660 Duke St.
Alexandria, VA 22314
(703) 549-1500

Nutrition Education Association
P.O. Box 20301
3647 Glen Haven
Houston, TX 77225
(713) 665-2946

Cirrhosis
Al-Anon Family Group Headquar-
   ters, Inc.
P.O. Box 862, Midtown Station
New York, NY 10018-0862
(212) 302-7240

Alcohol and Drug Problems
   Association of North America
1555 Wilson Blvd., Suite 300
Arlington, VA 22209
(703) 875-8684

Alcoholics Anonymous World
   Services
475 Riverside Dr.
New York, NY 10163
(212) 870-3400

Hepatitis
American Liver Foundation
1425 Pompton Ave.
Cedar Grove, NJ 07009
(201) 857-2626

Peptic ulcer disease
Digestive Disease National Coalition
507 Capital Court, NE
Suite 200
Washington, DC 20002
(202) 544-7497

National Digestive Disease
   Information Clearinghouse
Box NDDIC
2 Information Way
Bethesda, MD 20892-3590
(301) 654-3810

National Ulcer Foundation
675 Main St.
Melrose, MA 02176
(617) 665-6210

Nutrition Education Association
P.O. Box 20301
3647 Glen Haven
Houston, TX 77225
(713) 665-2946

NEUROLOGIC CONDITIONS

Alzheimer's disease
Alzheimer's Association
919 N. Michigan Ave.
Suite 1000
Chicago, IL 60611
(312) 335-8700; 1 (800) 272-3900

Cerebrovascular accident (stroke)
American Heart Association
7272 Greenville Ave.
Dallas, TX 75231-4596
(214) 373-6300

National Aphasia Association
156 Fifth Ave., Suite 707
New York, NY 10010
(212) 255-4329; 1 (800) 922-4622

National Easter Seal Society, Inc.
230 W. Monroe
Chicago, IL 60606
(312) 726-6200

National Institute of Neurological
    and Communicative Disorders
    and Stroke
31 Center Dr., MSC 2540
Building 31, Room 8A 06
Bethesda, MD 20892-2520
(301) 496-5924

Resources in Stroke Information and
    Care
Academy of Aphasia
Boston Veterans Administration
Medical Center 116B
150 South Huntingdon Ave.
Boston, MA 02130
(617) 495-4342

Parkinson's disease
National Parkinson Foundation Inc.
1501 NW Ninth Ave.
Miami, FL 33136
(305) 547-6666

Parkinson Disease Foundation
William Black Medical Research
    Building, Columbia-Presbyterian
    Medical Center
710 West 168th St.
New York, NY 10032
(212) 305-3480; 1 (800) 457-6676

Parkinson Support Groups of America
11376 Cherry Hill Rd., No. 204
Beltsville, MD 20705
(301) 937-1545

Seizures
Epilepsy Foundation of America
4351 Garden City Dr.
Landover, MD 20785
(301) 459-3700; 1 (800) 332-1000

National Epilepsy Library Resource
    Center
1 (800) 332-4050

Traumatic brain injury
Brain Injury Association
1776 Massachusetts Ave., NW
Suite 100
Washington, DC 20036-1904
(202) 296-6443

MUSCULOSKELETAL CONDITIONS

Chronic back pain
International Association for the
    Study of Pain
909 NE 43rd St., Suite 306
Seattle, WA 98105-6020
(206) 547-6409

National Committee on the
    Treatment of Intractable Pain
c/o Wayne Coy, Jr.
Cohn and Marks
1333 New Hampshire Ave., NW
Washington, DC 20036
(202) 452-4836

Osteoarthritis
Arthritis Foundation
1314 Spring St., NW
Atlanta, GA 30309
(404) 872-7100

(continued)

Osteoporosis
National Osteoporosis Foundation
1150 17th St., NW, Suite 500
Washington DC 20037
(202) 223-2226

Sprains and strains
American College of Sports
 Medicine
P.O. Box 1440
Indianapolis, IN 46206-1440
(317) 637-9200

American Physical Therapy
 Association
1111 North Fairfax St.
Alexandria, VA 22314
(703) 684-2782

SKIN CONDITIONS

Dermatitis
American Dermatologic Society of
 Allergy and Immunology
Mayo Clinic
Department of Dermatology
Rochester, MN 55905
(507) 284-2555

Dermatology Foundation
1560 Sherman Ave., Suite 302
Evanston, IL 60201-4802
(708) 328-2256

Herpes simplex
American Social Health Association
 (Herpes Resource Center)
P.O. Box 13827
Research Triangle Park, NC 27709
(919) 361-8400

Latex allergy
Latex Packet Practice Department
American Association of Nurse
 Anesthetists
222 South Prospect Ave.
Park Ridge, IL 60068-4001
(708) 692-7059, Ext. 305

Psoriasis
National Psoriasis Foundation
6600 SW 92nd, Suite 300
Portland, OR 97223-7195
(503) 244-7404

ENDOCRINE CONDITIONS

Diabetes mellitus
American Diabetes Association
National Service Center
P.O. Box 25757
1660 Duke St.
Alexandria, VA 22314
(703) 549-1500

American Dietetic Association
216 West Jackson Blvd., Suite 800
Chicago, IL 60606-6995
(312) 899-0040; 1 (800) 366-1655

Juvenile Diabetes Foundation
120 Wall St.
New York, NY 10005-3904
(212) 899-7575; 1 (800) JDF-CURE

Hyperthyroidism
National Institutes of Health
Institute of Diabetes, Digestive, and
 Kidney Disorders
31 Center Dr., MSC 2560
Building 31, Room 9A 04
Bethesda, MD 20892-2520
(301) 496-3583

Hypothyroidism
National Institutes of Health
Institute of Diabetes, Digestive, and
  Kidney Disorders
31 Center Dr., MSC 2560
Building 31, Room 9A 04
Bethesda, MD 20892-2520
(301) 496-3583

IMMUNE AND HEMATOLOGIC CONDITIONS

AIDS
National AIDS Network
2033 M St., NW, Suite 800
Washington, DC 20036
(202) 293-2437

National HIV and AIDS Hotline
Centers for Disease Control and
  Prevention (CDC)
1 (800) 342-AIDS

UCSF AIDS Health Project
Box 0884
San Francisco, CA 94143-0884
(415) 476-6430

Anaphylaxis
Asthma and Allergy Foundation of
  America
1125 15th St., NW, Suite 502
Washington, DC 20005
(202) 466-7643

Aplastic anemia
Aplastic Anemia Foundation of
  America
P.O. Box 613
Annapolis, MD 21404
(410) 867-0240; 1 (800) 747-2020

Hemophilia
National Hemophilia Foundation
110 Green St., Suite 303
New York, NY 10012
(212) 219-8180

Rheumatoid arthritis
American College of Rheumatology
60 Executive Park South, Suite 150
Atlanta, GA 30329
(404) 633-3772

Arthritis Foundation
1330 W. Peachtree St.
Atlanta, GA 30309
(404) 872-7100

Sickle cell anemia
Sickle Cell Research Foundation
(213) 299-3600

Systemic lupus erythematosus
Lupus Foundation of America
1300 Piccard Dr., Suite 200
Rockville, MD 20850
(301) 670-9292

URINARY CONDITIONS

Chronic renal failure
National Kidney Foundation
30 E. 33rd St., Suite 1100
New York, NY 10016
(212) 889-2210

Neurogenic bladder
United Ostomy Association
19972 MacArthur Blvd., Suite 200
Irvine, CA 92612-2405
(714) 660-8624; 1 (800) 826-0826

REPRODUCTIVE CONDITIONS

Benign prostatic hyperplasia
Recovery of Male Potency
27211 Lahser Rd., No. 208
Southfield, MI 48034
1 (800) TEC-ROMP

(continued)

Endometriosis
Endometriosis Association
8585 N. 76th Pl.
Milwaukee, WI 53202
(414) 355-2200

Fibrocystic breast changes
American Cancer Society
1599 Clifton Rd., NE
Atlanta, GA 30329
(404) 320-3333

<u>CANCER</u>

Bladder cancer
American Cancer Society
1599 Clifton Rd., NE
Atlanta, GA 30329
(404) 320-3333; 1 (800) ACS-2345

United Ostomy Association
19972 MacArthur Blvd., Suite 200
Irvine, CA 92612-2405
(714) 660-8624; 1 (800) 826-0826

Breast cancer
American Cancer Society
1599 Clifton Rd., NE
Atlanta, GA 30329
(404) 320-3333; 1 (800) ACS-2345

Reach to Recovery
c/o American Cancer Society
1599 Clifton Rd., NE
Atlanta, GA 30329
(404) 320-3333; 1 (800) ACS-2345

Cervical cancer
American Cancer Society
1599 Clifton Rd., NE
Atlanta, GA 30329
(404) 320-3333; 1 (800) ACS-2345

Colorectal cancer
American Cancer Society
1599 Clifton Rd., NE
Atlanta, GA 30329
(408) 320-3333; 1 (800) ACS-2345

United Ostomy Association
19972 MacArthur Blvd., Suite 200
Irvine, CA 92612-2405
(714) 660-8624

Laryngeal cancer
International Association of
  Laryngectomies
3340 Peachtree Rd., NE
Atlanta, GA 30029
(404) 320-3333

Leukemia
National Leukemia Association
585 Stewart Ave., Suite 536
Garden City, NY 11530
(516) 222-1944

Lung cancer
American Lung Association
1740 Broadway
New York, NY 10019-4374
(212) 315-8700; 1 (800) LUNG-USA

Testicular cancer
American Cancer Society
1599 Clifton Rd., NE
Atlanta, GA 30329
(404) 320-3333, 1 (800) ACS-2345

Suggested readings

Aigotti, R. *The People's Cancer Guide Book: Practical Information to Help You Understand Cancer.* South Bend, In.: Belletrist, 1995.

Baiilod, R. "Home Dialysis: Lessons in Patient Education," *Patient Education Counselor* 26(1-3):17-24, September 1995.

Bartkiw, T.P., et al. "Innovations in Prostate Disease Education," *Urology Nursing* 15(4):117-22, December 1995.

Canobbio, M. *Mosby's Handbook of Patient Teaching.* St. Louis: Mosby–Year Book, Inc., 1996.

Clark, C. *Wellness Practitioner: Concepts, Research and Strategies.* New York: Springer Publishing Co., 1996.

Clement, S. "Diabetes Self-Management Education," *Diabetes Care* 18(8):1204-14, August 1995.

Cochrane, J. "Patient Education: Lessons from Epilepsy," *Patient Education Counselor* 26(1-3):33-6, September 1995.

Giger, J., and Davidhizer, R. *Transcultural Nursing,* 2nd ed. St. Louis: Mosby–Year Book, Inc., 1995.

Handbook of Diagnostic Tests. Springhouse, Pa.: Springhouse Corp., 1995.

Kaufman, M.W., et al. "Raynaud's Disease: Patient Education as a Primary Nursing Intervention," *Journal of Vascular Nursing* 14(2):34-39, June 1996.

Naftulin-Madsen, A. "COPD — The Client's Perspective," *Home Health Focus* 1(10):6-7, March 1995.

Rodman, K. "Strategies in Patient Teaching," *Gynecologic Oncology Nurse* 6(1):26, Winter 1996.

Superio-Cabuslay, E., et al. "Patient Education Interventions in Osteoarthritis and Rheumatoid Arthritis: A Meta-Analytic Comparison with Nonsteroidal Anti-inflammatory Drug Treatment," *Arthritis Care Research* 9(4):292-301, August 1996.

Index

i refers to an illustration; t refers to a table.

i refers to an illustration; t refers to a table.

i refers to an illustration; t refers to a table.